Practice of Sleep Medicine

Boris A. Stuck
Joachim T. Maurer
Angelika A. Schlarb
Michael Schredl
Hans-Günter Weeß

Practice of Sleep Medicine

Sleep Disorders in Children and Adults

Springer

Boris A. Stuck
Dept. of Otorhinolaryngology, Head and Neck Surgery
University Hospital Marburg, Philipps-Universität Marburg
Marburg, Germany

Angelika A. Schlarb
Department of Psychology
Bielefeld University Department of Psychology
Bielefeld, Germany

Hans-Günter Weeß
Sleep Disorders Centre
Pfalzklinikum Klingenmünster
Klingenmünster, Germany

Joachim T. Maurer
Division of Sleep Medicine, Dept. of Otorhinolaryngology, Head and Neck Surgery
University Hospital Mannheim
Ruprecht-Karls-University Heidelberg
University of Applied Sciences Mannheim
Mannheim, Germany

Michael Schredl
Sleep Laboratory, Central Institute of Mental Health
Medical Faculty Mannheim/Heidelberg University
Mannheim, Germany

ISBN 978-3-030-17411-8 ISBN 978-3-030-17412-5 (eBook)
https://doi.org/10.1007/978-3-030-17412-5

This Springer imprint is published by the registered company Springer Nature Switzerland AG.
The registered company address is: Gewerbestrasse 11, 6330 Cham, Switzerland

Contents

About the Authors

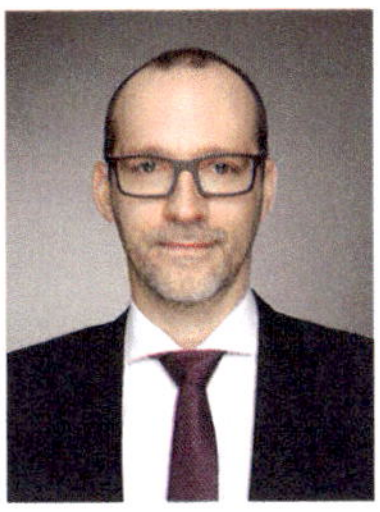

Boris A. Stuck

Dr. Stuck has been working in the field of sleep medicine since 1999. In 2009, he received his Ph.D. degree in otorhinolaryngology for his thesis on sleep-related breathing disorders. Until 2014, he was executive senior physician of the Department of Otorhinolaryngology of the University Hospital of Mannheim and vice-chairman of the Sleep Center. Since April 2017, he has been professor and chair of the Department of Otorhinolaryngology of the University Hospital of Giessen and Marburg (UKGM), Campus Marburg. He has the additional qualification of sleep medicine and is qualified in somnology (DGSM) and is section editor of the scientific journal *Somnology*. He is the responsible author of the German guidelines on the *Diagnosis and Treatment of Snoring in Adults* and *Sleep-Related Breathing Disorders in Adults*. Since 2018 he has been a board member and since 2020 the Executive President of the German Sleep Society.

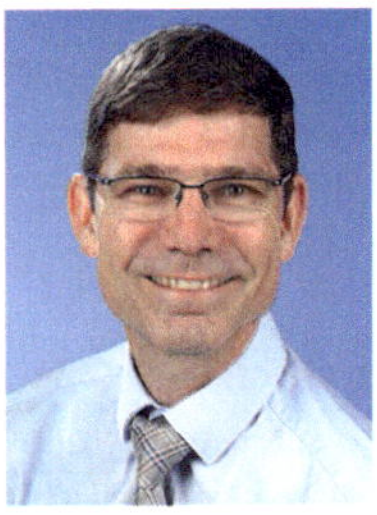

Joachim T. Maurer

A specialist in otorhinolaryngology, Dr. Maurer has been director of the Sleep Center at the University Hospital Mannheim since 1995 and of the Division for Sleep Medicine since 2019. He is qualified in sleep medicine and somnology (DGSM) and is a member of the Audit Committee, the Accreditation Commission for Sleep Centers, the Committee on Continuing Medical Education, and the Objection Committee in Sleep Medicine of the State Medical Chamber of Baden-Württemberg. He is honorary professor at the University of Applied Sciences, Mannheim.

Since 1996, he has organized several courses on diagnostics and therapy as well as the surgical therapy of sleep apnea. He is section editor of the scientific journal *Somnology*, coeditor of *Sleep and Breathing*, and coauthor of the German guidelines *Diagnosis and Therapy of Snoring in Adults* and *Sleep-Related Breathing Disorders in Adults*. Also, he is president of the Association of Somnologists of Baden-Württemberg.

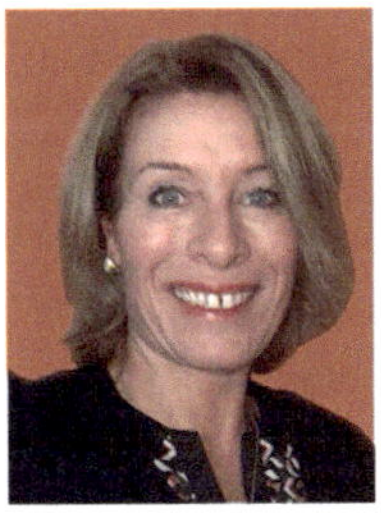

Angelika A. Schlarb

Dr. Schlarb is a certified psychologist and psychological psychotherapist and has an additional qualification in psychotherapy of children and adolescents, group therapy with focus on behavioral therapy, and hypnotherapy. She received her Ph.D. degree with contributions about therapy of sleep disorders in adults, children, and adolescents and holds the professorship for Clinical Psychology and Psychotherapy of Children and Adolescents of the University of Bielefeld, Germany. She is director of the University Outpatient Department for Children and Adolescents and of the Sleep Research Lab of the University of Bielefeld, member of the German Sleep Society (DGSM), and deputy speaker of the Research Team of Pediatrics. Furthermore, she is a member of the European Sleep Research Society (ESRS) and the International Pediatric Sleep Association (IPSA), editor of several scientific special issues on the topic of sleep medicine and therapy, and coeditor of the scientific journals *Somnology* and *Journal of Sleep Research (JSR)*. She contributed to the German guideline "*Nonrestorative Sleep/Sleep Disorders: Insomnia*" and co-coordinated the revision of the German guideline on "*Insomnia in Pediatric and Adolescent Patients*". Her scientific and clinical focus is on the diagnosis and therapy of sleep disorders in pediatric, adolescent, and adult patients; chronotype research; love, relationships, and sleep; chronic diseases and sleep; and sleep disorders associated with psychiatric diseases.

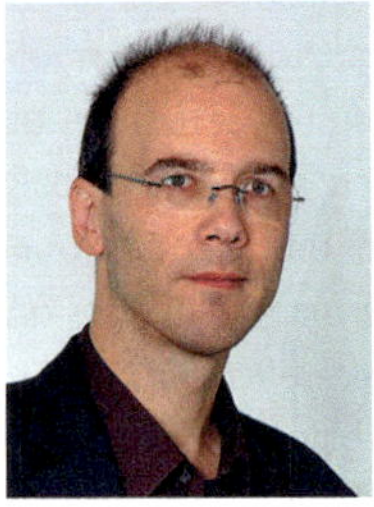

Michael Schredl

Dr. Schredl is a certified psychologist with a degree in electrical engineering, a somnologist (DGSM), and director of the Sleep Lab of the Central Institute of Mental Health in Mannheim, Germany. Since 1990, he has performed research in sleep and dreaming with a focus on factors of dream recall, the impact of wakefulness on dream contents, nightmares, dreams and psychic disorders, memory consolidation during sleep, stress systems, and sleep disorders. He is associate professor at the Faculty of Social Sciences of the University of Mannheim and leader of the working group "Dreaming" within the German Sleep Society (DGSM). Furthermore, he is a member of the International Association for the Study of Dreams and the European Sleep Research Society and editor of the open-access journal *International Journal of Dream Research*.

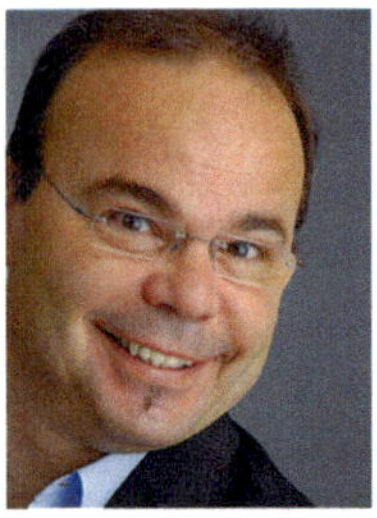

Hans-Günter Weeß

Dr. Weeß is a certified psychologist, psychological psychotherapist, and somnologist and since 1991 has served as director of the Interdisciplinary Center of Sleep Medicine at the Pfalzklinikum Klingenmünster. In addition, since 1992, he has been a lecturer at the University of Koblenz-Landau, Germany. Since 2009, he lectures in the context of the postgraduate program of psychological psychotherapy of the University of Koblenz-Landau and, since 2017, at the Institute of Further Education and Training in Clinical Psychology (IFKV). Since 2008, he is a member of the Management Board of the German Sleep Society (DGSM) and the Commission for Accreditation and Quality Management, which is responsible for the accreditation in the southwestern part of Germany, and is commission manager QN of Somnology for Physicians, Psychologists, and Scientists and Head of the Sleep Medicine Training Commission of the German Sleep Research Society.

He is coeditor of the journal *Somnologie* and a member of the scientific council of the journals *Schlaf* and *Schlafmagazin* and of the expert commission of the Federal Highway Research Institute in the context of daytime sleepiness for expert opinion on driving ability. In addition, he is author of several publications, including the *European Guideline for the Diagnosis and Treatment of Insomnia* developed by the European Sleep Research Society and holds the mandate of the DGSM for the guideline on shift work of the German Society for Occupational and Environmental Medicine (DGAUM).

His scientific and clinical focus is the diagnosis and therapy of daytime sleepiness, insomnia, narcolepsy, parasomnias, and other rare sleep-related diseases, methods of sleep medicine, training and further education in sleep medicine.

Physiological Basics of Healthy and Disturbed Sleep

J. T. Maurer, H.-G. Weeß and M. Schredl

B. A. Stuck et al., *Practice of Sleep Medicine*, https://doi.org/10.1007/978-3-030-17412-5_1

In contrast to wakefulness, sleep is characterized by very low motor activity and responsiveness. Body functions and hormone secretion are modulated during sleep. Core body temperature and cortisol secretion are markers of the endogenous rhythm that is synchronized by the suprachiasmatic nucleus with the 24-h-day rhythm. The change of sleep and wakefulness is controlled by a homeostatic and a circadian process (approximately 24 h) and the change between REM and non-REM sleep by an ultradian process (<24 h). The importance of sleep for physical and mental recuperation, thermoregulation, the immune system, memory consolidation, and ontogenesis is discussed. In healthy sleepers, non-REM sleep (N1, N2, N3), REM sleep (R), and wakefulness (W) are distinguished based on EEG, EOG, and submental EMG. In the third version of the *International Classification of Sleep Disorders* (ICSD-3, 2014), seven main groups are differentiated.

1.1 History of Sleep Medicine

Since humans have started thinking about themselves and their lives, they have also reflected upon sleep and dreaming. For a long time, sleep was considered to be a passive and inactive condition. In Greek mythology, this idea was personified by Hypnos, the god of sleep, who had a close relationship to his twin brother Thanatos, the god of death. Passiveness and inactivity were also included in the Proto-Germanic origin of the word "sleep" (or "schlafen" in German), which originally had the meaning of becoming relaxed ("schlaff/schlapp werden").

In ancient times, Aristotle, and later Galen, assumed that sleep was caused by changes in the brain, such as thickening of the blood. They interpreted the role of sleep as restoration of the brain and for regeneration of mental perceptiveness as well as internal heat. In later times, medical research on the context of sleep was based only on ancient manuscripts and their interpretation.

Only in the second half of the nineteenth century was sleep investigated with an experimental approach. In 1863, Kohlschütter was the first who tried to assess the waking level at different phases of sleep by applying acoustic stimuli of various volumes. In this way, he wished to determine the depth of sleep. The experiments performed by Jouvet and by Moruzzi and Magoun in the first half of the twentieth century showed sleep to be a highly active process of the human brain.

In 1929, the psychiatrist Hans Berger published his invention of electroencephalography (EEG), which allowed measuring brain electrical activity at the intact skin in the waking state as well as during sleep. A first classification of sleep in different stages was performed by Loomis in 1937 based on EEG. With the detection of rapid eye movements (REM) in 1953 by Aserinsky and Kleitman, it was possible for the first time to describe REM sleep.

Based on EEG, electrooculography (EOG), and electromyography (EMG), a group of experts with Rechtschaffen and Kales published criteria for the evaluation of sleep stages in humans. However, these criteria were based exclusively on the examinations of healthy individuals and could not always be suitably applied into the sleep disorders that were increasingly described in the following years. This situation only changed with the publication of the new standards of the American Academy of Sleep Medicine (AASM) in 2007, which were revised several times in some aspects until today.

1.2 Classification of Sleep Disorders

The possibility to register many biosignals during sleep completed the merely subjective description of the symptoms of sleep disorders by the patient or an observer. Sleep disorders could be characterized, defined, and differentiated more precisely. In the past decades, this was the basis of developing different classifications of sleep disorders.

In a first classification, in 1979 sleep disorders were differentiated only based on the predominant symptoms into these:

- Disorders of initiating and maintaining sleep (insomnias)
- Disorders with excessive sleepiness (hypersomnias)
- Disorders of the sleep–wake rhythm
- Disorders in relationship with sleep, sleep stages, or partial awakening (parasomnias)

In 1990, a classification based on the etiopathogenesis of sleep disorders was published

(*International Classification of Sleep Disorders*, ICSD), which differentiated:
- Disorders regarding the quantity, quality, or the time of sleep (dyssomnias)
- Parasomnias
- Disorders related to physical or psychiatric diseases
- Proposed sleep disorders

Dyssomnias were classified into these categories:
- Intrinsic sleep disorders (e.g., narcolepsy; see ▶ Chap. 5)
- Extrinsic sleep disorders (e.g., environment-related sleep disorders; see ▶ Chap. 9)
- Circadian rhythm sleep disorders (e.g., advanced sleep phase syndrome; see ▶ Chap. 6)

In most cases, the diagnosis required polysomnography (PSG) (see ▶ Sect. 2.6), which made it impossible to assign a complained sleep disorder to one of the four main groups based only on the symptoms.

In 2005, the American Academy of Sleep Medicine (AASM) published the second version of the *International Classification of Sleep Disorders* (ICSD-2), which was revised in 2014 (ICSD-3). ICSD-2 and ICSD-3 not only included new findings about sleep disorders and thus specified the diagnoses, but in some aspects returned to a phenomenological classification, as is elucidated in the following overview of ICSD-3.

Main Groups of Sleep Disorders According to the American Academy of Sleep Medicine (AASM) from 2014
- Insomnias
- Sleep-related breathing disorders
- Hypersomnias of central origin
- Circadian rhythm sleep–wake disorders
- Parasomnias
- Sleep-related movement disorders
- Other sleep disorders

Sleep-related organic and neurological disorders are listed in an appendix.

The outline of the present manual and the mentioned diagnostic criteria of sleep disorders follow the ICSD-3.

Practical Tip

The current classification of sleep disorders (ICSD-3) consists of seven main groups. The disorders were classified according to etiological and also phenomenological aspects as far as possible. The main groups were completed by explicitly sleep-related organic and neurological disorders. Sleep disorders observed in the context of organic or psychiatric diseases are not described separately.

1.3 Phenomenology of Sleep

According to the criteria of the AASM of 2020, four different stages of sleep and wakefulness (◘ Fig. 1.1) can be defined as of the age of 2 to 6 months (see also ▶ Chap. 11, Sleep disorders in children). Their properties with regard to EEG, EOG, and EMG are partly different in children and adults (◘ Table 1.1). Sleep is divided into epochs of 30 s that are assigned to the stages based on the following criteria:
- *Sleep stage N1* (◘ Fig. 1.2) describes the transition from wakefulness to sleep, that is, a kind of dozing.
- *Sleep stage N2* (◘ Fig. 1.3) describes stable sleep.
- *Sleep stage N3* (◘ Fig. 1.4) is deep sleep.
- *Sleep stage R* (◘ Fig. 1.5), REM sleep, is often called—even if it is not really correct—the dream sleep phase or also paradoxical sleep. In this stage, the most intensive dreams take place (see ▶ Sect. 1.8); when awakened in this phase, people often remember the contents of their dreams. Furthermore, despite high EEG activity, which is similar to stage N1 or W, the arousal threshold is paradoxically highest.

The percentage of the sleep stages N1 and N2 in the entirety of the sleep of an adult healthy sleeper, about 30 years old, amounts to about 55–60%. The deep, or also slow-wave, sleep is described by sleep stage N3; its percentage is about 15–25%. REM sleep generally encompasses 20–25% of the total sleep time. The percentage of wakefulness is typically less than 5% of the sleep period.

The sequence of the single sleep stages results in a profile, the so-called *hypnogram*. The

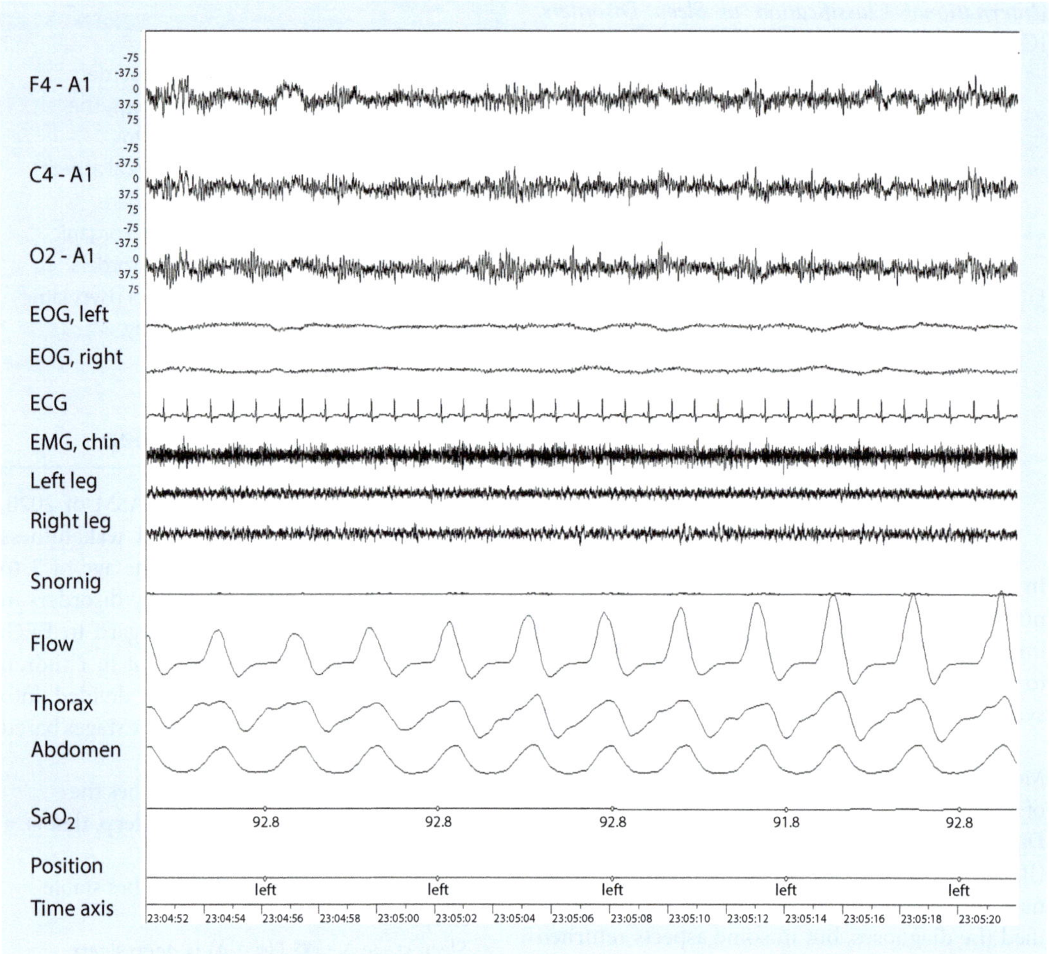

Fig. 1.1 Typical stage of wakefulness within a 30-s epoch of polysomnography in a 40-year-old male individual. In the EEG, an alpha rhythm is found with a frequency of 8–12 Hz. In the second half of the epoch, the EOG reveals low-amplitude, slow eye movements

sequence of sleep stages reveals a characteristic pattern over the sleep period. The first sleep cycle starts with superficial sleep (N1) after falling asleep, followed by stable sleep (N2) and deep sleep (N3). Finally, REM sleep can be observed, which completes every sleep cycle. Each sleep cycle has a duration of about 90 to 110 min. Depending on the duration of sleep and interindividual variance four to seven sleep cycles can be observed in healthy sleepers. The amount of deep sleep decreases with the number of sleep cycles within a sleep period, and the percentage of REM sleep increases continuously (Fig. 1.6).

The duration of the nighttime sleep period is intraindividually rather stable; however, in the interindividual context, the durations may vary greatly and are influenced by several factors.

Newborns (see ▶ Sect. 11.1) sleep for about 16 h, distributed over four or five sleep phases; about half the sleep time is REM sleep (so-called polyphasic sleep pattern).

In prepubertal schoolchildren, generally day sleep or a power nap is no longer observed, and the night sleep amounts to approximately 10 to 11 h (so-called monophasic sleep pattern). REM sleep is now reduced to less than 35% of the total (see ▶ Chap. 11).

In later ages, again increasingly polyphasic sleep patterns are found, although the total sleep time over 24 h neither increases nor decreases. Besides the increase of organic and psychic diseases (see ▶ Chap. 10), in particular the loss of social factors determining a rhythm (e.g., work, children) and the reduction of the endogenous rhythm (see ▶ Sect. 1.5) are responsible. Generally,

Table 1.1 Characteristics of the sleep stages in adults according to the American Academy of Sleep Medicine (AASM) scoring manual (V2.6 2020)

Stage	EEG	EOG	EMG
W	Dominating alpha and beta activity	Eyeblinks, rapid eye movements, sometimes even slow, partly rolling eye movements at the transition to N1	High tone, movement artifacts
N1	Theta activity (vertex spikes)	Slow, partly rolling eye movements	Reduction of muscle tone (<W)
N2	Theta activity, K complexes, sleep spindles	No eye movements, EEG artifacts, sometimes even slow, partly rolling eye movements at the transition from N1	Reduction of muscle tone (<N1)
N3	Delta waves <2 Hz (slow waves): >20%	No eye movements, EEG artifacts	Reduction of muscle tone (<N2)
R	Theta (also slow alpha) activity, sawtooth waves	Conjugated, rapid eye movements (REM)	Lowest muscle tone (≤N3), partly phasic activation

W wake, *R* REM (rapid eye movements)
Only stage W and N1 are differently defined in children (► Chap. 11)

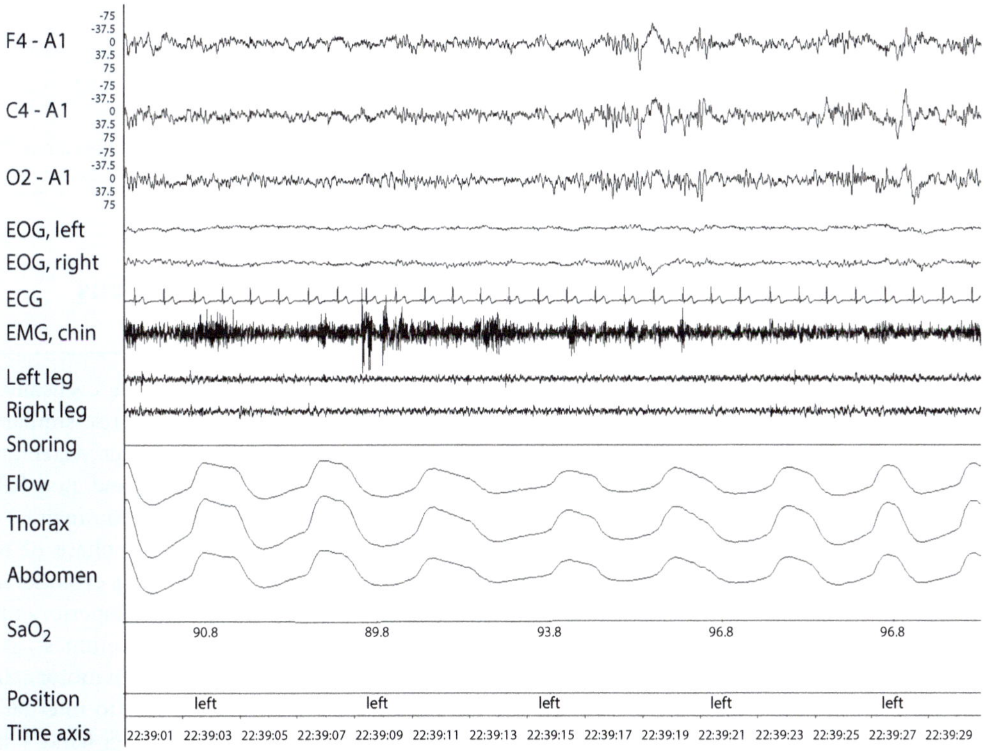

Fig. 1.2 Typical stage N1 within a 30-s epoch of polysomnography in a 40-year-old man. In the EEG, predominantly a theta rhythm (low amplitude, mixed frequency) is found with a frequency between 3 and 7 Hz. In the second half of the epoch, an abortive sleep spindle is seen that does not lead to the assignment of N2 because of its phenomenology, but in particular because of its occurrence in the second half of the epoch

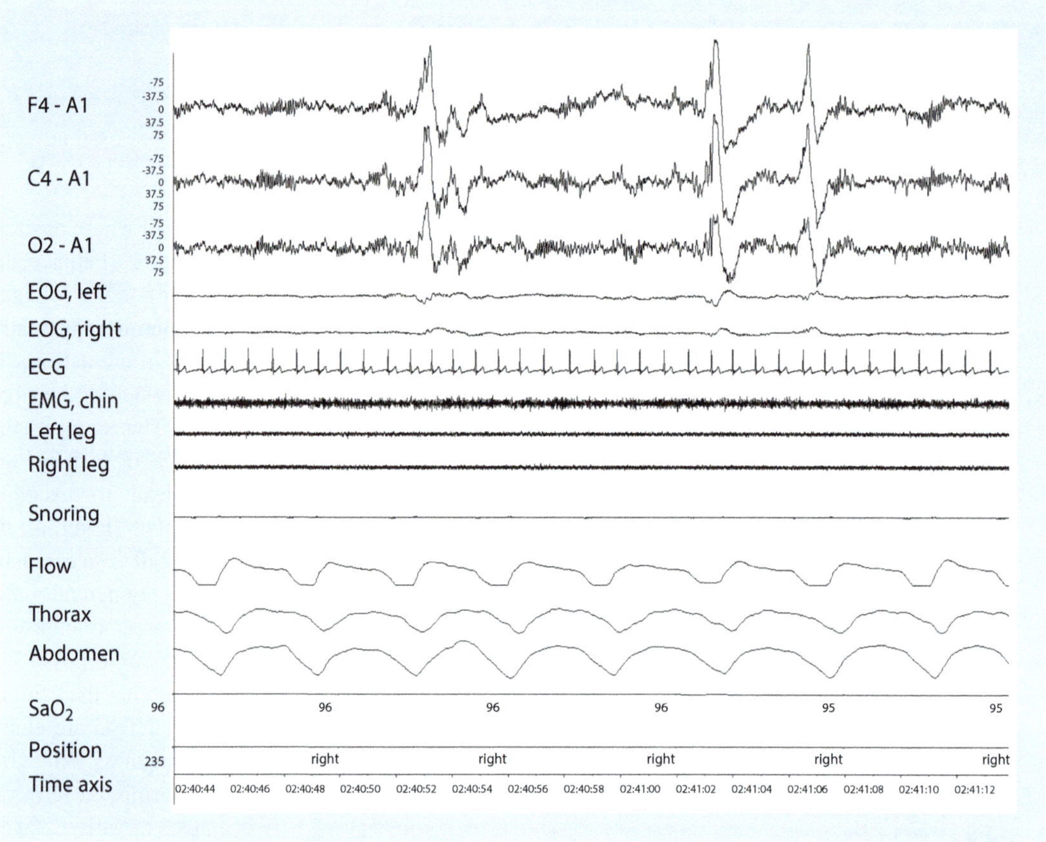

Fig. 1.3 Typical stage N2 within a 30-s epoch of polysomnography in a 40-year-old man. The EEG is similar to that of stage 1 (theta rhythm with low amplitude and mixed frequency); additionally, sleep spindles can be observed with a typical frequency between 12 and 14 Hz (maximum, 11–16 Hz) and K complexes

a sleep duration between 7 and 9 h is considered as healthy. Variations in duration of sleep between 4 and 12 h, however, can be observed, and there is no reason to directly classify them as pathological.

Correlations between duration of sleep and life expectancy are discussed, but because of the methodical limitations of single studies, no clear statements can be given. There are hints that an average duration of sleep of more than 9 or less than 6 h is associated with a slightly reduced life expectancy. However, it must be taken into account that the average genetic sleep quantity was taken as the basis for the risk estimation in those studies. According to this assumption, deviations of more than 1–2 h from the individually genetic sleep quantity would have to be evaluated as pathological.

For the assessment of sufficient sleep quantity at night, it is less the absolute quantity that is decisive but rather the alertness of the individual during the day.

1.4 Physiological Alterations During Sleep

Times of rest and activity alternate cyclically in nearly all creatures. Conditions of rest similar to sleep are already found in the lower vertebrates, although sleep with clear REM and non-REM phases is only found in birds and mammals.

Sleep is a particularly intense phase of rest with high vulnerability, such that its evolutionary advantages must have been highly superior to the disadvantages. In contrast to wakefulness, it is characterized by a nearly nonexistent motor activity and a very low responsiveness to internal as well as external stimuli. On the other hand, it is a complex, highly active condition, which is seen in the determined sequence of non-REM and REM sleep with its partly high neuronal activity and modulation of nearly all body functions during sleep. If sleep is interrupted, consciousness and

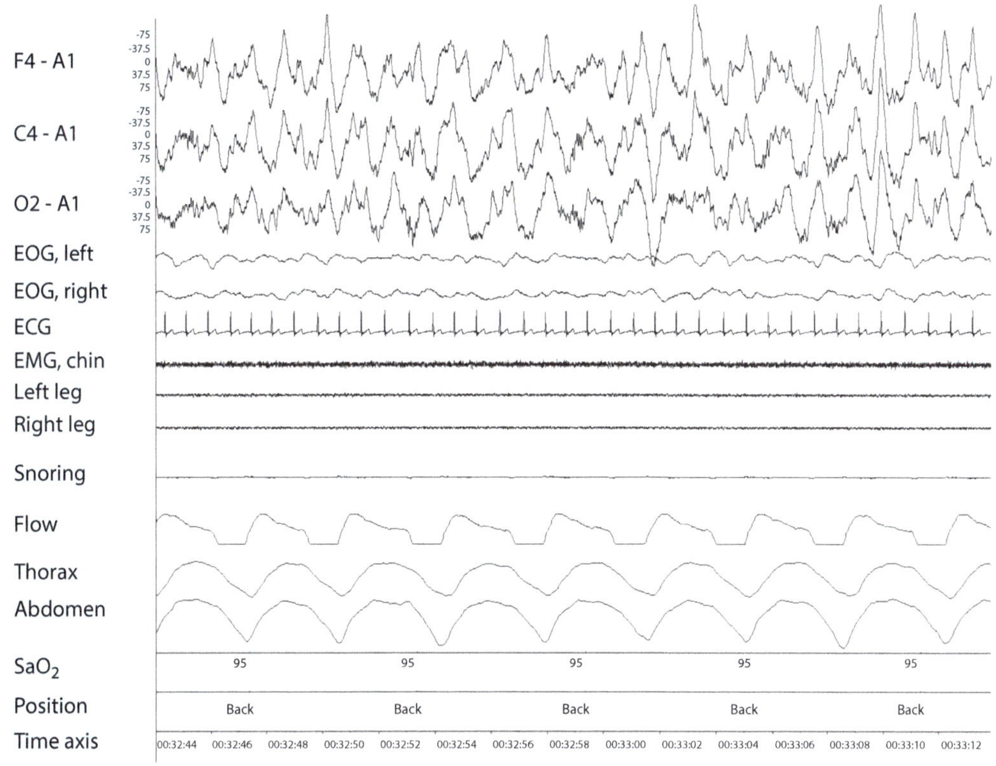

Fig. 1.4 Typical stage N3 (deep sleep) within a 30-s epoch of polysomnography in a 40-year-old man. In the EEG, delta waves are found in more than 20% with frequencies between 0.5 and 2 Hz (slow waves)

body functions return completely to the level of normal wakefulness within a very short time. However, sleep is subjectively only perceived when it lasts for 10 to 20 min without interruption, that is, without significant awakening or arousal (see ▶ Sect. 2.7.2.2).

Practical Tip

Based on motor activation, electric brain activity, cerebral neurotransmitter activity, and autonomous activity, three conditions can be differentiated: wakefulness, non-REM sleep, and REM sleep.

- Wakefulness is characterized by a high motor and cortical activation.
- During non-REM sleep, motor and cortical activation are greatly reduced.
- During REM sleep, minimal motor activation is associated with a high cortical activity.

Manifold physiological changes during sleep generally concern all functional systems (◘ Table 1.2). Although many of those alterations have already been described in detail, very little is understood regarding pathogenetic processes. During non-REM sleep, anabolic processes are enhanced compared to wakefulness; especially, the inexact regulation of many body functions during REM sleep is apparent compared to non-REM sleep. The changes of the cardiovascular system, thermoregulation, and hormone secretion are specifically elucidated. Regarding changes in breathing, see ▶ Sect. 4.1.

1.4.1 Cardiovascular System During Sleep

Naturally, people sleep in a lying position. The increased venous backflow from peripheral vessels leads to increased filling of the right atrium and thus increased right ventricular stroke vol-

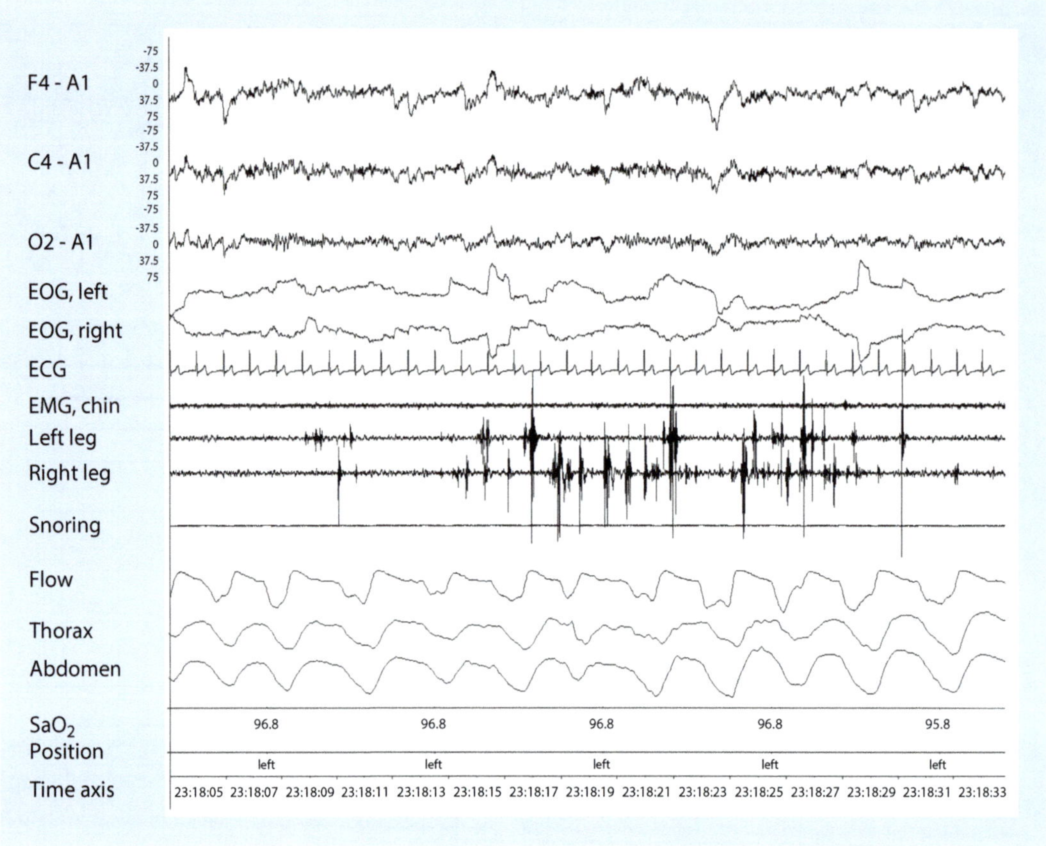

Fig. 1.5 Typical stage R (REM) within a 30-s epoch of polysomnography in a 40-year-old man. In the EEG, an alpha-theta rhythm is found similar to stage 1. In the EOG, rapid conjugated eye movements are observed. In the EMG, typical phasic muscle twitches are seen

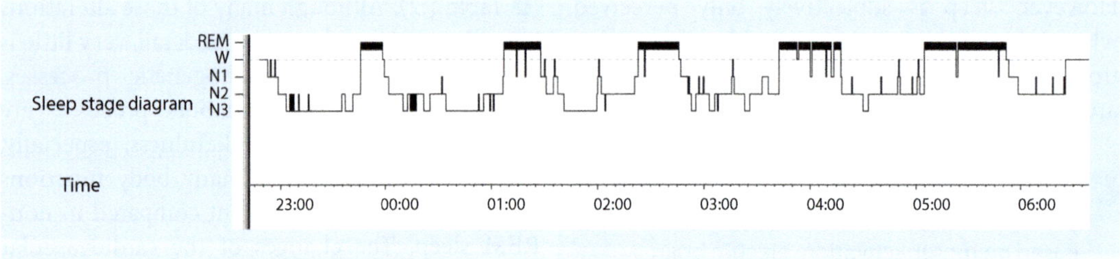

Fig. 1.6 Typical sleep profile of a healthy young man. Five sleep cycles have passed. It is clearly seen that the deep sleep is greatest in the first third of the night. In the last third of the night, increased REM sleep is observed. Further explanations are found in the text

ume. As a consequence, the atrial natriuretic peptide is increasingly and renin decreasingly secreted. During sleep, this position-related diuretic effect is reversed so that finally no volume deficit occurs.

When falling asleep, the sympathetic tone is reduced and the parasympathetic tone raises. Overall, this leads to an increasing reduction of the cardiac output from light sleep over deep sleep to REM sleep. The decreasing heart rate and left ventricular stroke volume are assumed to be responsible for this effect. In connection with the decreased total peripheral resistance, the systemic arterial blood pressure decreases during non-REM sleep with increasing sleep depth. However, so far no consistent explanation exists for the

Table 1.2 Physiological changes during sleep

Parameter	Transition from wakefulness → non-REM	Transition from non-REM → REM	Difference wakefulness → sleep
Cardiovascular system	–		
– Heart rate	10–20% ↓	↑ to ↓, variability ↑	10–20% ↓
– Conduction system	AV transition ↓	AV transition ↓	AV transition ↓
– Stroke volume	5–10% ↓	Variable	↓ to →
–Cardiac output	↓	↓	Up to 25% ↓
– Total peripheral resistance	↓	↑ to →	15–20% ↓
– Systemic arterial blood pressure	↓	↑	10–20% ↓
– Pulmonoarterial pressure	↓	?	2–4 mmHg ↑
– Cerebral blood flow	↓	↑	↓
Gastrointestinal tract	–		
– Swallowing rate	↓	?	↓
– Gastrointestinal mobility	↓	↓ to →	↓
– Salivary secretion	↓	?	↓
Gastric acid secretion	↑ to ↓	?	↑ to ↓
– Sphincter pressure (esophagus, anus)	→	?	→
Urogenital system	–		
– Urine production	↓	↓	20–50% ↓
– Urine osmolality	↓	↓	↓
– Erection (penile and clitoris)	↓	↑	→

proven increase of the blood pressure, the total peripheral resistance, and the heart rate during REM sleep to a level of sleep stage N2.

1.4.2 Thermoregulation

Body temperature as a key variable of the circadian rhythm varies as much as 1 °C during 24 h. It reaches its maximum directly before going to bed and decreases during nighttime to its minimum in the early morning hours (Fig. 1.7a). On one hand, the greatest sleepiness is associated with minimal temperature; on the other hand, it is most probable to reach REM sleep about 30–90 min after the temperature minimum. During REM sleep, mammalians show a poikilotherm behavior; in this sleep stage, they are able to control only their core body temperature: neither sweating for heat loss nor trembling for heat generation is sufficiently possible. In particular for infants, this phenomenon bears the risk of hyperthermia or hypothermia. During non-REM sleep, the body temperature may be controlled in the same way as in the stage of wakefulness, even if it occurs in a slightly reduced way.

1.4.3 Hormone System and Sleep

Many endocrine systems are determined by a more or less strict circadian rhythm. The effects of sleep and the circadian rhythm on hormone

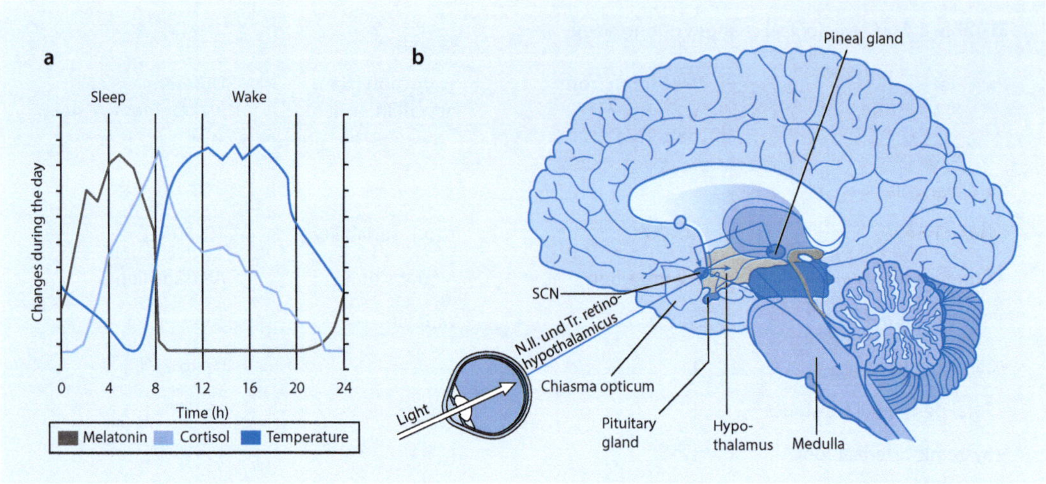

Fig. 1.7 **a** Circadian course of the body temperature and selected hormones. **b** Significant anatomical structure of the sleep–wake regulation (**b** modified according to Birbaumer N, Schmidt RF (2006) *Biologische Psychologie*, 6th Edition, Springer, Berlin)

secretion typically overlap, and it is not easy to separate one from the other.

However, it was possible to prove that the release of growth hormone is enhanced particularly by deep sleep, which is apparent in a maximal blood level about 1 h after falling asleep, independent from the time of falling asleep (Fig. 1.7a).

Similarly, prolactin release increases during sleep and decreases rapidly after waking up.

In contrast, the hypothalamic-pituitary-adrenal axis (HPA) is difficult to stimulate during deep sleep, which leads to a low cortisol value at the beginning of sleep. Only with increasing duration of sleep and the decreasing part of deep sleep does the concentration of cortisol increase.

The ACTH concentration clearly increases about 1 h before awakening and reaches its maximum directly after waking up. The time of the maximum value seems to depend rather from the time of the anticipated awakening than from the real time of awakening. Further, there are hints that the course of the cortisol level is relevant for sleep-associated memory formation.

Also, the regulation of body weight seems to be influenced by sleep. Concentration of the appetite suppressant leptin increases with increasing duration of sleep whereas the level of the appetite-stimulating ghrelin decreases.

Interactions with sleep are described for different cytokines; for example, increased sleepiness is induced by interleukins and tumor necrosis factor, which is important in the context of infections and cancer diseases.

1.5 Circadian Rhythm

All biological processes are subject to a rhythm, wherein the rhythms of 1 day ("circadian") are most obvious. From single-cell organisms to humans, rhythms are already present on the cellular level in the form of so-called clock genes. In mammalians, they are coordinated by the suprachiasmatic nucleus (SCN) in the hypothalamus, which is the master timer (called Zeitgeber) or pacemaker. In humans, the endogenous rhythm of the SCN amounts on average to a bit less than 25 h, which could be detected in volunteers who spent several weeks in a bunker without any contact with the outside world. The endogenous rhythm is only synchronized to 24 h by further zeitgebers. Besides social factors (time of the day, working times, etc.), this is mainly the change between light and dark (Fig. 1.8).

Besides the rods and cones that are responsible for eyesight, special ganglion cells are found in the retina that contain the photosensitive protein melanopsin. The axons of those retinal ganglion cells are directly connected with the SCN via the retinohypothalamic tract. If melanopsin is missing, synchronization is still possible via rods and cones, although less precise, because they dispose themselves of synapses to the ganglion cells.

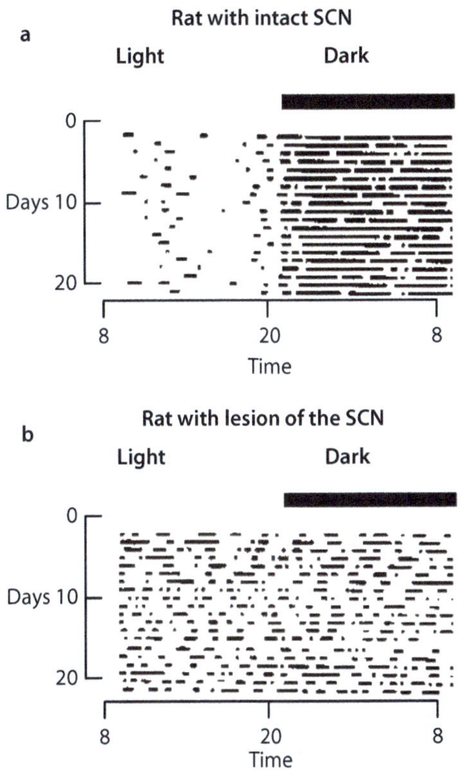

Fig. 1.8 **a, b** Activity profile of a rat with intact suprachiasmatic nucleus (SCN) (**a**) and after lesion of the SCN (**b**). As nocturnal animals, healthy rats show high activity during nighttime and long resting phases during daytime. After lesion of the SCN, their rest–activity pattern completely lost its circadian rhythm

Without retinal ganglion cells, synchronization with light–dark alternation is no longer possible (Fig. 1.7b).

In the ventrolateral area of the SCN, the neurotransmitters vasoactive intestinal peptide (VIP) and neuropeptide Y are especially relevant. Synchronization of the cells of the SCN is then mediated via vasopressin-controlled efferences to subordinate systems of the hypothalamus and other brain structures. In this context, in particular the epiphysis (pineal gland) must be mentioned. Its melatonin secretion is inhibited by light, which leads to a feedback for the SCN with regard to the day–night alternation. In nocturnal as well as in diurnal mammalians, the maximum melatonin level is measured at night. The relevant markers of the endogenous rhythm are the core body temperature and the cortisol level (Fig. 1.7a). This rhythm is missing in VIP-deficient mice, for example.

1.6 Sleep Regulation

As a model, sleep is described by three basic mechanisms:

- A *homeostatic process*, wherein the previous sleep and wake times determine the pressure to sleep
- A *circadian process* that defines the circadian oscillating degree of wakefulness
- An *ultradian process* that controls the alternation of REM and non-REM sleep within the sleeping period

The first two processes determine the time and duration of sleep and influence the ultradian process.

In 1982, Borbély developed the "two-process model" for the aforementioned ideas with the process S (homeostatic) that approaches asymptotically a maximum during wakefulness and is then reduced during sleep, and the process C (circadian) as the degree of wakefulness that tends to its lowest values in the evening (Fig. 1.9).

Simply put, the *process S* can be compared with the intensity of the delta waves (delta power) because delta power depends on the previous wake time more than the duration of deep sleep. Recent investigations show an accumulation of adenosine and the associated receptors in the basal forebrain during wakefulness and an increasing degradation with increasing duration of sleep. Adenosine itself triggers the ventrolateral preoptic region (VLPO) that is discussed as the "door to sleep" because it blocks cholinergic, adrenergic, serotonergic, and histaminergic arousal systems (see the following chapter) and thus induces non-REM sleep.

For *process C*, the SCN is responsible for sending arousal signals that continuously increase until the early evening hours. Afterward, they decrease rapidly, which relevantly increases the individual's readiness to sleep.

To describe the *ultradian rhythm* of non-REM-REM sleep cycles, by 1975, Hobson and McCarley had developed their model of reciprocal interaction of aminergic and cholinergic neurons in the mesopontine crossing of the brainstem. Based on recent neurophysiological examinations, this

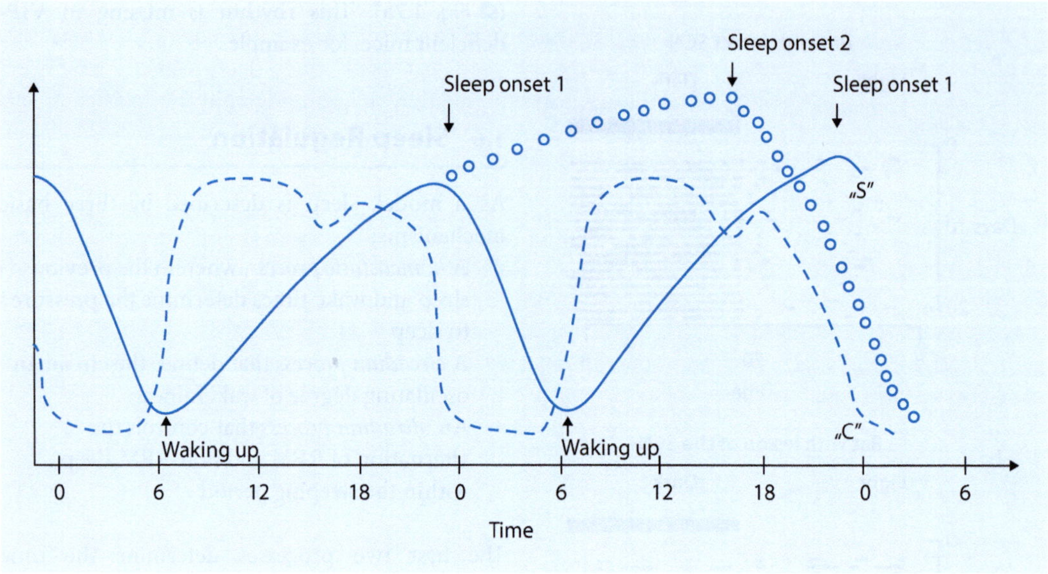

Fig. 1.9 Model of sleep regulation according to Borbély. *C* circadian degree of wakefulness, *S* endogenous "sleep substance" accumulating in the wake phase. Sleep onset occurs when *C* is low and *S* is high (sleep onset 1). *Dotted line* is the course of *S* when sleep was missed for 1 night; sleep onset then typically occurred in the afternoon (sleep onset 2)

model was modified but generally confirmed: a dopaminergic (tuberomammillary nucleus), serotonergic (raphe nuclei), and adrenergic (locus coeruleus) activity that decreases from wakefulness via non-REM sleep and is almost completely suppressed during REM sleep is opposed to a high cholinergic (laterodorsal tegmentum, pedunculopontine nuclei) activity during wakefulness as well as during REM sleep. Accordingly, pharmaceuticals with a cholinergic or anticholinergic profile mostly have significant impacts on the parameters of REM latency, percentage, and density.

The condition of wakefulness is furthermore actively maintained by predominantly glutamatergic, besides also cholinergic, neurons of the ascending reticular activating system (ARAS) in the brainstem. An electrophysiological correlate of the diffuse tonic and phasic activation is the low-amplitude, high-frequency activity in the EEG. Sleep is induced by an active GABAergic decline of the tonic activity level of the ARAS during wakefulness. GABA is the most important and most broadly distributed inhibiting transmitter in the CNS. It binds to $GABA_A$ and $GABA_B$ receptors, whereof the $GABA_A$ receptors mediate the relevant sedating and sleep-promoting as well as anxiolytic and muscle-relaxing effects.

Although serotonin shows activating and even mood-lifting effects during the daytime, it is significantly responsible for the overall development of sleep and especially for deep sleep regulation. The serum concentration of serotonin during sleep correlates directly with the percentage of deep sleep. The peptide hormones hypocretin 1 and 2 (orexin A and B) originate from a precursor protein exclusively produced in maximally 100,000 neurons of the dorsal, lateral, and posterior hypothalamus as well as the perifornical nucleus. Hypocretinergic neurons seem to have a mainly excitatory effect on systems stimulating wakefulness. Their activity continuously increases during the day with a maximum in the evening.

1.7 Functions of Sleep

Simply put, the condition of wakefulness is considered as a temporary hyperactive catabolic phase serving as time for food intake and reproduction. Different functions are assigned to sleep; the most important of these are explained in the following paragraphs.

The *function of recovery* seems to be clear for everybody from their own experience. This concept is supported by the increased level of growth hormone directly after sleep onset, the restoration of cerebral glycogen as well as enhanced delta power, and the prolonged sleep phase after sleep deprivation. Opposed to these are the reduced protein synthesis during sleep, the unchanged duration of sleep despite physical stress, and the unchanged mitotic rate during sleep.

Another hypothesis states that sleep has the function of *saving energy*. Energy consumption actually decreases during sleep by about 10%, and body temperature is reduced. The evidence of neurons in the anterior hypothalamus that contribute to thermoregulation as well as sleep regulation supports the concept that sleep and thermoregulation are closely linked.

In addition, sleep is considered as being relevant for a *well-functioning immune system*. This idea, however, is generated exclusively from investigations with sleep-deprived laboratory animals or patients. Sleep deprivation led to an increased susceptibility for infections and a reduced vaccination response. In cases of extreme sleep deficit, an animal experiment with rats even revealed a collapse of the immune system with fatal outcome.

The *ontogenic theory* attributes an important function to REM sleep for the differentiation of the brain, especially during the first months of life. In terms of this model, the atony of the skeletal muscles during REM sleep allows stimulation of the brain without the necessity of movements that would have to be actually performed. In the fetal stage, for example, breathing movements are neuronally executed during REM sleep. Furthermore, certain behavioral patterns that are necessary to conserve the species are regularly trained and presented to a potential mating partner: these include the erection of men that is closely linked to REM sleep and the increased vaginal blood flow of women. During REM sleep, primarily processes occur that are associated with psychic well-being and intellectual performance (see ▶ Sect. 1.8). REM deficiency in children may lead to later developmental problems, behavioral disorders, permanent problems with sleep, reduced brain mass, and an extraordinarily high neuronal cell death (see ▶ Chap. 11).

The *consolidation of memory and acquired knowledge and skills* during sleep is scientifically proven. In 1924, it could already be confirmed that simple learning tasks (declarative learning) that were offered immediately before a sleep period were better retained than tasks before a wake period of the same duration. In particular, studies of recent times reveal the probability of a correlation between non-REM sleep and the declarative memory. REM sleep, however, seems to have a key role for procedural memory (e.g., riding a bike) and emotional memory (emotion-related content). These findings are not only academically relevant, but they may also confirm the impaired memory that is a frequent complaint of patients with sleep disorders.

1.8 Dreaming

1.8.1 Definitions

In everyday language, the term dream is used with many meanings, in such expressions as being a dreamer, dream house, or the woman of my dreams. Approaching the phenomenon of dream from a scientific perspective requires clear definitions for dreaming as process as well as for dreams (dream reports):

- *Definition I*: Dreaming is subjective experiencing that occurs during sleep.
- *Definition II: A dream or a dream report is the recollection of subjective experiences that occurred during sleep after waking up.*

The term 'subjective experiences' intends to elucidate the fact that dreaming is a holistic experience with sensory impressions, emotions, and thoughts, that is, we experience ourselves in dreams in the same way as in the state of wakefulness. Sleep physiology (EEG, eye movements, heart rate, etc.) can be assessed and measured, but the subjective experiences can only be accessed by means of interviews after awakening. For sleep and dream research, it is important to distinguish both levels, the physiological and the psychological level.

The second definition illustrates one aspect very clearly. Dreaming is not directly accessible, either for the dreamer nor for the researcher. Two transitions have to be made to obtain a dream report: first, the individual has to awaken (sleep–wake transition), and, second, the individual has to recall what happened before waking up (dimension of time). So, the question has to be asked to what extent the dream report reliably reflects the experiences that occurred during sleep.

Table 1.3 Different types of dreams

Term	Definition
REM dreams	Recalling the subjective experiences that occurred during REM sleep
Non-REM dreams	Recalling the subjective experiences that occurred during non-REM sleep
Sleep-onset dreams	Recalling the subjective experiences that occurred during non-REM sleep stage 1
Nightmares	REM dreaming with strongly negative emotions that typically cause awakening
Night terror (pavor nocturnus)	Abrupt arousal from slow wave sleep associated with panic, might be accompanied by non-REM dreams
Posttraumatic replications	REM or non-REM dreams that realistically replicate a traumatic event
Lucid dreams	REM dreams associated with the awareness that the current experiences are dream experiences

Dreams can be classified into different groups (Table 1.3).

In the first sleep lab studies on dreams, the participants were woken up from REM sleep, and the researcher received reports about vivid and colorful dreams with very high probability (more than 80%). After awakenings from non-REM sleep, however, dreams were reported very rarely. In 1962, David Foulkes highlighted the fact that the definition of dreaming play a major role in this context: He did not ask specifically about vivid dreams but generally about what went through the participant's mind before the awakening. Applying this approach, he obtained report rates of more than 50% even for non-REM awakenings. Even if non-REM dreams are often shorter, less emotionally intense, and more comparable to thoughts than REM dreams, the distinction is not clear-cut. About 25% of non-REM dreams cannot be differentiated from REM dreams based on their content.

Sleep-onset dreams occur in non-REM stage 1 and are typically forgotten when the sleeper is not awakened by noise during the process of falling asleep. Mostly sleep-onset dreams are a continuation of the thoughts one has prior to sleep onset; sometimes these thoughts can become very bizarre. However, there are also many people who experience single images and also sequences of images during sleep onset, so that the distinction to REM dreams is not clear-cut.

The classification of dreams based on sleep stages emphasizes the current view that dreaming takes place during the entire time of sleep. The brain and consciousness never sleep.

The following three dream phenomena are associated with fear: nightmares, night/sleep terror (pavor nocturnus), and posttraumatic replications.

Nightmares are REM dreams in which the strong negative affect causes awakening. Nightmares are differentiated from distressing or "bad" dreams that also contain strong negative emotions such as fear, disgust, or grief but that do not result in awakening (see ► Chap. 7).

In the context of *night terror* or sleep terror (pavor nocturnus), the individual abruptly arouses from slow wave sleep with intense panic, but the person is not really fully awake and often cannot recall the incident (see ► Chap. 7).

Posttraumatic replications originate from traumatic events such as sexual abuse or war experiences and may occur during REM or non-REM sleep. Even during daytime, such posttraumatic repetitions may appear, these are called "flashbacks." These three dream phenomena (nightmares, night terrors, posttraumatic replications) are forms of parasomnias (see ► Chap. 7).

During *lucid dreams*, the dreamer is aware of the fact that s/he is dreaming. This state is highly interesting to researchers but also for the individual himself/herself because of the manifold possibilities to influence the dream according to one's own intentions.

In other states of consciousness, dreamlike imagery is experienced, for example, under anesthesia or in the context of near-death experiences. Even during wakefulness, dreamlike phenomena may occur; these are called daydreams or mindwandering.

1.8.2 Dream Recall

Although it is currently assumed that every individual dreams every night, recalling the events experienced during sleep after waking up varies a great deal. Some people are able to report a dream nearly every morning, whereas others state that they have not dreamt for many years or - to be correct - that they do not remember any dream for a long time. The basic factors for those inter-individual differences in dream recall are not yet fully understood.

Regarding dream recall, a stable gender difference have been found. The findings that women showed a higher rate of dream recall than men could be explained by a study showing that girls talk more often about their dreams during childhood and adolescence compared to boys, which might indicate a gender-specific dream socialization; that is, talking about dreams and the interest in dreams has been promoted in girls but not so much in boys. Findings showing that dream recall decreases with age in cross-sectional studies have to be viewed with caution because there are no longitudinal studies (investigations of a individuals from young adulthood to older ages), and a high constancy of the dream recall over this period can be expected from retrospective studies.

Regarding personality factors, most studies did not find correlations between dimensions such as repression, extraversion, and anxiety and dream recall frequency. Similarly, cognitive factors such as general intelligence are not relevant with regard to dream recall. Personality dimensions such as "thin boundaries" that are related to creativity and vivid fantasy life had a significant but small influence. The fact that the ability to recall dreams can be significantly increased with simple means (preparing pen and paper, focusing on dream recall when waking up) indicates that trait factors may only explain a small portion of the inter-individual differences in dream recall.

Regarding sleep parameters, it was found that people who have poor sleep quality and often awaken at night remember their dreams more frequently. Also, insomnia patients have a higher frequency of dream recall than healthy individuals. This difference is plausible: the higher the frequency of nocturnal awakenings, the greater the chance to recall a dream.

Today, empirical findings are best fit in with the arousal-retrieval model of dream recall. Two steps are important in this context: first, one has to be awake after the dream experience so that it can be stored into the long-term memory, and, second, the awakening process should contain few interferences, and the dream should have a significance and/or emotional intensity so that it will be well remembered.

Practical Tip

Tips to increase dream recall
- Prepare pen and paper in the evening on the night table before going to bed.
- Make up your mind before falling asleep to recall a dream in the morning.
- After waking up, take some time, think back and rehearse all that you can recall (like learning a poem by heart).
- Take at least some notes of the dream actions.
- Record your dreams regularly.

Table 1.4 Reality character of diary dreams (*n* = 365)

Category	Incidence
Possible in wakefulness, normal everyday experiences	29.3%
Possible in wakefulness, but unusual elements	39.5%
One or two bizarre (impossible) elements	27.4%
Several bizarre elements	4.1%

1.8.3 General Characteristics of Dreams

In more than 90% of dreams the dream-self is involved in the dream action, i.e., most dream experiences are holistic in a similiar way as we experience wakefulness. Dreams that the dreamer watches like a movie and in which the dream-self remains totally passive are very rare.

Regarding the reality character of dreams, the general public often assumes that most dreams are bizarre, that is, contain elements that are not possible in the physical reality of our waking world. This concept is probably explained by the fact that in most cases only exciting, interesting and/or extraordinary dreams are shared with others or published. An content analysis of dreams that had been recorded for 2 weeks by participants on a regular basis (see ◘ Table 1.4), however, showed that only about 30% of the dreams actually contain elements that are impossible in waking life. In this context, the definition of bizarreness is of importance. Some authors already consider abrupt scene shifts or inconsistencies (the apartment from one's childhood is located in another city) as bizarre, so that according to this definition nearly all dreams contain bizarre elements.

In laboratory dreams as well as diary dreams, healthy individuals showed a balanced proportion of positive and negative dream emotions. However, in the laboratory, more neutral dreams occur, i.e., lab dreams are less intensive than home dreams.

The common view that dreams are predominantly negative is probably explained by the fact that negative dreams, in particular when they are recurring, are more easily recalled even after several years. Further, positive dream emotions are less frequently described explicitly in the dream report, so that studies that do not assess the dreamers' subjective ratings but only analyze the dream reports are subjected to bias, that is, a preponderance of negative emotions is then found.

All dreams contain visual perceptions. In individuals who are congenitally blind, these visual perceptions in dreams are completely missing. Visual dream content, even decades after the loss of sight, can be found in individuals who lost their vision after the age of 7.

Auditory perception also plays an important role in dreams, whereby language is more prominent than noises.

Kinesthetic experiences (sensations that originate from movement) occur now and then, for example in the context of flying dreams, but also in the context of other types of movement. Tactile, gustatory, and olfactory experiences and pain only rarely occur in dreams.

1.8.4 Correlation Between Wakefulness and Dream

Before addressing possible functions of dreams in the next paragraph, the question if and how waking-life experiences influence the dream content is discussed. To study this topic, different methodical approaches have been applied.

For determining temporal references of dream elements, the participant is asked - typically after reporting or recording the dream(s) - when a certain event that occurred in the dream had happened in waking life the last time, for example, seeing one's mother. Even if such studies frequently showed a very plausible exponential decrease with increasing time interval to the matching waking-life experience (comparable to other memory processes), the results have to be evaluated with caution. The main problem is that it is nearly impossible for participants to remember all waking-life events and thoughts of the last days, weeks, or years. Another difficulty is that many events take place over and over again in waking life. For example, the mother in the dream might be associated with the telephone call from the previous evening with her but also might be linked to a childhood memory. These types of studies may provide interesting ideas for hypotheses, but the findings have to be confirmed by experimental and field studies.

For experimental manipulation, the pre-sleep experiences of the participants are influenced, for example, by showing movies, reading stories, or letting the participant carry out specific activities. In many studies films were used in the evening before the participant went to bed in the sleep lab. Overall, the studies on experimental manipulation showed that specific film elements were rarely found within subsequent dreams, but the emotional quality of dreams were affected by the experimental conditions, i.e., a stressful film was followed by dreams with more negative emotions.

Because experimental manipulation did not show large effects on dreams, *field studies* tried to investigate the effects of real stressors and life events on dreams. Field studies are performed outside the artificial lab environment and assess waking-life events and dreams by means of diaries, questionnaires, or interviews. Daytime events and dreams can be assessed on a day-to-day basis (or from night to night) to test how many days it will take until a specific event actually show up in the dream. This approach can be used to assess intraindividual fluctuations of dream content over time.

Life events such as divorce and pregnancy have shown clear influences on the dream content of the individuals. The strong effects, are especially obvious in traumatic events such as sexual abuse, war experiences, or natural disasters. Our own data indicated that participants who had experienced the Second World War reported, even in 2000 more frequently war dreams than younger participants. The field studies demonstrated impressively that dramatic and stressing life events have a strong and sometimes long-lasting influence on dreaming.

In summary, the empirical results support the *continuity hypothesis* stating that dreams directly reflect the waking life. However, further research efforts are necessary to exactly assess the factors such as emotional intensity of waking-life experiences, personality of the dreamer, etc. that moderate the relationship between dreaming and waking.

1.8.5 Function of Dreams

The question arises if dreaming defined as subjective experiences during sleep has a function that goes beyond the function(s) of sleep (see ► Sect. 1.7). Memory consolidation during sleep, for example, takes place on the cellular level and system level so that it is not very likely that dreams are involved in these processes; they probably just reflect those processes. Practicing simple motor abilities during lucid dreams such as throwing darts with the nondominant hand, showed a positive effect on performance on the next morning. This effect is comparable with the effect of mental training carried out in the waking state, which has already been applied in sports for many years. Research still has to demonstrate the function or positive effects of dreams on wakefulness in an experimental setting. One problem is that dreaming can only be accessed via the dream report (recall of the dream experience after waking up); possible positive effects may be explained by sharing the dream or reflecting on the dream content and is not necessarily causal to the dream experience itself. Unfortunately, one cannot study the effects of unrecalled dreams on waking life. Over the years, many functions of dreaming have been proposed, for example, the dream as the guardian of sleep (Sigmund Freud). Today, many researchers assume that dreaming has a problem-solving function because elements from memory (waking-life experiences of the past) are mixed with new input of current wakefulness within dreams in a creative way—a kind of brainstorming at night. Research efforts are still needed to answer the question of the function of dreaming.

1.9 Questions

1. Please describe and define the sleep stages according to the AASM criteria.
2. Which physiological changes during sleep do you know?
3. Please describe the sleep–wake regulation taking into account chronobiological aspects.
4. Which findings indicate that dreaming takes place during the entire sleep?

Further Reading

1. American Academy of Sleep Medicine. International classification of sleep disorders, vol 3. Aufl. Darien: American Academy of Sleep Medicine; 2014.
2. Berry RB, Brooks R, Gamaldo CE, Harding SM, Lloyd RM, Marcus CL Vaughn BV, for the American Academy of Sleep Medicine. The AASM manual for the scoring of sleep and associated events: rules, terminology and technical specifications, version 2.6. www.aasmnet.org. Darien: American Academy of Sleep Medicine 2016.
3. Czeisler CA, Gooley JJ. Sleep and circadian rhythms in humans. Cold Spring Harb Symp Quant Biol. 2007;72:579–97.
4. Dijk DJ, Lockley SW. Integration of human sleep-wake regulation and circadian rhythmicity. J Appl Physiol. 2002;92:852–62.
5. Moore RY. Suprachiasmatic nucleus in sleep-wake regulation. Sleep Med. 2007;8(suppl 3):27–33.
6. Peter H, Penzel T, Peter JH. Enzyklopädie der Schlafmedizin. Heidelberg: Springer; 2007.
7. Schredl M. Researching Dreams: The Fundamentals. Cham: Palgrave Macmillan; 2018.
8. Walker MP. Why we sleep - The new science of sleep and dreams. New York: Scribner, 2017.

Diagnostic Methods

H.-G. Weeß

B. A. Stuck et al., *Practice of Sleep Medicine*, https://doi.org/10.1007/978-3-030-17412-5_2

At first sight only, sleep disorders are simple and easily accessible diseases. Actually, they are complex disorders that require intensive and thorough diagnostics. The genesis of sleep disorders, in particular in older individuals, is multifactorial, and so an interdisciplinary approach is necessary. According to the *International Classification of Sleep Disorders* revised in 2014 (ICSD-3), about 50 sleep disorders may be distinguished. Sleep disorders may be based on single medical, physiological, psychological, psychopathological, or pharmacological factors, but frequently they only become obvious through the interaction of different etiological conditions. The following chapter describes the whole spectrum of diagnostic methods in sleep medicine, starting with history taking and continuing to device-related diagnostics in adults. Herein, the description of the core elements of diagnostic methods in sleep medicine, that is, polygraphy and polysomnography, is the focus. The standard measurement parameters of polysomnography are defined based on the criteria of the DGSM (Deutsche Gesellschaft für Schlafforschung und Schlafmedizin, the German Society of Sleep Research and Sleep Medicine). These criteria are complemented by the scoring rules for polysomnography and polygraphy (home sleep apnea testing), which are revised by the American Academy of Sleep Medicine (AASM) almost yearly. The parameters to be reported for polysomnography and polygraphy as well as the indications of polysomnography are described for different sleep disorders according to the evidence-based criteria of the AASM. Further, typical polysomnographic particularities of different sleep disorders are depicted in detail. A description of Specific diagnostic methods for children is given in ▶ Chap. 11.

Regarding the interdisciplinary nature of sleep disorders in the diagnostic process knowledge of internal medicine, pneumology, cardiology, neurology, psychiatrie, psychology and otolaryngology (ENT) is essential. Often the most frequent sleep disorders, such as insomnia and sleep-related breathing disorders, coincide. A single-sided focus of diagnostics and therapy on only one disorder does not address the patients' complaints in these cases.

2.1 History Taking

Structured clinical interviews lead to a higher validity of the patient's history.

Free clinical interviews in the context of medical history taking may lead to underestimating or overlooking significant symptoms.

Also, *standardized sleep questionnaires* for self-assessment of the quality and quantity of sleep, daytime impairments, observations of the bed partner, as well as information about potential origins of sleep disorders allow objectifying the medical history and are suitable to facilitate the diagnostic process and to make it more economical (▶ Sects. 2.3 and 2.8).

Regarding the exploration of sleep disorders, five basic principles should be considered:

- Even seemingly harmless sleep disorders require diagnostic attention because, for example, severe sleep-related breathing disorders may cause only light symptoms during the day, or untreated chronified insomnia disorders can be associated with an increased risk for developing cardiovascular diseases, metabolic diseases, or psychiatric disorders.
- To establish a relationship of trust between the therapist and the patient, first a symptom-oriented approach is recommended. Trusting relationships require time on both sides.
- The patient should be involved as a "scientific coworker" in his own interest. Especially in cases of psychogenic sleep disorders, patients are prone to base their sleep problems on merely organic origins. Possible impairments of well-being or mood swings during the daytime are considered more as sequelae of the sleep problem and less as their origin. A sleep diary (▶ Sect. 2.3) might be helpful to explain the correlation between the patient's mental condition during the daytime and ability to sleep at night.
- In cases of psychogenic triggers, an empathic, respectful approach should be the focus. Confronting the patient with the psychological conditions that trigger or maintain the sleep disorder should be undertaken very carefully.
- The subjective symptoms are more important than the objective findings. Polysomnography (PSG) is an important diagnostic tool for identification of the origins of sleep disorders and their severity. Nonetheless, polysomnographic parameters do not always correlate directly with the experiences and complaints of the patient (▶ Sect. 2.7).

2

2.1.1 Sleep-Related Personal Anamnesis

The present chapter on history taking is mainly oriented toward the sleep disorders of adults. History taking for sleep disorders in pediatric patients may be significantly different, especially with the background that parents who are interviewed in the context of sleep disorders in children, in the sense of history compiling by a third party, have a central role. ► Chapter 11 provides the necessary information for the special methods of history taking in children,.

The medical personal history is the beginning of the diagnostic process of sleep disorders. Intensive data collection strengthens the patient's impression of being taken seriously and increases the understanding of the diagnosing physician. Even at the beginning of the diagnostic process, structured sleep diaries may be helpful (► Sect. 2.3).

Assessment of Sleep-Related Complaints

- Bedtimes and their regularity
- Behavior and conditions before going to bed and after getting up in the morning
- Subjective duration of sleep onset
- Subjective extent and characteristics of wake time after sleep onset
- Particular phenomena such as snoring, sleep apnea (► Chap. 4), or sleepwalking (► Chap. 7) that occur during sleep should be reported by the bed partner as a third party (► Sect. 2.1.2)
- Sleep–wake structure, especially sleep-promoting or sleep-disturbing behavior during daytime and at night
- Particular life situations or diseases at the onset of the disorder
- Duration of the complaints
- Chronic or temporary occurrence of the complaints
- Psychophysiological arousal during and before the sleep phase (► Sect. 3.2.2)
- Cognitive and emotional arousal preceding and during the sleep period (► Sect. 3.2.2)
- Anticipatory anxiety regarding sleep and focusing on the sleep problem (► Sect. 3.2.2)
- Other factors concerning sleep hygiene (► Sects. 3.1.6 and 3.2.1)
- Movement of the extremities (► Chap. 8)
- Nightmares and nighttime arousal (► Chap. 7)

Assessment of General Daytime Complaints

Mental condition such as irritability, depression, anxiety, etc. (► Chap. 10 and ► Sect. 0):

- Anticipatory fears regarding sleep and focus on the sleep disorder
- Monotony intolerance: assessing the proneness to fall asleep with potentially circadian or ultradian rhythms (► Chaps. 1 and 6), if needed, by means of a sleep diary (► Sect. 2.3)
- Sleepiness and fatigue during the day (► Sect. 2.1.3)
- Subjective impairments in daytime performance, such as memory impairments, concentration deficits, reduced driving ability, and social life impairments (► Sect. 2.8)

Further, the exploration of factors involved in the onset of the sleep disorders is essential. Psychosocial stress (divorce, job change, death of a closely related person, etc.), medical conditions (thyroid disorder, pain syndrome, pharmaceutics, hospital stays, menopause, etc.), lifestyle changes (weight gain, etc.), and sleep-incompatible behavior are frequent origins of sleep disorders.

Analysis of the patient's behavior and general condition, as well as observations by third parties during sleep with regard to snoring, apnea, sleepwalking, or restless legs, may provide important information about the genesis of a sleep disorder.

2.1.2 Sleep-Related History Compiled by Third Parties

The diagnostic process of sleep-related history taking by interviewing third parties includes observers (partners, other patients, nursing staff, etc.) to confirm and describe sleep-related symptoms. In cases of diagnostically unclear complaints, the observations of others may sometimes provide surprising information facilitating the diagnosis or at least a probable diagnosis. Generally, these observations include symptoms that a patient does not perceive consciously. In children, history taking by interviewing others is mandatory (▶ Chap. 11). Based on the suspected diagnosis, the observer may be involved in systematic observations of the behavior. Especially for the differentiation of pavor nocturnus, nightmares, sleepwalking, nighttime enuresis, nighttime movement disorders (including jactatio capitis nocturna), sleep-talking, bruxism, and neurological sleep disorders [such as Rapid Eye Movement (REM) behavior disorder, and nocturnal cerebral seizures], systematic observation by third parties is indicated.

2.1.3 History Taking Regarding Sleepiness, Fatigue, and Daytime Performance

Daytime impairments associated with fatigue and sleepiness are frequently observed symptoms of sleep disorders; however, they may also occur in the context of other medical conditions or psychiatric disorders. Such symptoms can significantly reduce the patients' quality of life and impair their daytime performance. As a consequence, fitness for work and ability to drive is frequently reduced. Social interactions can be disturbed by sleepiness and also fatigue to the extent that the affected individuals withdraw from their usual social contacts. Hobbies, club activities, and activities with family and friends are given up. The feeling of insufficiency and the lack of self-confidence caused by these missing performances are often triggering factors and the base of developing psychasthenia and depressive disorders.

Although all patients complain about *fatigue* or *daytime sleepiness*, a more detailed exploration reveals differences regarding the quality of sleepiness- or fatigue-related impairments.

Practical Tip

Fatigue describes the subjective feeling of tiredness and exhaustion as it rather occurs in the context of psychosomatic disorders.

Sleepiness, however, has no psychiatric correlation. It often occurs as a sequela of nonrestorative or reduced sleep. Hereby, the increased proneness to fall asleep is characteristic, especially in monotonous situations.

Patients with *psychogenic insomnia disorders* (▶ Chap. 3) primarily describe the symptoms of fatigue, but they may also suffer from sleepiness. They experience rather the feeling of psychiatric exhaustion that is often enhanced in stress situations. This feeling may be understood as an expression of the chronically increased level of stress. More frequently, a feeling of overstrain occurs. The fatigue-related impairments rarely correlate with situational conditions such as driving a car, meetings, sports, or other activities. Moreover, intrapsychiatric conditions such as increased stress perception can be found. Important differences depending on the time of the day are rarely observed. In situations where sleeping is allowed, sleep onset does not occur.

Thus, the specific examination procedures for assessment of daytime sleepiness such as the multiple sleep latency test (MSLT), the maintenance of wakefulness test (MWT), or also the pupillographic sleepiness test (▶ Sect. 2.8.1) do not reveal pathological sleepiness values. The nighttime sleep quantity is often reduced because of the longer sleep-onset latencies and frequent wake times during the sleep period.

In cases of *medical sleep disorders* without psychogenic triggers and without increased levels of tension, another clinical picture of daytime sleepiness develops, frequently the result of nonrestorative sleep. It is characterized by a significantly increased proneness to fall asleep during daytime. If daytime sleep is possible, it occurs within a very short time.

In these patients psychological stress leads rather to a reduction of sleepiness. Furthermore, interestingly, motivating tasks or situations may reduce the sleepiness. In monotonous and low-stimulus situations, for example, driving on the

2

highway, watching TV, or cinema or theater, lectures, or long meetings, sleepiness is observed more frequently. Often significant circadian variations occur with increased sleepiness in the morning after getting up (hangover) and the early afternoon and evening hours. The quantity of night sleep is unchanged or even prolonged. Especially in the evenings and during holidays, longer sleep durations are observed.

In examinations of daytime sleepiness (MSLT, MWT, ▶ Sect. 2.8.1), very often reduced sleep-onset latencies and a pathological test value (pupillary unrest index, PUI) are found. Polysomnography often reveals increased sleep fragmentation with frequent changes of the sleep stages as well as increased percentages of light sleep and reduced percentages of deep sleep.

Of course, many variations exist between the seemingly diametric types of sleepiness and fatigue wherein medical and psychogenic proportions are mixed and interdependent (▶ Chap. 10). The characteristics described here, however, are not only theoretical observations; they also indicate different therapy approaches. Regarding the qualities of sleepiness- and fatigue-related impairments, see ◘ Table 2.1.

◘ **Table 2.1** Characteristics of fatigue and sleepiness

Fatigue	Sleepiness
Subjective feeling and perception of reduced performance in physically, psychologically, and mentally demanding situations	Reduction of the central nervous system alertness, i.e., wakefulness
Intrapsychic correlation of fatigue: exhaustion, feeling of overstrain, increase in stressful situations	Urge to sleep, no intrapsychic correlate, under stress, reduction of the sleepiness
In situations where sleep is possible or desired, it does not occur; no daytime sleep episodes	In situations where sleep is possible or desired, sleep occurs; daytime sleep episodes
No intolerance of monotony	Intolerance of monotony
No distinct circadian rhythm	Circadian rhythm
Monotonous situations do not stimulate sleep	Monotonous situations stimulate sleep
Sleep duration at night is normal or reduced	Sleep duration at night is normal or increased, sometimes with sleep fragmentation
Sleep-onset latency during daytime and at night is inconspicuous or prolonged	Sleep-onset latency during daytime and at night is unchanged or reduced
Sleep quantity on weekends or holidays is mostly unchanged	Sleep quantity on weekends or holidays is mostly increased

Fatigue and sleepiness are internationally used terms

2.1.4 Further History Taking for Differential Diagnostic: Assessment of Possible Origins of Sleep Disorders

General practice (GP)-based, psychiatric, neurological, and drug- and substance-related history taking includes current and former complaints, diseases, and substance consumption that might have triggered and maintained the sleep disorder.

In the context of *GP-based history taking*, in particular somatic diseases (endocrine, cardiovascular, neurodegenerative) are interesting as a possible origin of secondary sleep disorders (see ▶ Box 3.2).

The psychiatric history is relevant to assess psychiatric disorders that are frequently characterized by sleep disorders (▶ Chap. 10). About 80% of psychiatric diseases are accompanied by sleep disorders and about 30% of insomnias are based on psychiatric disorders. Special attention should be paid to these conditions:

- Mono- or bipolar affective diseases
- Prepsychotic conditions
- Chronified mood swings
- Substance abuse
- Intrapsychic conflicts
- Social stress situations

Insomnias are often prodromal characteristics of depressive disorders and are also frequently considered as the last symptom to disappear after remission of the depression. In the diagnostic process, the focus is on differentiating subtypes of chronic insomnia to find an adequate indication for therapeutic measures.

History taking and examination with regard to *neurological disorders* aim at assessing possible diseases of the central and peripheral nervous system. Most interesting are the following:

- Dementing processes
- Lesions of the central and peripheral nervous system
- Inflammatory processes
- Systemic diseases
- Other diseases affecting the nervous system

If a respective diagnosis is suspected, further examination such as electroencephalogram (EEG), long-term EEG, evoked potentials, imaging techniques, and laboratory examinations may be required. The indication must not be too strict in this context.

In particular, in cases of neurodegenerative diseases affecting the hypothalamus including the suprachiasmatic nucleus and the subcortical cholinergic, dopaminergic, and serotonergic pathways involved in sleep–wake regulation, important sleep disorders may be observed up to the dissolution of the sleep–wake rhythm. In more than 50% of the cases, dementia is associated with sleep disorders. The severity of dementia and the dissolved daytime rhythm are closely interrelated. A high discrepancy between the objective sleep disorder and the subjective sleep evaluation can be noted. In the context of dementia of Alzheimer's type (DAT), sleep disorders are more frequent than in the context of Lewy body dementia (LBD).

Many pharmaceuticals and medical substances affect sleep. The *drug-related history* includes all drugs available on prescription or obtainable without prescription. Several pharmaceuticals such as beta blockers, contraceptives, some antidepressants, appetite suppressants, or hypnotics may have a negative impact on sleep. Hence, many substances may cause insomnia as well as hypersomnia complaints. Even low doses of stimulants and addictive substances such as alcohol, tobacco, and other drugs may significantly impair sleep ability. The consumption of those substances even additionally and often persistently impairs the sleep ability of patients with sleep disorders compared to healthy individuals.

Practical Tip

The time of the first drug intake is of particular importance because the sleep quality changes in the further course following and might give indications for drug-related sleep disorders.

In the context of medical certificates, for example, on the fitness to drive or to work, urine screening is indicated with regard to stimulating and sedating substances to avoid simulation or dissimulation in the diagnostic process.

2.2 Laboratory Parameters for Sleep Disorders

Because numerous somatic and psychiatric diseases are secondarily associated with sleep disorders, screening regarding defined laboratory parameters is indicated in cases of respective anamnestic indications (◘ Table 2.2). When the

◘ **Table 2.2** Laboratory screening in cases of suspected secondary sleep disorders (further diagnostics and GP-based or internal examination if necessary)

Basic parameter	Additional parameters in cases of respective clinical suspicion
Blood count	Synthesis output by the liver (albumin, cholinesterase, INR)
BSG, CRP	Kidney values (creatinine, urea)
Electrolytes (sodium, potassium, calcium)	Vitamin B_{12}, folic acid, iron metabolism (transferrin situation, ferritin)
Glucose	Daily blood sugar profile, glucose tolerance test, HbA1c
Thyroid parameters (TSH)	–

differential diagnosis of single sleep disorders and their symptoms is established, the determination of further laboratory parameters may be indicated, for example, the values of iron, folic acid, and vitamin B_{12} for the differentiation between idiopathic and secondary restless leg syndrome (RLS). In the context of hypersomnia disorders, the determination of vitamin B_{12} and vitamin D may also be useful.

2.3 Sleep Questionnaire

Validated questionnaires are an important diagnostic tool. The results are relatively independent from the examiner (objectivity) and make the diagnostic process more efficient. In the waiting room, the patient may fill out the questionnaire and the receptionists or nursing staff may evaluate the forms after relevant instruction. The therapist must interpret these questionnaires, including all other findings.

For assessment of daytime sleepiness, the Epworth Sleepiness Scale (► Sect. 2.8.1) is applied as a generally accepted procedure in routine diagnostics.

The sleep diary is completed in the evening before going to bed and in the morning directly after arising to assess the patient's subjective quality of sleep and sleep-disturbing behavior. These data are collected:

- Sleep–wake disorder of any origin
- Subjective ability to sleep
- Sleep hygiene (lifestyle habits and behavior with regard to sleep)
- Sleep-disturbing behavior before and during the sleep period
- Condition before and during the sleep period
- Nocturnal particularities
- Consumption of substances

All bedtimes and sleep times, including those occurring during the daytime, should be noted. The estimation of the restorative quality of sleep has to be documented by the patient, as well as sleep-disturbing problems in the job-related and private environment. The consumption of coffee or tea or alcohol, and drug intake, as well as sleep-promoting activities such as use of relaxation techniques, need to be documented.

Practical Tip

The sleep diary is a basic standard for the diagnosis of sleep disorders. It should be kept for a period of at least 2 weeks.

For reasons of the initially enhanced self-observation with regard to sleep behavior and the resulting irritations and secondary increase of tension in the bed situation, the first 7 days are included in the analysis to only a limited extent.

2.3.1 Insomnia Questionnaire

Questionnaires on insomnia inform about the presence, the severity, and the course of an insomnia disorder. Because of the last-mentioned aspect, they are also suitable for therapy evaluation.

The Pittsburgh Sleep Quality Index (PSQI) contains 19 items on self-assessment and 5 questions on observations of third parties, such as the bed partner. Based on the replies, statements can be given on these points:

- Subjective quality of sleep
- Sleep-onset latency
- Sleep efficiency
- Consumption of hypnotics
- Daytime sleepiness
- Incidence of different sleep disorders within the previous 4 weeks

The PSQI validly differentiates between good and poor sleepers. It may indicate the severity of the disorder and thus evaluate the therapy.

Practical Tip

The PSQI is a standard procedure for the routine diagnostics of sleep disorders and provides information about the subjective quality of sleep.

The Insomnia Severity Index (ISI) consists of seven items assessing the type and severity of insomnia complaints of the previous 2 weeks based on a five-step rating scale. Insomnia is valued according to its severity, its impact on the psychosocial performance level during the day, and the subjectively experienced impairments. Furthermore, subjective satisfaction with one's own ability to sleep is assessed.

A score between 0 and 28 is calculated. Between 0 and 7, it is considered as clinically inconspicuous; a score of 8–14 indicates a subliminal insomnia, a score of 15–21 describes a moderate insomnia, and scores beyond 22 are considered as severe. The advantage of this procedure is that it is standardized and a theoretically validated test.

Numerous questionnaires have been developed to assess etiological factors and other aspects of insomnia. A widely distributed tool for the assessment of cognitive misconceptions and misbehavior is the "Dysfunctional Beliefs and Attitudes about Sleep Scale." It refers mainly to individual cognitions that maintain sleep disorders. Other procedures such as the "Presleep Arousal Scale" or the "Glasgow Sleep Effort Scale" assess the psychophysiological level of excitement in the bedtime situation. For better understanding of the impairment of the functional level during daytime, questionnaires assessing sleepiness and fatigue are recommended (▶ Sect. 2.8.1.3.2). Because of the high association of insomnia disorders with psychiatric diseases, psychiatric and psychological questionnaires may contribute to a better understanding of the etiology as well as the impact of an insomnia disorder: these include the "Beck Depression Inventory" as well as the "State-Trait Anxiety Inventory."

2.3.2 Questionnaires for the Assessment of Sleep-Related Breathing Disorders

Various questionnaires have been developed aiming at assessing the risk of sleep-related breathing disorders.

The STOP-Bang questionnaire consists of eight items and is a validated screening tool for the assessment of obstructive sleep apnea. Initially, it was developed for preoperative screening regarding obstructive sleep apnea. It is also validated for the general population. The questionnaire is based on six questions and two measurable values.

- S: Snoring (yes/no)
- T: Tiredness (yes/no)
- O: Observed/observed apnea (yes/no)
- P: Pressure/hypertension (yes/no)
- B: Body mass index (>35 kg/m^2?)
- A: Age (>50 years?)
- N: Neck/circumference at the level of Adam's apple (>43 cm in males and >41 cm in females)
- G: Gender (male yes/no)

Together with the Berlin Questionnaire, the STOP-Bang questionnaire is the most frequently recommended screening tool for obstructive sleep apnea (OSA). Compared to other screening questionnaires, the STOP-Bang questionnaire has the highest sensitivity and specificity for moderate and severe obstructive sleep apnea. A meta-analysis could confirm the high predictive value of the questionnaire. For the general population, a score of 0–2 means a low risk of OSA, with a moderate risk for scores of 3–4 and a high risk for scores of 5–8.

The Berlin Questionnaire supports the identification of obstructive sleep apnea. It is more suitable for exclusion diagnostics than for the assessment of the severity of possibly existing obstructive sleep apnea. Based on 11 items, the patient is classified in categories of high or low risk for obstructive sleep apnea. A review of 19 trials revealed a significant number of false-negative diagnoses based on the Berlin Questionnaire, which limits its application as a diagnostic tool. Furthermore, it was considered as being unsatisfactory regarding a sensitivity of 0.76 and a specificity of 0.45. The accuracy of the questionnaire was valued as too low, with 56% to 70%.

The NAMES test (Neck circumference, Airway classification, coMorbidities, Epworth scale, and Snoring) assesses the neck circumference, an examination of the upper airways, comorbidities, the Epworth score, and nighttime snoring to evaluate the risk of a possible sleep-related breathing disorder in a multidimensional way and to increase the validity of the information. The NAMES2 further includes body mass index (BMI) and gender.

2.3.3 Questionnaire Regarding Restless Legs Syndrome

To support the diagnostic process in the context of the restless legs syndrome (RLS), the RLS diagnose index (RLS-DI) has been developed. This tool constitutes diagnostic and additional criteria of RLS with five questions, each on a three-point rating scale. The overall score allows statements on the probability of the diagnosis. An RLS-DI overall score of more than 11 means a high probability of RLS, and more than 16 means a confirmed diagnosis.

2

Practical Tip

To assess the severity of RLS, most frequently the International RLS Study Group Rating Scale (IRLS) is used.

The IRLS is a self-assessment questionnaire. It includes ten items that evaluate the severity of the complaints and their impact on the daytime condition. The answers can achieve scores between 0 and 4 each, with higher scores representing more severe conditions and complaints.

Based on the sum score, the severity is defined as follows:

- 0: symptom-free
- 1–10: mild RLS
- 11–20: moderate RLS
- 21–30: severe RLS
- 31–40: very severe RLS

A large international validation trial showed very good test-theoretical quality criteria for the IRLS. the IRLS should only be applied in patients who have a confirmed diagnosis of restless legs syndrome because, in the context of psychiatric and neurological disorders, patients report higher IRLS scores even without the presence of RLS.

2.4 Physical Examination

Regarding all sleep disorders, the physical examination is an important element of the diagnostic process when a medical origin is assumed or has to be excluded. Based on the suspected diagnosis, examination of the head and neck area, heart and lungs, or the neurological system has a major role. The physical examination is indicated in particular in the context of sleep-related breathing disorders (▶ Chap. 4), movement disorders in sleep (▶ Chap. 8), and sleep disorders caused by medical diseases (▶ Chap. 9). It is described in the respective chapters.

2.5 Actigraphy

For more than 30 years, actigraphy has been a method for objective measurement of movements that can be applied in a simple way over longer periods. The actigraph is a tool mostly worn at the wrist or the ankle that measures movement activity. The activity patterns, which are often registered and stored over several days, allow conclusions about the sleep–wake rhythm and also about leg activities during sleep (▶ Chap. 8.2).

Studies based only on the correlation between actigraphy data and polysomnographic data in young healthy individuals revealed a congruence of 91% to 93%. Validation studies mostly refer to correlations between the significant target parameters of polysomnography (PSG) and actigraphy, such as the overall sleeping time or sleep efficiency.

Actigraphy (◘ Fig. 2.1) allows statements about these concerns:

- Sleep habits
- Sleep disorders
- Daytime sleep episodes
- Therapy outcome

By means of keeping a behavior protocol at the same time, for example, the sleep-onset latency, nocturnal wake phases or a prolonged sleep duration may be estimated.

Despite these advantages, actigraphy may not replace PSG. The disadvantage of actigraphy is in particular the lack of precision because indirect measurements only roughly reflect sleep continuity. One frequently observed artifact is the removal of the tool, so that these phases may be misinterpreted as sleep, such as also calm phases during wakefulness, for example, when reading. Also overlapping movements that are externally induced, as, for example, when sitting in a car, may be misinterpreted. The management of the artifacts is only possible with the simultaneous application of a behavioral protocol.

Practical Tip

If periodic limb movements in sleep (PLMS) are confirmed, actigraphy may be applied for diagnostics and therapy because it can provide information about the incidence of periodic limb movements during sleep. Times of going to bed and of getting up should be exactly documented.

In the context of outpatient insomnia diagnostics, actigraphy may provide important information on disturbed sleep–wake rhythm, irregularities of bedtimes, and nighttime behavior.

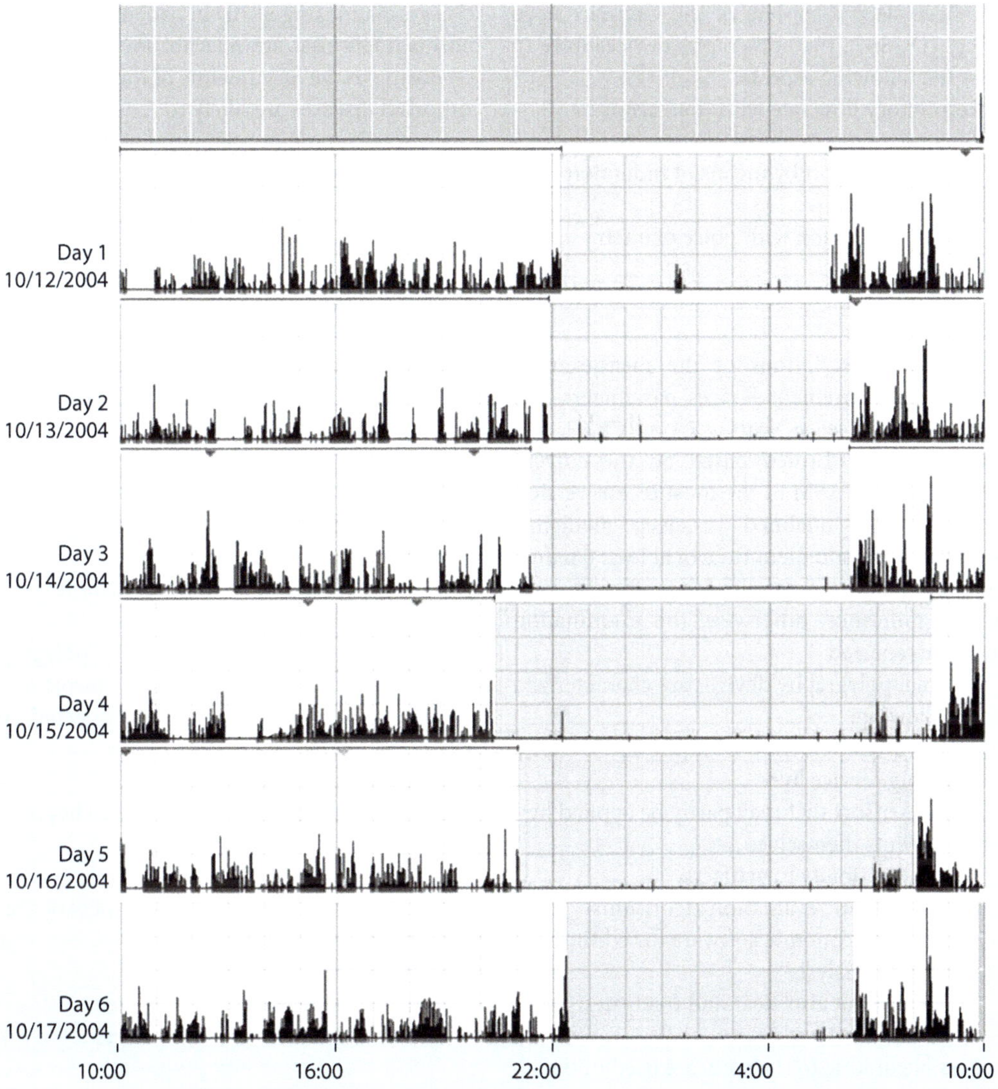

Fig. 2.1 Actigraphy. Measurement during 6 days. Sleep periods are shown in *light gray*

2.6 Outpatient Step-by-Step Diagnostics for Sleep-Related Breathing Disorders and Polygraphy Systems

The necessity of device-related diagnostics in cases of sleep-related breathing disorders (SRBD) is obvious after positive anamnesis of the respective symptoms. The more characteristic symptoms that are found, the more likely is the suspected diagnosis that has to be verified. According to the recommendations of the American Academy of Sleep Medicine (AASM) from 2017 as well as the S3 guideline on non-restorative sleep/sleep disorders—"Sleep-related breathing disorders"—of the German Society of Sleep Research and Sleep Medicine (DGSM, Deutsche Gesellschaft für Schlafforschung und Schlafmedizin), the monitored cardiorespiratory polysomnography is considered as the gold standard of device-related sleep medical diagnostics in the sleep lab. For limited diagnostics of sleep-related breathing disorders, simpler, portable polygraphy systems are also available.

According to the S3 guideline on nonrestorative sleep/sleep disorders of the German Sleep Society (DGSM), the polygraphy devices have to assess the following aspects:

- Respiratory flow rate with thermistor or dynamic pressure sensor
- Respiratory effort by means of induction plethysmography
- Oxygen saturation with pulse oximetry
- Pulse rate
- Body position

For detailed descriptions of the measurement technique, measurement devices, parameters, and their definition, see ► Sects. 2.7.1 and 2.7.8. The evaluation is performed based on the current schemes of the AASM in the most recent version by a physician qualified in sleep medicine. Generally, a measurement time of at least 6 h during the sleep period is required for sufficient diagnostic significance; otherwise, the examination should be repeated.

Optimal polygraphy devices are characterized by the following:

- Robust measurement techniques and sensors with long service lives
- Simple sensors that may partly be applied by the patients themselves
- Low susceptibility to artifacts
- Valid automatic evaluation algorithms
- Simple and economic software for editing the automated analysis
- Exhaustive but also clear and freely designable automated findings
- Possible linking to the software used in the practice or the hospital information system by means of different interface technologies (e.g., HL7 interface)

According to the already cited S3 guideline of the DGSM as well as recommendations of the AASM from 2017, the diagnosis of SRBD with unattended polygraphy systems is possible in cases of moderate to strong suspicion and to determine the severity of SRBD. The evaluation should be performed visually by qualified staff. Evaluation by only software-inherent algorithms cannot be recommended. For exclusion diagnostics of SRBD, PSG is recommended because polygraphy is not considered as sufficiently valid for this purpose.

Generally, polygraphy should not substitute PSG for diagnosing SRBD in patients with comorbid disorders that are relevant for this question. According to the S3 guideline of the DGSM, some comorbid diseases are likely to reduce the significance of polygraphy systems and require diagnostic polysomnography:

- Pulmonary diseases
- Psychiatric disorders
- Neurological disorders
- Neuromuscular diseases

In the same way, polygraphy is not recommended for the comorbid appearance of sleep disorders such as these:

- Central sleep apnea
- Insomnia
- Periodic movement disorders in sleep
- Narcolepsy
- Circadian sleep–wake rhythm disorders

The AASM recommends unattended polygraphy in cases of moderate to strong suspicion of obstructive sleep apnea without suspected concomitants:

- Central sleep apnea
- Hyperventilation and sleep-related hypoxemia
- Cardiopulmonary disease
- Significant neuromuscular weakness of the respiratory muscles
- Hypersomnia
- Parasomnia
- Sleep-related movement disorders

Furthermore, it is not recommended when the patient's history reveals stroke or current chronic opiate medication. The AASM also recommends PSG when unattended polygraphy despite strong clinically suspected diagnosis was negative, contradictory, or technically inadequate. In addition, the AASM requires that the evaluation of unattended polygraphy is performed by a physician qualified in sleep medicine, a certified sleep laboratory, or a comparable institution.

It must be realized that, in cases of predominant hypopnea, polygraphy systems are not always able to validly differentiate between obstructive and central sleep apnea (► Sect. 2.7.8). Because of the missing EEG channels, they are less exact for the definition of the severity of sleep apnea compared to polysomnography. Furthermore, the lack of an EEG may lead to the wrong classification of apnea when physiological irregularities of breathing occur during the wake-sleep transition (sleep-onset apnea) and thus provide false-positive results. These limited systems do not provide differential diagnoses of sleep apnea.

In Germany, the healthcare institutions have defined an outpatient stepped care model for the diagnosis of SRBD that seems to be suitable for application in other countries also because of its clear structure and efficiency.

Outpatient Stepped Care Model for the Diagnosis of SRBD

- Step 1: standardized questionnaires regarding specific symptoms and comorbidities of SRBD (▶ Sects. 2.3 and 2.8.1).
- Step 2: clinical examination with sleep anamnesis (▶ Sect. 2.1).
- Step 3: outpatient examination of the patient at home by means of eight-channel polygraphy.
- Step 4: in case of clearly positive outpatient polygraphy findings, therapy by means of nocturnal ventilation or other procedures may be introduced in an outpatient or inpatient sleep lab with polysomnographic monitoring. If the polygraphy findings are not clear, especially with regard to the presence of SRBD or missing differential diagnostic significance, diagnostic polysomnography is performed in the sleep lab in an inpatient or outpatient context.

Taking into account the mentioned limitations of the significance of polygraphy, relevant biosignals of sleep-related breathing disorders are assessed depending on the measurement system during one night at the patient's home (step 3).

The results are usually evaluated on the next day by means of computer-based analysis (◻ Figs. 2.2 and 2.3). In this regard, the American Academy of Sleep Medicine defined algorithms for the standardized evaluation of polygraphic examinations (◻ Tables 2.5 and 2.6).

According the S3 guideline on non-restorative sleep/sleep disorders [chapter "Sleep-Related Breathing Disorders" of the German Society for Sleep Research and Sleep Medicine (DGSM) and the recommendations of the American Academy of Sleep Medicine (AASM)], positive unattended polygraphic findings at home may lead directly to the initiation of a nocturnal ventilation therapy in a sleep lab under polysomnographic conditions (step 4). In case of inconclusive polygraphic results diagnostic polysomnography is performed prior to the beginning of therapy.

Recently, randomized controlled trials have been published on the initial therapy induction showing that CPAP/APAP adaptation may be performed in certain subgroups even without polysomnographic monitoring in a sleep lab. The expenses for an outpatient initial titration on nocturnal ventilation might be lower, but the consecutive costs in cases of reduced compliance are higher. This procedure can only be discussed for simple, uncomplicated cases of obstructive sleep apnea. Further studies are necessary to identify predictors of the treatment success even in the long-term course.

Follow-up and therapy controls may take place by means of polygraphy systems. In patients with unclear therapeutic success, and high cardiovascular risk, and patients with other sleep disorders in comorbidity, PSG controls might be indicated.

More recently, further outpatient examination procedures have been developed that seem to be suitable to provide diagnostic information to the presence of sleep-related breathing disorders, as, for example, peripheral arterial tonometry (PAT) and pulse transit time or pulse wave analysis.

Peripheral arterial tonometry (PAT) assesses variations of the vascular tonus at the finger during sleep. The peripheral vascular tonus and the peripheral vascular resistance are influenced by the sympathetic nerve activity. Hereby, the respiratory indices (desaturation index, AHI, RDI) measured by means of PAT correlate significantly positively with the sleep-related parameters assessed by polysomnography. In the current version, dated 2020, the AASM describes PAT as an

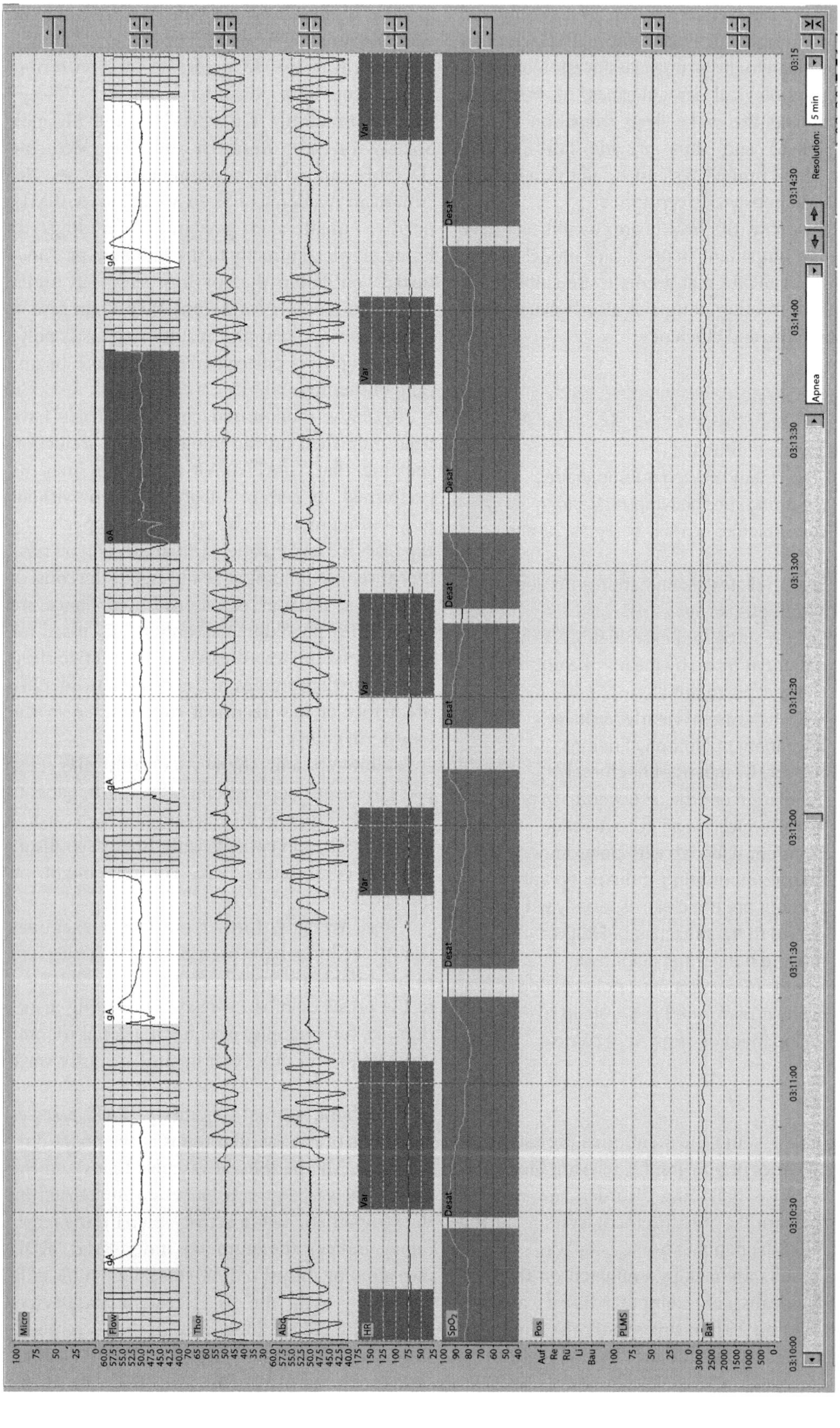

■ **Fig. 2.2** Depiction of 5 min of polygraphy measurement for obstructive sleep apnea. Repeated mixed and obstructive apneas (see figure, *Flow*), associated O_2 desaturations (see figure, *SpO₂*), and apnea-terminating accelerations of the heart rate are found as expression of arousals

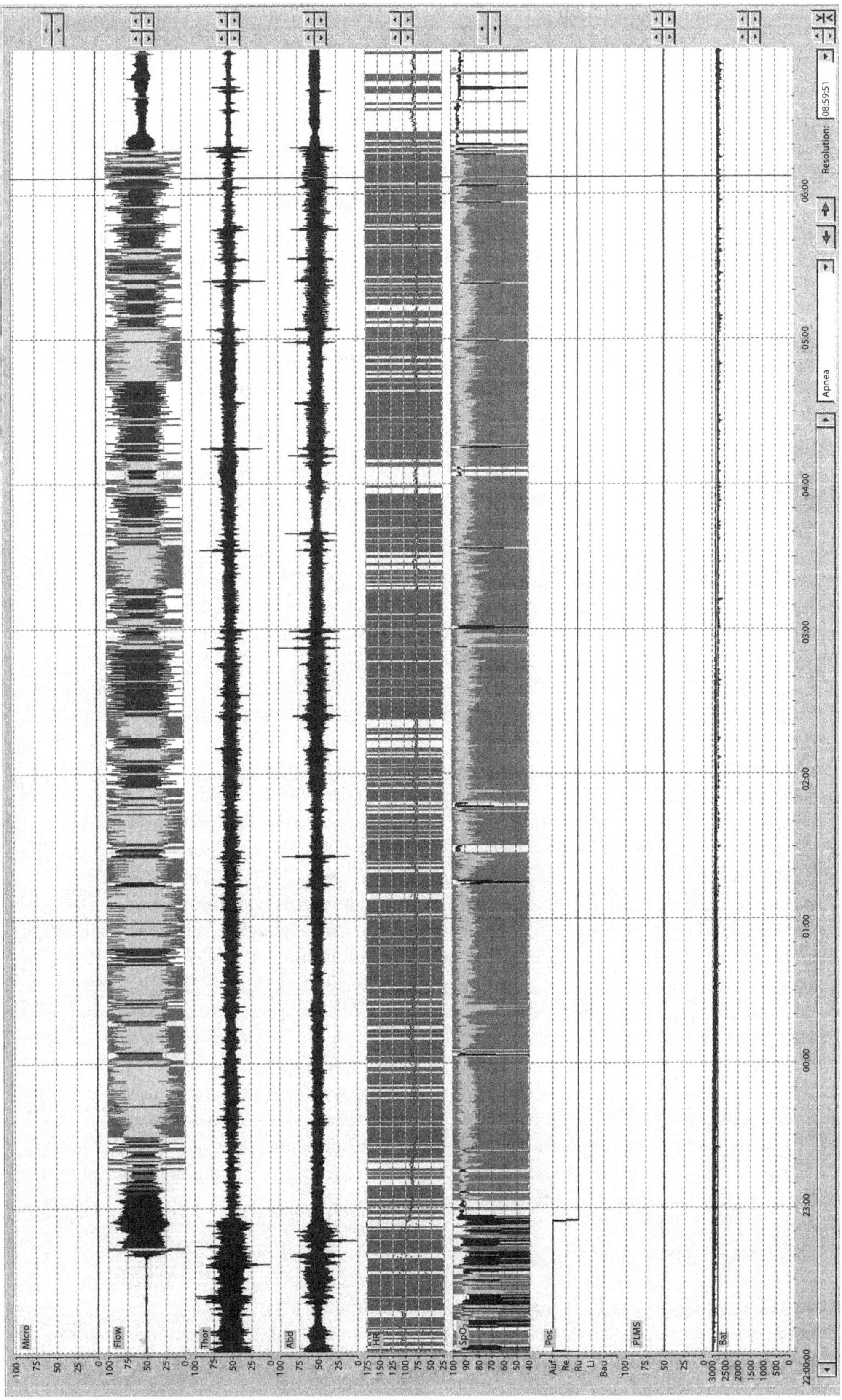

Fig. 2.3 Depiction of an entire night of polygraphic examination for obstructive sleep apnea. Obstructive, mixed, and central apneas in the oronasal airflow are assessed (see figure, *Flow*). Furthermore, repetitive HbO_2 desaturations (see figure, *SpO_2*) and variations of the heart rate are seen. The patient has a respiratory disturbances index (RDI) of 46.2/h and a desaturation index of 62.1/h

alternative to traditional polygraphic systems provided that these concerns among others are addressed:
- Oximetry and heart rate are documented.
- Raw data are retrievable.
- Automated analysis can be retrieved and edited.

In the future, PAT might be taken into consideration also outside the sleep lab as a method to assess sleep-related breathing disorders.

2.7 Polysomnography (PSG)

Polysomnography (PSG) is the gold standard in the diagnosis of sleep disorders because it can assess sleep and its pathological changes in an objective manner. By means of PSG, the origins of sleep disorders, for example, sleep apnea, periodic limb movements in sleep, or even sleep perception disorders, may be identified and verified that cannot be assessed by any other diagnostic procedure.

Numerous investigations show that the percentage of outpatient diagnoses had to be changed or completed in up to 50% of the cases after performing a PSG. In particular, in sleep-related breathing disorders, the diagnoses had to be modified, or a relevant sleep-related secondary diagnosis had to be added.

Since an expert group of the American Academy of Sleep Medicine (AASM) has published a new classification system (*International Classification of Sleep Disorders*, 3rd Edition; ICSD-3), there is the hope now for an extensive and generally accepted classification system for clinical and scientific sleep medicine, supported by the fact that the ICD-11 provides a separate chapter for sleep disorders.

The *AASM Manual for the Scoring of Sleep and Associated Events* – Rules, Terminology, and Technical Specifications (2007–2020) – is mainly based on those established by Rechtschaffen and Kales [13], in particular with regard to the selection of biosignals for the description of sleep. The arousal classification of an earlier group of the American Sleep Disorders Association (ASDA) is completely included. Independent scoring criteria for the sleep of children and outpatient examinations in cases of suspected sleep-related breathing disorders have been elaborated. The criteria were completed by standardized recommendations for amplifier settings, standardized user interfaces of PC-based systems, data formats, and visual evaluation and diagnosis of PSG. All statements of the AASM were based on empirical evidence, literature reviews, or consensus procedures.

Compared to the criteria of Rechtschaffen and Kales, the scoring rules for sleep were partly simplified. First, the number of the sleep stages to be evaluated was reduced. Rechtschaffen and Kales differentiated deep sleep stages 3 and 4 that were summarized to the sleep stage N3. The sleep stage "movement time" was eliminated. The interval evaluation in blocks of 30-second epochs is maintained. An automated analysis of the sleep stages alone is explicitly not desired. The rules for the first occurrence of a sleep stage at sleep onset (sleep-onset latency) were specified, the less economic 3-min rule for the evaluation of the sleep stages N2 and REM (R) was eliminated, and the definitions of *graphoelements* (K complexes, sleep spindles, vertex waves) for the assessment of single sleep stages was simplified. Graphoelements are characteristic phenomena of EEG patterns that are typical for certain sleep stages. K complexes and spindles, for example, determine the sleep stage N2, while vertex waves are characteristic for the sleep stage N1. Compared to Rechtschaffen and Kales, the classification of the single sleep stages was also modified, probably for better differentiation of both scoring systems. The most important modification is the classification of the numeric sleep stages with an "N" for the new criteria: Rechtschaffen and Kales [13] used an "S" before the numeric sleep stage. For example, stage "S1" (R&K) is now stage "N1."

It must be mentioned critically that precise definitions for the graphoelements are still absent, or their definitions do not always meet the criteria of scientific verification; for example, the time criteria of the AASM for a vertex wave. Generally, the efforts of the AASM with regard to standardization, simplification, and scientific justification of the scoring rules are very welcome; however, they require regular development and revision based on newly acquired scientific knowledge and technical options.

The following paragraphs describe these criteria:
- The basics of the current classification of sleep stages
- The standard biosignals that have to be measured by PSG
- The evaluation and scoring of the results of PSG in the context of most frequently observed disorders

The German Society for Sleep Research and Sleep Medicine (DGSM) has developed quality criteria for the performance of polysomnographies. This publication partly modified and further developed criteria of other European sleep societies. Those criteria refer to the structural aspects of a sleep center, technical- and staff-related equipment, and processes in a sleep center accredited by the DGSM. The criteria of the DGSM may be retrieved on the homepage of the DGSM (▶ www.dgsm.de) and those of the European Sleep Research Society (ESRS) on ▶ www.esrs.org.

Each polysomnographic measurement has to be preceded by technical and biological calibration.

The *biological calibration* is necessary for these considerations:

- Delimitation between physiological events during sleep and artifacts
- Verification of the amplifier settings and polarities of the single measurement channels
- Allocation of specific behaviors during sleep to respective measurement patterns

Biological Calibration

- Open versus closed eyes for 20 s each (alpha blockage effect)
- Blinking
- Eye movements to the left and to the right with straight head position
- Rolling of the eyes
- Swallowing
- Clenching the teeth
- Snoring
- Counting to 5 (differentiation between speech and snoring with use of a snoring microphone)
- Forced inspiration
- Forced expiration
- Holding the breath; Müller's maneuver (negative Valsalva maneuver) for assessment of paradox respiratory excursions
- Extension of the left and right big toe

For biological calibration, the patient is lying on his bed and is asked via a bidirectional intercom to perform the aforementioned actions under continuous documentation of the respective biosignals in the PSG.

According to the applicable rules for documentation, the biological calibration with exact labeling is then archived for 10 years together with the polysomnographic measurements of the corresponding night.

Thorough documentation of the polysomnographic files is of high clinical relevance. The night protocol written by the medical staff has to allow a rapid and clear assignment to the patient and the measured night.

The documentation includes these aspects:

- Medication
- Type of therapy
- Biological calibration
- All particular events such as technical defects, artifacts, etc.

Furthermore, it should include detailed observation of the behavior:

- Time of getting up
- Emotional condition
- Sleepwalking, etc.

Medical emergency situations, such as epileptic seizures or cardiac arrhythmia, can be immediately recognized by the measurement and documentation of numerous vital parameters and the presence of qualified personnel. Thus, the sleep lab environment very closely resembles the supervision in an intensive care unit. During measurement, qualified staff is already in a position to eliminate emerging error sources such as electrode and sensor artifacts. In cases of therapeutic PSG with adaptation of ventilation therapy for sleep-related breathing disorders, the medical staff assesses a *titration protocol.*

Practical Tip

The titration protocol includes the type of therapy device and the mask that is used. The applied pressure, ventilation mode, and its modifications are exactly documented, and changes of the ventilation mode are justified by emerging respiratory events, O_2 variations, and cardiac parameters.

Regarding diagnostic and therapeutic options and precision, inpatient PSG is superior to outpatient measurements at the patient's home.

2

2.7.1 Standard Parameters of Polysomnography (PSG)

According to the criteria of the AASM for the assessment of sleep, the polysomnographic standard biosignals for diagnostic PSG include three measurements of the EEG based on the international ten-twenty system with measurements of F4-A1, C4-A1, and O2-A1. As backup or for better detection of the differences, the measurements of F3-A2, C3-A2, and O1-A2 are also recommended (◘ Fig. 2.4): these are unipolar measurements. The longitudinal rows allow the clear identification and definition of graphoelements that show specific patterns in the EEG. Over the frontal measurements, K complexes and delta waves are defined, over the central measurements sleep spindles and vertex waves, and over the occipital measurements alpha waves that are relevant for the definition of the sleep-onset process and arousal reactions.

In addition, the standard PSG includes two measurements of electrooculography (EOG) and electromyography (EMG).

The *EOG* electrodes are placed about 1 cm from the left and right orbita edge of the respective eye, whereby the electrodes in the vertical line are shifted about 1 cm (◘ Fig. 2.5). Beside the registration of slow eye movements (slowly rolling eyes), the electrodes also allow the registration of horizontal and vertical eye movements with lower amplitudes.

Electromyography of the mental and submental muscles ensures an optimal identification of the atony of the skeletal muscles during REM sleep and describes stage-related variations in the amplitude of the muscle tension. One electrode is placed 1 cm above the midline of the chin, and two electrodes are placed 2 cm below the point of the chin (one is placed 2 cm to the right, the other one 2 cm to the left). Bipolar measurement of the mental and submental muscles is performed. The remaining electrode at the submental muscle is used as reserve in cases where the contact impedance of one electrode during measurement decreases (◘ Fig. 2.6).

To identify cardiac events, at least one-channel ECG is registered. As the typical measurement II uses electrodes of the right shoulder and the left

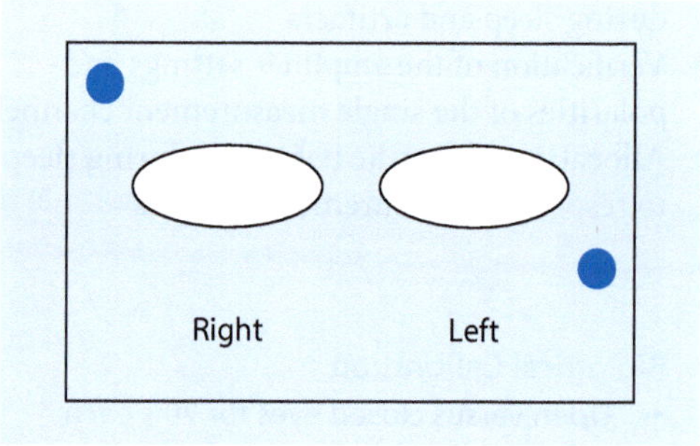

◘ **Fig. 2.5** Electrooculography (EOG) Abstand, Leereichen electrode positions

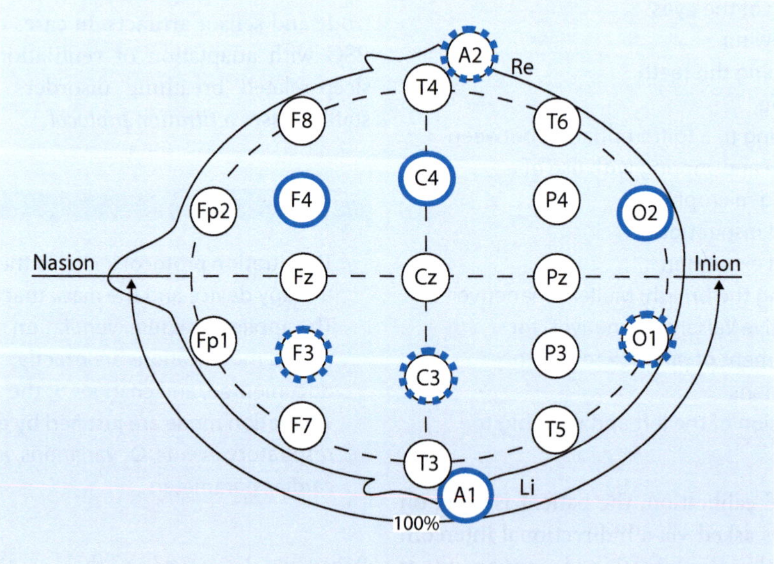

◘ **Fig. 2.4** EEG standard electrode positions according to the ten-twenty system. *Dotted circles* represent substitute or backup electrodes

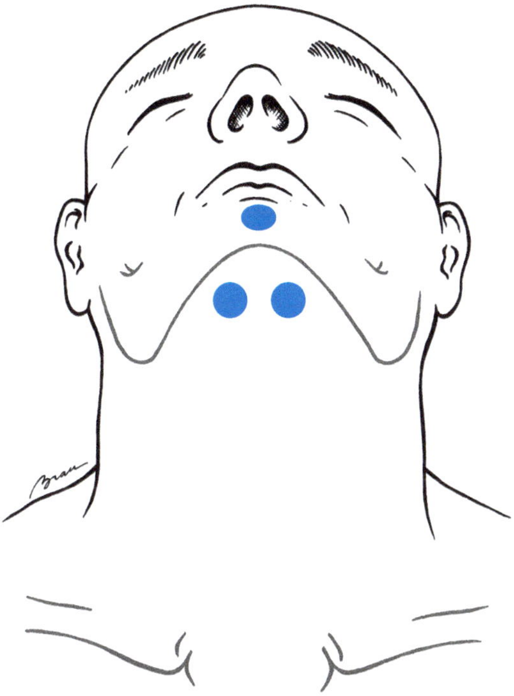

◘ **Fig. 2.6** Electomyography (EMG) electrode positions (courtesy of Dr. G. Bran)

leg, the electrodes are applied at the trunk parallel to this axis. This measurement mainly serves for detection of changes of the heart rhythm and their correlation with other PSG parameters (e.g., apneas).

Furthermore, the airflow of mouth and nose are registered separately, and thoracic and abdominal excursions during respiration, arterial HbO_2 saturation by means of pulse oximetry, a (snoring) microphone, and positional sensors are added. These devices serve for assessment of respiratory events and their allocation to the body position during sleep.

Based on the AASM criteria, the registration of the *oronasal airflow* is performed to detect apneas by means of thermistors (thermo-sensors) and hypopneas by means of dynamic pressure measurement (◘ Fig. 2.7). For practical reasons, dynamic pressure measurement has prevailed as diagnostic standard in many institutions. However, the classic nasal cannulas of dynamic pressure measurement usually only allow registration of nasal respiration. Thus, it is recommended in cases of clear mouth breathing to also register the oronasal airflow by means of thermistor. The AASM recommends the use of a combined sensor

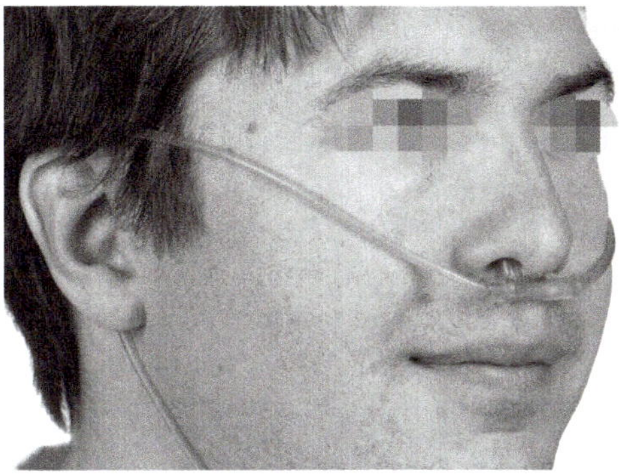

◘ **Fig. 2.7** Dynamic pressure measurement by means of nasal cannula

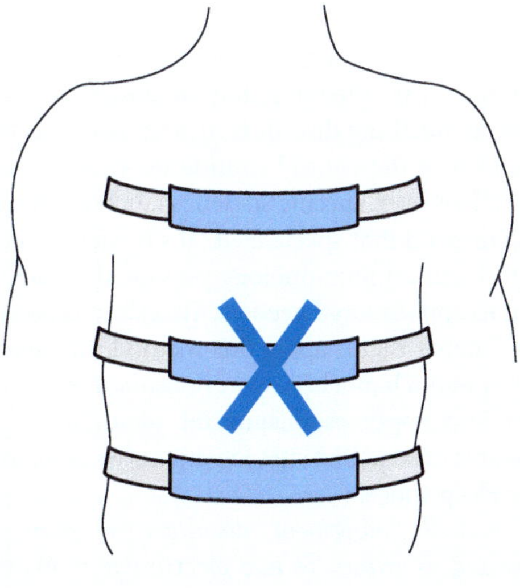

◘ **Fig. 2.8** Positioning of the sensors for thoracic and abdominal respiratory excursions

that provides dynamic pressure measurement for the identification of hypopneas and thermistor measurement for the detection of apneas. According to the AASM criteria, it is currently also possible to estimate the oronasal airflow by thoracic and abdominal sensors for inductance plethysmographic measurement (see following).

To assess the *respiratory effort*, piezoceramic sensors with elastic bands are applied at the rib cage and the abdomen (◘ Fig. 2.8). As they do not provide a quantitative signal because of their punctual measurement technique and are suitable only to a limited extent to differentiate central and obstructive hypopneas, inductance plethysmographic sensors are recommended: these are sensors for thorax and abdomen involving the entire circumference. The signal in this case does not depend on the length and the tension of the sensor but is proportional to the surface that the sensor includes.

During titration or for therapy evaluation in the context of nocturnal ventilation therapy, a device-inherent flow sensor may also be applied.

Esophageal pressure measurement is the gold standard for assessing the respiratory effort. Hereby, one or more pressure sensors placed in a thin and flexible tube at various positions are inserted in the esophagus. The first pressure sensor is placed above and the second below the diaphragm, and the pressure difference sets the signal. In this way, the intrathoracic pressure changes resulting from the respiratory efforts can be quantitatively measured.

The application of an esophageal pressure sensor for clear differentiation of obstructive and central breathing disorders in sleep is not recommended in the clinical routine for practical reasons. However, specific societies (such as DGSM) recommend that specialized labs or sleep centers with focus on pulmonology provide this method and its application if needed. Also, sleep centers in ENT departments apply this method, in particular as multichannel pressure sensors in the pharynx and upper esophagus for identification of possible obstruction sites in patients with obstructive sleep apnea.

Periodic movement disorders in sleep are assessed by means of two electromyograms that are measured at the respective anterior tibialis muscles: these are bipolar measurements. The first electrode is placed four fingerbreadths below the tuberosity of the tibia and one fingerbreadth lateral to the tibia edge. To allow for specific anatomical particularities, the first position should be determined by the patient as instructed by the staff. The second measurement point is about 5 cm in the distal direction. The tibial electrodes should be well fixed to avoid removal by nighttime leg movements (◘ Fig. 2.9)

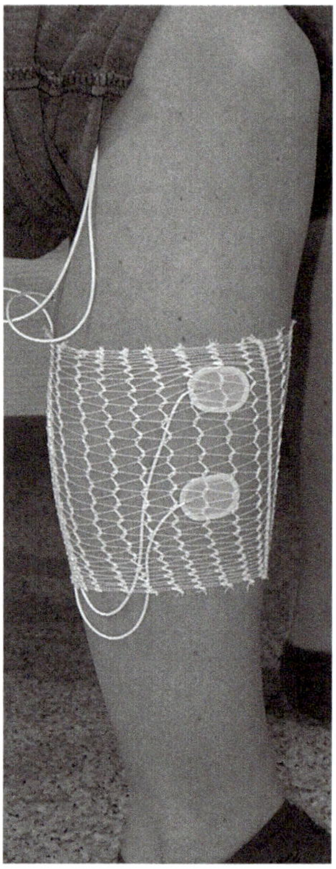

◘ **Fig. 2.9** EMG electrodes placed at the anterior tibialis muscle

2.7.1.1 Measurement of Blood Pressure During Sleep

Sleep disorders, in particular sleep-related breathing disorders (SRBD), may negatively influence the cardiovascular system. SRBD are associated with hypertension, heart attack, and stroke. For diagnosis of arterial hypertension, measurement of blood pressure at night is crucial (dipper/non-dipper). The diagnosis is recognized eight times more easily by means of nocturnal blood pressure measurement than with a one-time measurement during the day. The nearly exclusively applied means of blood pressure measurements with cuffs are less suitable because of the sleep-disturbing pumping during polysomnographic examination of sleep. Alternative, continuously measuring procedures according to Penaz (Portapres) or invasive arterial blood pressure measurements are generally appropriate for assessing nocturnal blood pressure fluctuation, but the methods are very expensive and thus not applicable for standard polysomnography (PSG) or polygraphy (PG).

The method of pulse transit time (PTT) is a parameter in sleep diagnostics that has been known for several decades. Changes of PTT have been used as markers for autonomous arousals, but the application of PPT for blood pressure assessment is new. It is determined by the time the pulse wave of a cardiac cycle needs to run from a central point of the arterial system into the periphery. Often the R-wave of the ECG is used as

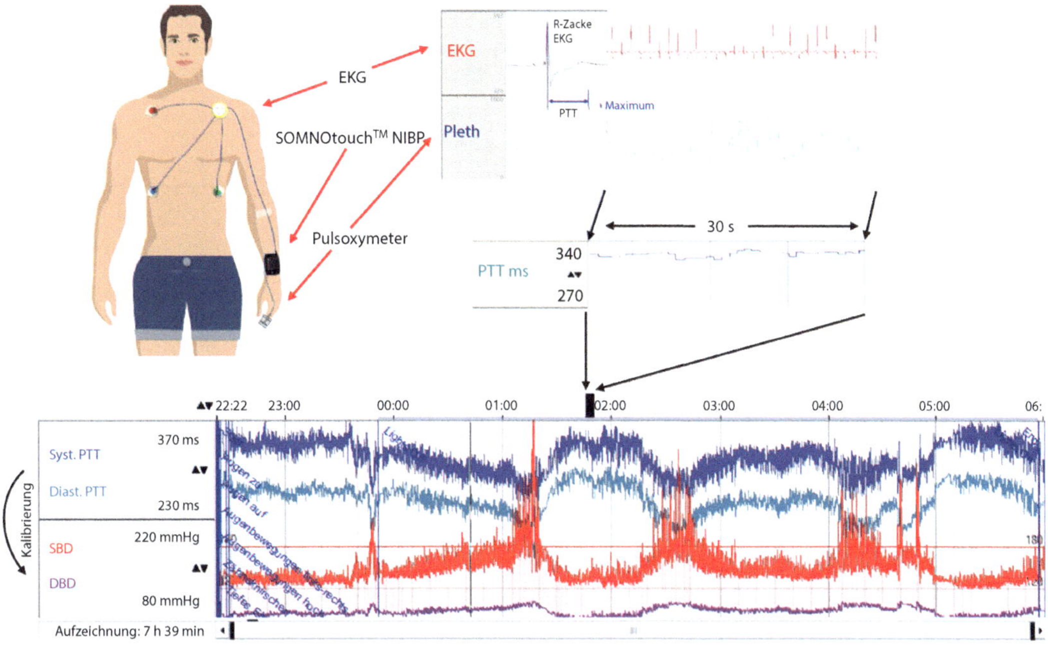

Fig. 2.10 Measurement of the blood pressure based on the pulse transit time (PPT) principle. *Top left:* Scheme for placing the electrodes for continuous blood pressure measurement based on the PPT principle. *Top right:* From the time delay between the R-wave of the ECG and the peripheral pulse wave, PPT can be defined (and documented) for every heart cycle. From the one-point calibration and the nonlinear model, an exact systolic and diastolic pressure can be computed for every PPT value. *Bottom:* Continuous measurement of the PPT or the systolic and diastolic pressure during the entire sleep duration. *PPT* pulse transit time, *SBP* systolic blood pressure, *DBP* diastolic blood pressure, *Pleth* plethysmogram, *ECG* electrocardiogram

the starting time, and the arrival time of the pulse wave in the periphery is measured by means of pulse oximetry. Both signals are assessed in PG or PSG by default. The velocity of the pulse wave is correlated directly with the elasticity or rigidity of the vessel. The elasticity is crucially influenced by the blood pressure. So, considering individual mechanical properties of the vessels, the pulse wave velocity allows drawing conclusions about the blood pressure. Because the central vessels have a different wall structure compared to peripheral vessels, a different elasticity results: the distinction is made between central and peripheral pulse wave velocity.

The individual properties of the vascular elasticity are assessed by means of cuff measurements (calibration), and the blood pressure changes are calculated with sufficient exactness with a patented nonlinear mathematical model [8] (see Fig. 2.10).

Thus, the PPT blood pressure method allows measuring the blood pressure during sleep in a reactionless and continuous way, that is, from beat to beat. During sleep, suprathreshold intrinsic or extrinsic disturbances may generate arousals; as a consequence, a fluctuating increase of the systolic pressure may occur in response to a transitory reduction of the parasympathetic tonus and subsequent heart rate increase (NBPF, nocturnal blood pressure fluctuation). These NBPFs amount to 10–20 s and an average of 29 mmHg ([5]; $n = 878$ NBPFs; see Fig. 2.11).

With an AHI of 60/h, these NBPFs trigger an increase of the average arterial blood pressure of about 10 mmHg at night, which counteracts or even avoids the natural reduction (dipping). In cases of severe SRBD characterized by long apnea/hypopnea and short breathing periods, higher NBPFs may also be generated in REM sleep. A continuous increase of the systolic blood pressure during these periods is characteristic. After an apnea-related increase, blood pressure does not return to its original value. As a consequence, the blood pressure increase potentiates (superposition) and reaches extremely high apnea-correlated values of more than 200 mmHg.

The continuous and disturbance-free measurement of the blood pressure during sleep is a

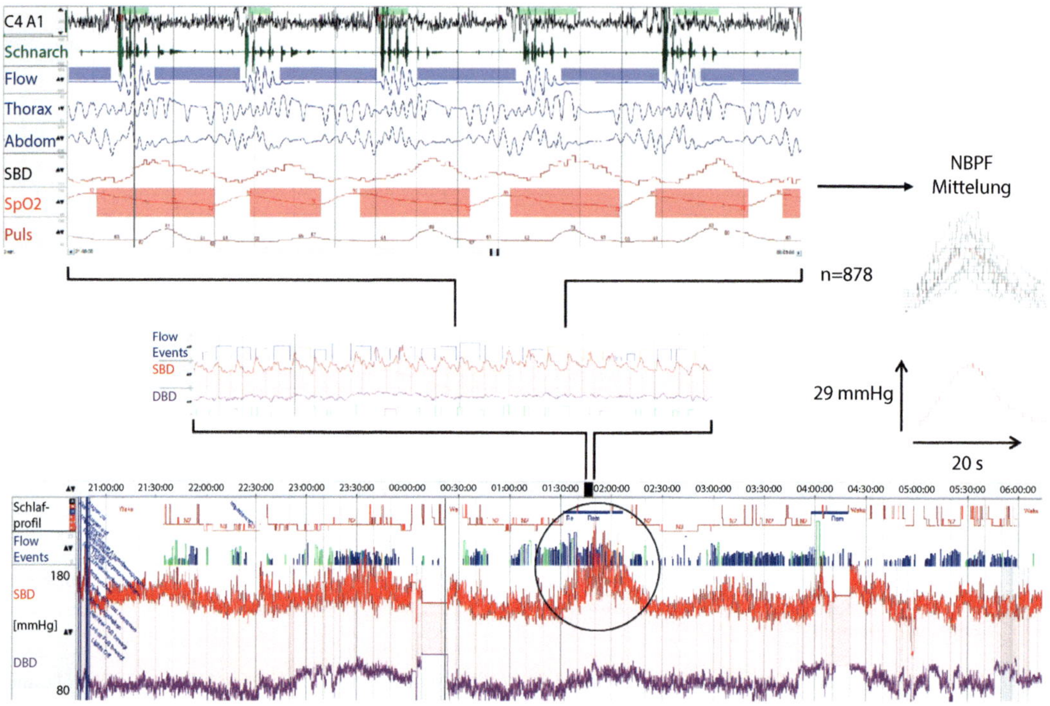

Fig. 2.11 Nocturnal blood pressure fluctuations (NBPFs). *Top left:* NBPFs following obstructive apneas (*green*, arousals; *blue*, apneas; *red*, desaturations). *Top right:* NBPFs averaged over $n = 878$; the average increase is 27 mmHg and the average duration is 20 s. *Bottom:* Blood pressure during the night with REM sleep-related pressure increase over 200 mmHg (superposition, *black circle*; artifact, *gray*). *SBP* systolic blood pressure, *DBP* diastolic blood pressure

clinically significant and, in the future, an indispensable tool to determine the severity of the disease or the severity of the sequelae regarding the cardiovascular system [10].

Digital videometry serves for registering the body position, but mainly also for assessing behavioral particularities during sleep. In this way, especially in cases of parasomnia and epileptic events during sleep, valid statements on the differential diagnosis can be made.

The standard parameters of polysomnography are summarized in Fig. 2.12.

Parameters and Measurements of Standard PSG

- Three EEG: F4-A1, C4-A1, and O2-A1 (as backup measurements or for better detection of lateral differences; also F3-A2, C3-A2, and O1-A2)
- Two EOG: left and right orbital edge
- One EMG: three electrodes (one mental muscle, two submental muscles)
- (Snoring) microphone
- Body position sensor
- Oronasal airflow, with mouth and nose separately assessed (thermistors, dynamic pressure measurement)
- Thoracic and abdominal respiratory excursions (piezo-ceramic elastic belt, induction plethysmography)
- Two EMG, anterior tibialis muscles
- One ECG, at least single channel
- Pulse oximetry, HbO2 saturation
- Videometry with zoom and panning head technique or high resolution for digital zooming

2.7.2 Parameters to Be Reported for Polysomnography (PSG)

In the morning following the nocturnal measurement, the PSG is evaluated by a somnologist or sleep physician or verified if the assistant staff has

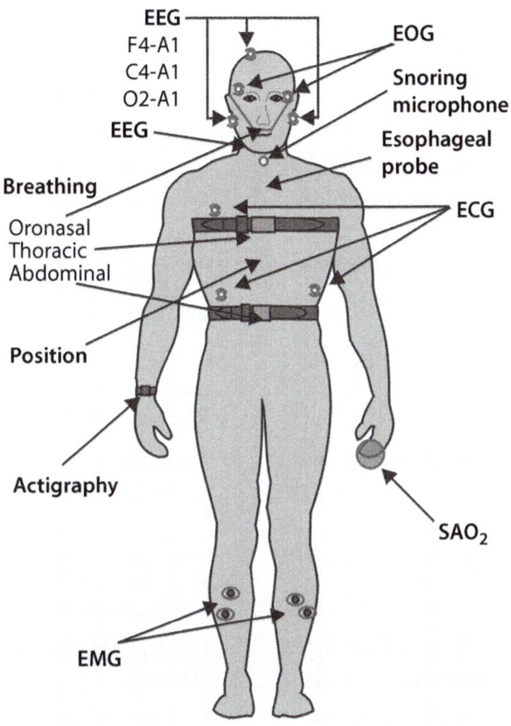

Fig. 2.12 Schematic depiction of the measurement of some parameters of polysomnography, modified according to Weeß [Steinberg R, Weeß H-G, Landwehr R (2010) Schlafmedizin. Grundlagen und Praxis. Uni-Med, Bremen]

preevaluated the files. The evaluation is based on the AASM criteria (▶ Sect. 1.3). In addition, motor (e.g., PLMS, periodic limb movement in sleep), respiratory (e.g., apneas), EEG-related (e.g., arousal), and other important events are differentiated. Evaluation via only software-inherent algorithms without verification by a specialist is not accepted because of the missing validity.

2.7.2.1 Sleep Scoring Data

Based on the classic sleep parameters (EEG, EOG, EMG), the quality of night sleep can be described by means of descriptively statistical parameters.

These statistical values refer to these characteristics (Table 2.3):

- Ability to initiate sleep
- Sleep ability at night
- Qualitative composition of night sleep
- Physiological, cyclic sequence of the sleep stages (sleep fragmentation)

The *sleep period time* (SPT) describes the interval from sleep onset to waking up in the morning.

The *total sleep time* (TST) refers to the actual time slept during the sleep period. Nocturnal wake phases are subtracted from the sleep period time.

The *sleep efficiency* describes the relationship of the time spent in bed sleeping to the overall bedtime given in percentages. Together with the total sleep time (TST) and the sleep period time (SPT), the sleep efficiency is considered as a specific parameter of the nocturnal sleep ability.

The *sleep-onset latencies* for the sleep stage N1, and in particular for stage N2, describe the ability to initiate sleep. It is defined as the time from turning off the light (alternatively, the start of the measurement) to the occurrence of the first epoch N1 or N2. More strict interpretations of sleep onset require the linked occurrence of three epochs of sleep stage N2 for the sleep-onset latency.

The *REM latency* (time between the first occurrence of N1 to the first occurrence of R in minutes) gives information about disorders of the non-REM/REM organization as it may be observed, for example, in the context of narcolepsy and impairments of some psychiatric sleep disorders. Significantly shorter REM latencies, usually of 90 ± 20 min to less than 10 min (so-called sleep-onset REM, SOREM) are an indicator for narcolepsy. Some authors also define SOREM with a latency of 15 or 20 min. In cases of depression, the average REM latency may amount to 50 min, but also to less.

The percentage of single sleep stages, referring to the sleep period time or the *time in bed* (TIB), changes with increased age. The percentage of deep sleep and that of REM sleep are of particular interest in this context.

Although deep sleep seems to have an important restorative function, REM sleep is considered to be highly important for intellectual performance, learning and memory processes, and emotional condition (see ▶ Chap. 1). The percentage of wakefulness during the sleep period is important in the context of insomnia disorders because it describes the extent of the difficulty maintaining sleep in a characteristic way. The percentage of light or superficial sleep (N1, N2) is increased in many sleep disorders with repetitive arousals or in cases of chronic application of hypnotics.

Table 2.3 Statistical parameters of polysomnography evaluation according to AASM (2020)

Sleep parameter	Calculation	Function/significance	Reference values
Time in bed or measurement time	Time span from turning off the light to turning it on (in minutes)	Bedtime, insomnia disorders, sleep deficit syndrome	–
SPT 1	Sleep period time 1: interval from the first N1 to definite waking up (in minutes)	Sleep ability, insomnia disorders	High interindividual variation, 5–9 h, age-dependent
SPT 2	Sleep period time 2: interval from sleep onset (N2) to definite waking up (in minutes)	Sleep ability, insomnia disorders	High interindividual variation, 5–9 h, age-dependent
TST 1	Total sleep time 1: SPT 1 without wake phases (in minutes)	Sleep ability, insomnia disorders	High interindividual variation, 5–9 h, age-dependent
TST 2	Total sleep time 2: SPT 2 without wake phases (in minutes)	Sleep ability, insomnia disorders	High interindividual variation, 5–9 h, age-dependent
SEI	Sleep efficiency index: TST1/TIB × 100	Sleep ability, insomnia disorders	Age-dependent; >85–90%
SOL 1	Sleep-onset latency 1: interval from turning off the light to first occurrence of N1 (in minutes)	Ability to initiate sleep, sleep-onset disorders	<30 min
SOL 2	Sleep-onset latency 2: interval from turning off the light to first occurrence of N2 (in minutes) or N2 linked over 3 epochs	Ability to initiate sleep, sleep-onset disorders	<30 min
SOL N3	Sleep-onset latency 3: interval from first occurrence of N1 to first occurrence of N3 (in minutes)	Sleep quality, sleep cycles, non-REM/REM organization	–
REM latency	Interval from first occurrence of N1 to first occurrence of stage R (in minutes)	Sleep quality, sleep cycles, non-REM/REM organization, narcolepsy	90 ± 20 min
Percentage of wake phases: N1, N2, N3, R	Percentage of single sleep stages referring to TST 1	Sleep quality, physical and psychic restoration, disorders of maintaining sleep	Age- and gender-dependent (Table 2.6)
Arousal index (AI)	Average number of all arousals per hour, referring to TST 1	Sleep fragmentation, global	Age- and gender-dependent (males ↑)
Respiratory arousal index (RAI)	Average number of respiration-related arousals per hour, referring to TST 1	Sleep fragmentation, involvement of respiratory events, sleep-related breathing disorders	<10/h
PLMS arousal index (PLMS-AI)	Average number of PLMS-related arousals per hours, referring to TST 1	Sleep fragmentation, involvement of periodic leg movements, RLS, PLMD	<5/h, classification of the severity
			5 to ≤20/h: mild
			20–60/h: moderate
			>60/h: severe

Table 2.3 (continued)

Sleep parameter	Calculation	Function/significance	Reference values
Endogenous arousal index (EAI)	Average number of endogenous arousals per hour, referring to TST 1	Sleep fragmentation, involvement of endogenous events, insomnia, narcolepsy, etc.	Unclear, see Arousal Index (AI) for orientation
REM interval	Duration of one non-REM/REM cycle	Sleep cycles, non-REM/REM organization, narcolepsy, psychiatric sleep disorders	High interindividual variation, 90 ± 20 min

Table 2.4 Standard values of sleep stage percentages according to age and gender, based on a study by Redline et al. [14] including *n* = 2685 healthy sleepers as controls

Value	Stage 1		Stage 2		Stage 3/4		REM sleep	
Age (years)	Males	Females	Males	Females	Males	Females	Males	Females
37–54	5.8	4.6	61.4	58.5	11.2	14.2	19.5	20.9
95% CI	5.2–6.5	4.1–5.3	60.0–62.8	57.1–60.0	9.9–12.6	12.7–15.9	18.8–20.2	20.0–21.8
55–60	6.3	5.0	64.5	56.2	8.2	17.0	19.1	20.2
95% CI	5.6–7.0	4.4–5.7	63.2–65.9	54.5–57.8	7.1–9.5	15.2–18.9	18.4–19.8	19.3–21.1
61–70	7.1	5.0	65.2	57.3	6.7	16.7	18.4	19.3
95% CI	6.4–7.9	4.4–5.7	63.9–66.5	55.7–58.9	5.7–7.7	14.8–18.6	17.8–19.1	18.4–20.2
>70	7.6	4.9	66.5	57.1	5.5	17.2	17.8	18.8
95% CI	6.8–8.5	4.3–5.6	65.1–67.8	55.6–58.7	4.5–6.5	15.5–19.1	17.1–18.5	18.0–19.6

Evaluation based on the criteria of Rechtschaffen and Kales [13]
CI confidence interval

The standard percentages of the sleep stages (Table 2.4) reveal their dependence on age and show a clear gender effect to the disadvantage of older men regarding deep sleep (N3). It must be taken into account that these standard sleep scoring data are based on the original criteria of Rechtschaffen and Kales. However, the sleep scoring data established by the AASM (2007–2020) should not have resulted in a significant modification of the standard values. Possibly, a reduction of the sleep-onset latency, a slight increase of stage N2 to the disadvantage of stage N1, and a nearly unchanged percentage of REM and deep sleep may be expected. For the moment, more recent standard values based on the AASM criteria are not available.

2.7.2.2 Phenomenology and Classification of Arousals

An *arousal* is understood as sudden frequency change/acceleration of the EEG. It includes theta waves, alpha waves, or frequencies higher than 16 Hz. Sleep spindles with characteristic frequencies between 11 and 16 Hz (mostly 12 and 14 Hz) are excluded.

Arousals may lead to partial, temporary, or complete arousal; they always interrupt sleep and are a typical pathomechanism for many sleep disorders. Regarding diagnostics of sleep disorders, the etiology of the arousals (e.g., respiratory, motor, vegetative, endogenous) plays a major role.

Arousals during sleep are stimulus dependent. They may be triggered by interoception (psychophysical, sensor, neuronal, vegetative stimuli) or exteroception (acoustic, optic, tactile stimuli).

Regarding the diagnostics of sleep disorders, interoceptive arousals are critical.

- Interoceptive psychophysical arousals may occur in response to dream events, changed blood gas conditions, pH alterations, changes of the muscle elongation receptors, kinesthetic stimuli, or pain
- Interoceptive neuronal arousals develop in the cortex, the limbic system, the hypothalamus, or the reticular system of the brainstem

Arousals are seen in all age groups. As of the fourth decade, the incidence significantly increases; the development of the arousal frequency per hour of sleeping time depends on age. Male subjects show more arousals than females.

The *arousal index* (number of arousals per hour of sleep) describes the fragmentation of night sleep and the dissolution of the physiological sleep cycle. The higher is the fragmentation, the less differentiated or maintained are the sleep cycles. If the arousal index is correlated with motor, respiratory, or endogenous events, it allows conclusions about the contribution of comorbidity to the disorder of the physiological sleep cycle. Hence, the arousal index has a major role for determining the severity and evaluating the therapy success.

Currently, EEG-related arousal analyses are in the focus of polysomnographic diagnostics of sleep disorders. Compared to analytical methods of vegetative arousals, they are systemized, validated, and standardized. For improvement of arousal analysis during sleep, a systematic classification and validation of vegetative arousal reactions would be desirable.

In 1992, the American Sleep Disorders Association (ASDA) developed an upgraded EEG-related *arousal classification* that was internationally acknowledged as a standard. It is based on the classic measurements described by Rechtschaffen and Kales. Additionally, however, the measurement of occipital EEG measurement points (O1-A2, O2-A1, Oz-A1/A2) were recommended because the arousal frequencies can be better detected by occipital assessment. The analytical criteria of the AASM adopt the arousal classification of the ASDA. For classification of arousals according to the AASM [2], the information of frontal, central, and occipital measurements must be taken into account.

Arousal Criteria of the ASDA and the AASM [2]

An arousal is defined as an abrupt EEG frequency shift that may include theta, alpha, or frequencies higher than 16 Hz, except sleep spindles. The minimum length of the frequency acceleration is 3 s.

1. An arousal has to be preceded by at least 10 s of sleep. Arousals may also occur in a wake epoch if this epoch contains, for example, as much as 14 s of sleep. The AASM [2] indicates that arousals may generally also occur in a wake epoch between light out and light on and are included in the arousal index.
2. At least 10 s of sleep have to be registered between two arousals (◘ Fig. 2.13).
3. Arousals may be observed in non-REM sleep only in the EEG, that is, without increasing muscle tonus of the submental EMG. In REM sleep, the arousal has to be accompanied by a submental EMG increase of at least 1 s.
4. An increase of muscle tone alone does not suffice for classification as arousal.
5. Artifacts, K complexes, or delta waves are only considered as arousals when a frequency acceleration of more than 3 s is observed in at least one measurement channel.
6. "Pen blocking" artifacts (overregulation in one channel) are classified as arousals when a frequency acceleration follows.
7. Subsequent EEG and EMG changes with a respective duration of 3 s or less, but summarized as more than 3 s, are not classified as arousals.
8. Alpha interferences in non-REM phases with a length of 3 s or less and a frequency of more than 1/10 s (>0.1 Hz)

are not classified as arousals. Alpha interferences with a length more than 3 s are only classified as arousals when no other alpha interference has occurred in the previous 10 s.

9. Change in sleep stage is not a criterion of arousal.

The criticism regarding the described arousal classification primarily refers to the time criterion for the minimum length of an arousal. Numerous investigations could show that respiratory, motor, or endogenous arousals may also constitute shorter intervals; these are then sometimes called micro-arousals. In these cases, strict interpretation of the ASDA or AASM criteria leads to an underestimation of the arousal incidence and thus to an underestimation of the severity.

2.7.3 Polysomnography (PSG) in Patients with Insomnia

In many cases, but not in all, PSG has a key role in the diagnostics of insomnia. In our own patient cohort, the suspected diagnosis had to be modified after PSG in about 38% of cases. In 2003, the AASM established recommendations for the indication to perform PSG for the diagnostics and therapy of insomnia based on the evidence of scientific data.

According to the criteria of the AASM, insomnia is a relevant disease that requires accurate diagnostics and therapy. Primarily, the diagnosis of insomnia is based on the clinical symptoms by means of intensive medical, psychiatric, and pharmacological history taking and sleep anamnesis (evidence level 1).

Referring to the AWMF guideline on insomnia and the insomnia guideline of the ESRS, PSG is indicated when all other diagnostic measures are exhausted and the medical condition of

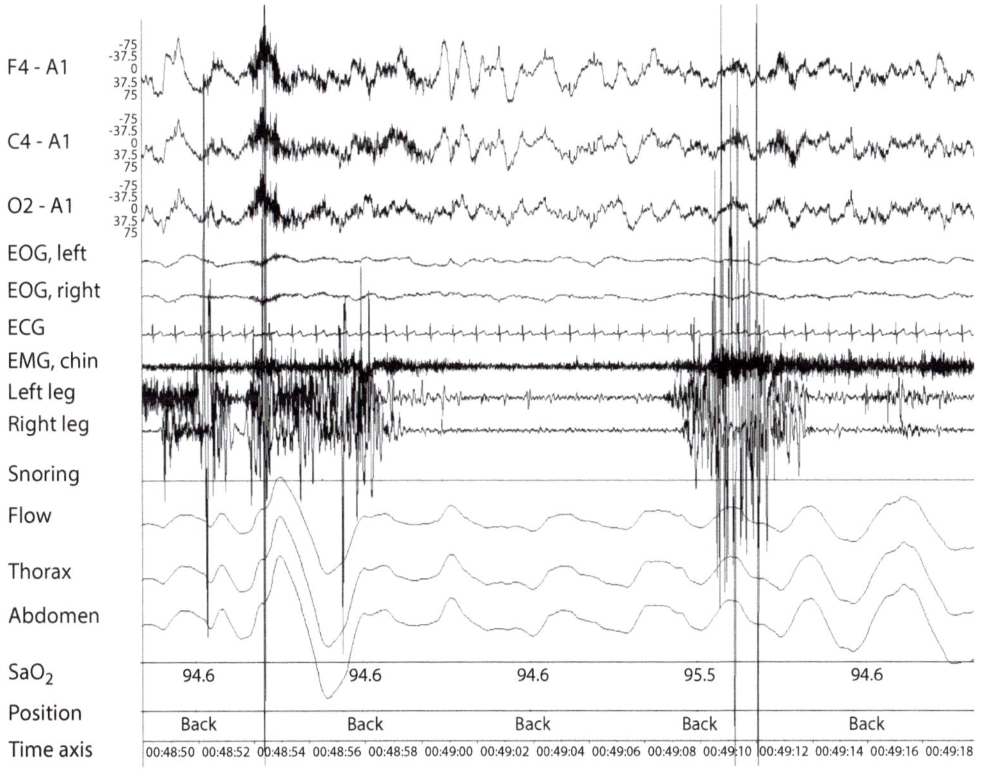

Fig. 2.13 A 30-s epoch of polysomnography. Two arousals with movement artifacts within 10 s. According to the AASM criteria, the second arousal is not counted. The frequency acceleration has to continue for at least 3 s

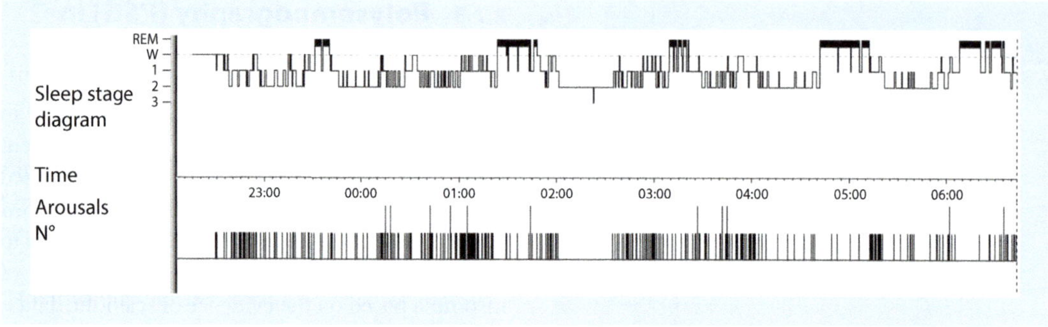

Fig. 2.14 Typical sleep profile of psychophysiological insomnia. It is clearly seen that the deep sleep phase is missing, with an increased number of changes of sleep stage and nocturnal wake phases (sleep stage diagram) resulting from a greater number of nocturnal arousals (arousal N0). It must be considered that the patient perceived sleep onset at 2 AM when the first sleep episode occurred without intermittent arousal. Because of the subsequently increased number of arousals, sleep afterward was not experienced as such, and the patient estimated the actual sleep quantity to be about 1 h in the morning protocol

insomnia is suspected, in particular in the context of sleep apnea syndromes or suspected periodic limb movements. According to the Association of Scientific Medical Associations (ASMA) guideline, PSG may also provide important diagnostic and therapeutic information in therapy-refractory cases as well as in high-risk groups associated with endangerment of self and others, such as professional drivers or subjects working with dangerous machinery. Polysomnography may also lead to further diagnostic and also therapeutic knowledge when a significant discrepancy is expected between the subjectively perceived severity of insomnia and the polysomnographic findings (see also Table 3.2).

The typical sleep profile of insomnia patients is characterized by these factors (Fig. 2.14):

- Prolonged sleep-onset latency
- Increased endogenous arousals
- Prolonged nocturnal wake phases
- Reduction of deep and REM sleep
- Modified sleep cycles

Often an alpha overlap is found in the sleep EEG, which is considered to be an expression of a chronically increased tension level. However, it is a nonspecific phenomenon that is also observed in other psychiatric disorders.

It is noteworthy that often a discrepancy is observed between objective polysomnographic findings and the patient's subjective perception of the ability to sleep. In these cases, frequently structural changes of sleep such as micro-arousals or the aforementioned alpha overlaps are found in the sleep EEG. Not least because of this fact, the evaluation criteria of PSG, even after revision by the AASM, are controversially discussed with regard to their clinical applicability, especially for insomnias.

The apparently disturbed perception of sleep, however, can also be explained based on several recent experimental findings in healthy sleepers and subjects suffering from disturbed sleep.

During the sleep-onset process, the probability of perceiving sleep onset is only clearly increased with the occurrence of the first sleep spindle. Subjects who were awakened before the first sleep spindle report significantly more often not to have slept at all. In the course of the night, the sleep perception depends not only on the depth of sleep but also on its continuity. Individuals who underwent experimental triggering of arousal in similar intervals as they occur in insomnia patients reported comparably linked wake phases as do insomnia patients even if objectively sleep could be seen between arousals. The human brain seems to need continuous sleep episodes of longer durations without arousals to perceive sleep.

2.7.4 Polysomnography (PSG) in Patients with Periodic Limb Movements in Sleep and Patients with Restless Leg Syndrome

Periodic limb movements in sleep (PLMS) and restless legs syndrome (RLS) are two independent, delayed, or even simultaneously emerging disorders with suspected central nervous system genesis.

According to the AASM recommendations [10], PSG is considered as the essential technical examination to confirm PLMS. RLS, in contrast, is primarily a clinical diagnosis. In the following cases, PSG is also indicated in this context:

- Cases with unclear diagnosis
- Children and adolescents with RLS
- Therapy-refractory RLS
- Persisting daytime sleepiness or sleep disorders under therapy
- Necessity of complex pharmaceutical strategies with opiates, anticonvulsants, or other atypical pharmaceutical treatment approaches

Furthermore, PSG is the most important criterion for verification of the effectiveness of therapeutic approaches to frequently associated nocturnal periodic arm and leg movements, especially for patients with persisting insomnia or daytime sleepiness under therapy (evidence level 1).

PLMS are characterized by episodes of periodic leg or, rarely, arm movements in sleep. They may be unilateral, bilateral symmetrical, or alternating (◘ Figs. 2.15, 2.16, and 2.17).

PLMS in combination with RLS are predominantly observed in the sleep stages N1 and N2: these occur less frequently in REM sleep. PLMS also emerge in wakefulness and at the transition between wake and sleep. PLMS increase with increased age. In healthy subjects aged between 30 and 50 years, the incidence amounts to about 5%; in 50-year-old individuals, PLMS is suspected in about 30% of the examined population.

Regarding diagnosis, PLMS must be differentiated from these events:

- Hypnagogic foot tremor
- Alternating leg muscle activation (ALMA)
- Excessive fragmentary myoclonus in non-REM sleep
- Phasic REM twitches
- Leg cramps
- PLMS associated with or terminating apnea

The last-mentioned symptoms are no longer observed in the context of sufficient ventilation therapy.

PLMS are often accompanied by other sleep disorders, frequently appearing in insomnia disorders, sleep apnea, narcolepsy, some psychiatric diseases, and REM behavior disorder.

The typical sleep profile with PLMS is significantly different from that of healthy sleepers. The sleep efficiency is relevantly reduced, more phases of light sleep (N1 and N2) are observed, and deep sleep and REM sleep are often reduced. The periodicity of the sleep cycles is significantly impaired or even disappears with the frequent arousals and the increased wake phases (◘ Fig. 2.14). In 1993, the Atlas Task Force of the American Sleep Disorders Association (ASDA) defined the duration, periodicity, and arousal reactions of rhythmic movements in sleep. In 2007, these criteria were substituted by those of the American Academy of Sleep Medicine (AASM). The original classification criteria, however, will probably be applied for a certain time until the computer-assisted analysis systems are able to implement the AASM criteria that are based on absolute signal properties.

AASM Criteria for the Classification of PLMS (2020)

- At least four consecutive contractions must be observed within an interval between 5 and 90 s (◘ Fig. 2.17). They are measured in all sleep stages and in wakefulness.
- The basic EMG signal should be measured with a relaxed anterior tibialis muscle and should not amount to more than 10 μV (between positive and negative amplitude, −5 μV to +5 μV). The application of 60 Hz (notch) filters should be avoided if possible. The impedances must be below 10,000 Ω; below 5,000 Ω is recommended. The measurement range should be between −100 and +100 μV.
- The duration of one leg movement (LM) is between (minimum) 0.5 s and (maximum) 10 s.
- The onset of LM is defined when the increase of the EMG is higher than 8 μV compared to the signal at rest. The end of LM is defined by a reduction of the EMG signal to <2 μV above the signal at rest for at least 0.5 s.

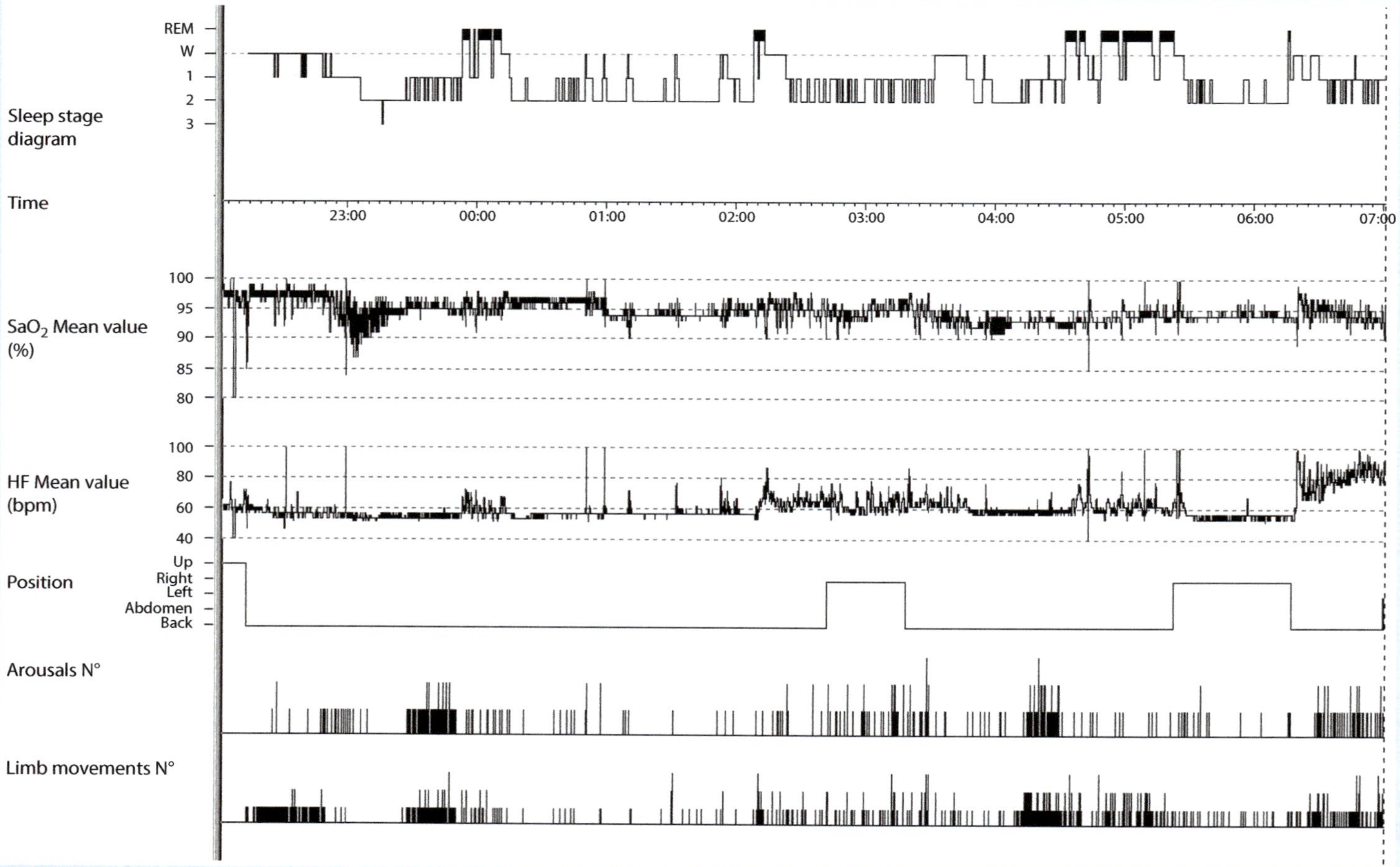

Fig. 2.15 Typical hypnogram in case of PLMS. The hypnogram shows the characteristic deep sleep suppression (stage N3) and the increased sleep stage change caused by repetitive arousals (arousal N0) in cases of periodic limb movements (limb movements N0). The increased sleep-onset latency is also striking. The increased number of arousals (arousal N0) is also seen in the increased heart rate variation (HF mean value, bpm) (N0 = number). The SaO_2 decrease at the beginning of the sleep period is still physiological and expresses the partially realized deep sleep. Note the scale of the *y*-axis, which shows a high resolution and suggests O_2 desaturation

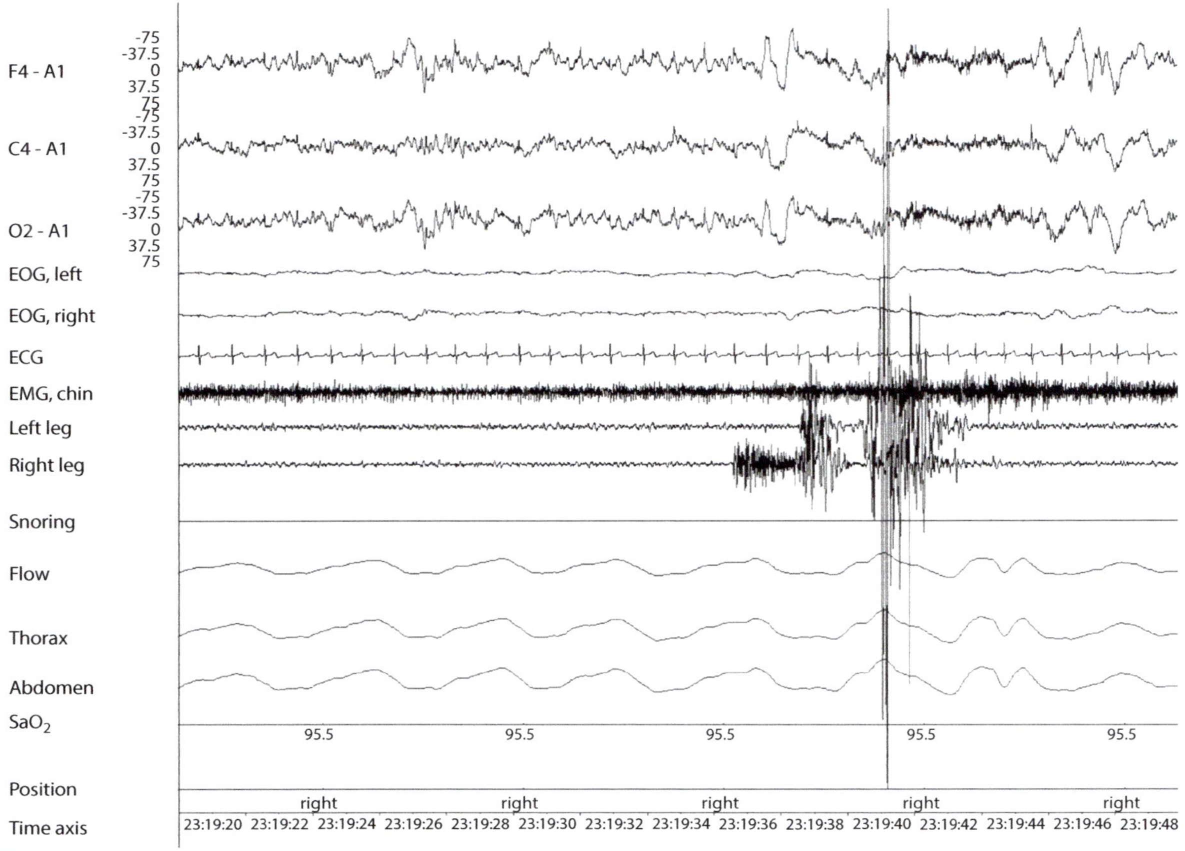

Fig. 2.16 Bilateral PLMS with arousal during a 30-s epoch of polysomnography. Arousals are classified as associated with leg movements if the interval between the end of the first event and the beginning of the second event is less than 0.5 s (independent from the order of the events). Leg movements of both legs are classified as one movement (LM) if less than 5 s is measured between the onsets of both movements

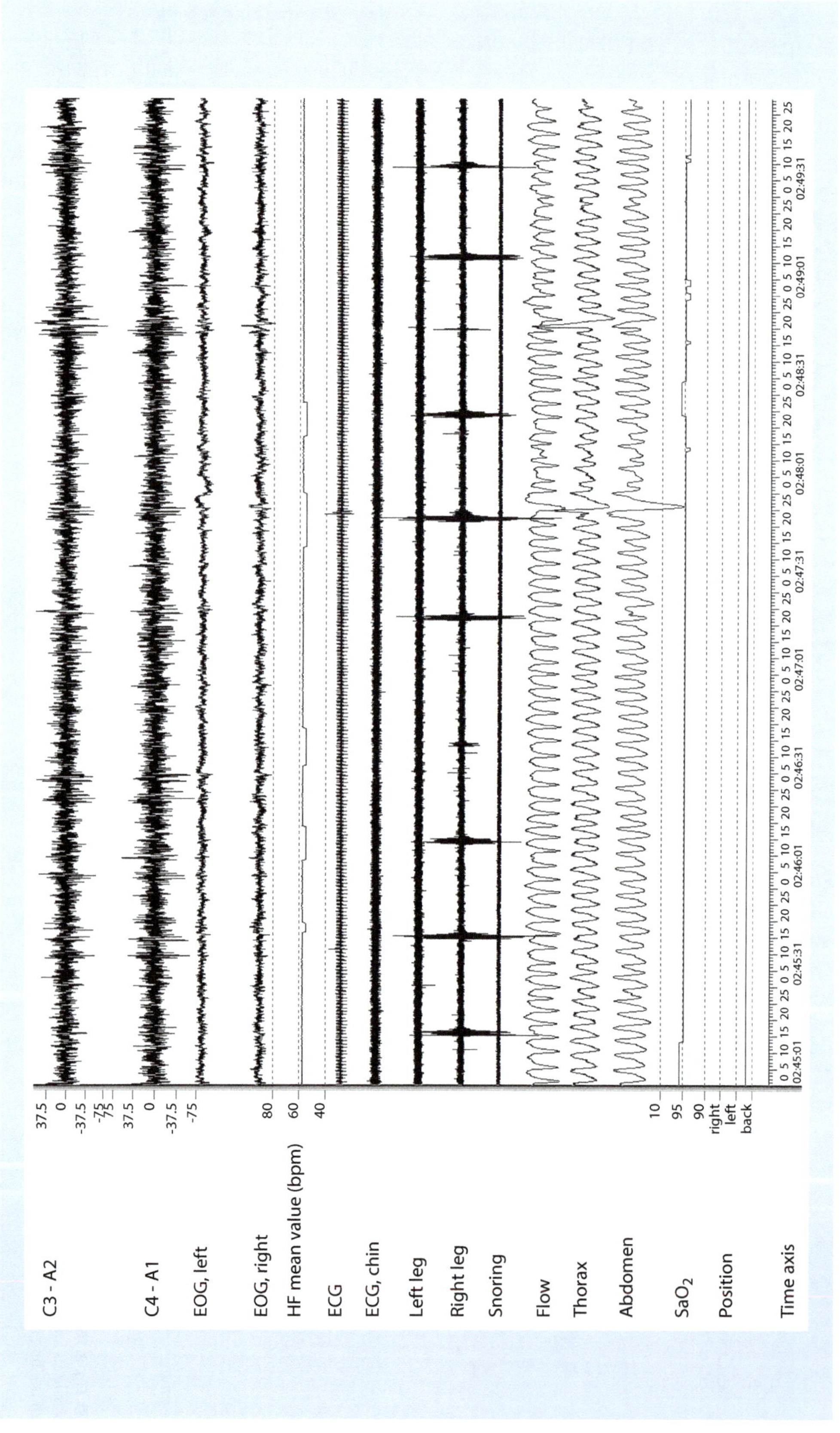

Fig. 2.17 PLMS of the right anterior tibialis muscle with arousals in the 5-min depiction of polysomnography. The associated arousals are no longer visible because of the time compression in the EEG. Amplitude increases in the EEG suggest the possible presence of an arousal

- Leg movements of both legs are classified as one leg movement (LM) if less than 5 s is measured between the onsets of both movements.
- According to the ASDA, leg movements at the end of an apnea or hypopnea that emerge together with an onset of hyperventilation are classified separately as breathing related. Today, they are no longer assessed based on the AASM criteria when they emerge in an interval that starts 0.5 s before the onset of apnea or hypopnea and ends 0.5 s after the end of apnea/hypopnea.
- Arousals are classified as associated with leg movements when the time interval between the end of the first event and the onset of the second event is less than 0.5 s (independent from the order of the events).

If a wake phase of less than 90 s separates a series of leg movements, the leg movements during the wake phase are not counted. However, the series of leg movements is assessed as such.

The AASM recommends the following parameters for analysis:

- Definition of the total number of PLMS during measurement and definition of the total number of PLMS with arousals.
- Assessment of a PLMS index (PLMSI) that is calculated by the following formula: total number of PLMS during TST × 60/TST (minutes).
- Definition of a PLMS arousal index (PLMSArl) calculated based on the formula: number of PLMS with arousal × 60/TST (minutes).
- Furthermore, it is recommended to differentiate between PLM in sleep and in wakefulness.

Practical Tip

PLMS index:
- Up to 5/h: inconspicuous
- Between 5/h and ≤20/h: mild disorder
- Between 20/h and 60/h: moderate disorder
- More than 60/h: severe disease

Besides the more exact specification, the advantage of the AASM criteria is the possibility to perform computer-based evaluation by an automated analysis systems. The AASM has also described the first criteria for other motor phenomena and disorders during sleep.

The AASM defines *hypnagogic foot tremor* (HFT) as EMG potentials occurring at the sleep-wake transition in a group of at least four events or as movements with lengths between 250 and 1000 ms and an incidence between 0.3 and 4 Hz without amplitude criteria. HFT is considered as a benign symptom without clinical relevance.

Alternating leg muscle activation (ALMA) emerges during sleep independently from sleep stages and is associated with arousals, and it is also described as a benign phenomenon with an increased probability of occurrence in the context of RLS, sleep apnea, and antidepressant medication. For identification, at least four side-alternating muscle activations are required, emerging with a minimum frequency of 0.5 Hz and a maximum frequency of 3 Hz. The duration of the single events amounts to 100–500 ms.

Excessive fragmentary myoclonus (EFM) in non-REM is characterized by EMG interferences, discharge of single motor neurons, with a maximum length of 150 ms. According to the AASM criteria, these must appear over at least 20 min in total with a frequency of at least 5/min. They are not associated with movements, and they have no clinical relevance even if they are more frequently observed in radiculopathies.

2.7.5 Polysomnography (PSG) in Cases of Bruxism

For the first time, the AASM formulated criteria for polysomnographic registration and evaluation of bruxism (▶ Chap. 8). Hereby, the criteria for analysis are applied to the submental EMG. However, additional measurements of the masseter muscle may also be performed. To confirm the diagnosis, an accompanying audiometric measurement may be performed in the PSG.

Phasic as well as tonic increases of the EMG activity of the submental EMG or the masseter muscle are measured that show at least twice the amplitude of the background EMG activity. Short (phasic) increases of the EMG activity are considered as bruxism episodes if their duration amounts to

0.25–2 s and at least three of such increases occur in regular intervals. Tonic increases of the chin activity are considered as bruxism at a length of more than 2 s. After a bruxism episode, a new episode may only be defined when the EMG has returned to the level of the background activity for at least 3 s. A second type of bruxism activity must not be forgotten. It is characterized by tonic increases that originate from the permanent clenching of the teeth.

The AASM does not give recommendations regarding the indication of PSG in the context of bruxism.

2.7.6 Polysomnography (PSG) in Cases of REM Behavior Disorders

For diagnosis of REM behavior disorder (RBD), one or both of the following phenomena have to be observed in the PSG.

- Tonic muscle activation in REM characterized by EMG activity emerging in at least 50% of the epoch that is above the lowest amplitude in non-REM.
- Excessive transient (phasic) muscle activation (ETM) during REM in the submental and tibialis EMG. Hereby, it is necessary that at least 5 mini-epochs occur with ETM in 5 of 10 mini-epochs (3 s) of the respective epoch (30 s). In the context of REM behavior disorders, ETMs have a length between 0.1 and 5 s, and their amplitude is at least four times higher than the background activity.

The AASM has not published any recommendations regarding the indication for PSG in cases of REM behavior disorders.

2.7.7 Polysomnography (PSG) in Cases of Rhythmic Movement Disorders in Sleep

Rhythmic movement disorders in sleep (jactatio capitis nocturna) are defined as movements of large muscle groups with a frequency between 0.5 and 2 Hz. It is recommended to summarize at least four movements to one episode or one cluster. For assessment, the EMG should show at least the double amplitude of the background activity. Accompanying videometry, as well as additional application of EMG surface electrodes on the muscle groups involved, is recommended to find an exact diagnosis.

The AASM has not published any recommendations regarding the indication for PSG in cases of rhythmic movement disorders in sleep.

2.7.8 Polysomnography (PSG) in Cases of Sleep-Related Breathing Disorders

Sleep-related breathing disorders (▶ Chap. 4) include:

- Obstructive sleep apnea syndrome
- Central sleep apnea syndrome
- Sleep-related hypoventilation syndromes
- Sleep-related hypoxemia

It is characteristic for these kinds of disorders that apnea or reduced breathing (hypopnea) or hypoventilations or hypoxemia occur during sleep. In association, O_2 desaturations and respiratory arousals may develop.

PSG is performed for diagnosis, differential diagnosis, assessment of the severity, and therapy monitoring of sleep-related breathing disorders. The S3 guideline on "Non-restorative sleep/sleep disorders" [chapter entitled "Sleep-Related Breathing Disorders" published by the German Society for Sleep Research and Medicine (Deutsche Gesellschaft für Schlafforschung und Schlafmedizin, DGSM] as well as the criteria for the indication of polysomnography for sleep-related breathing disorders of the AASM revised in 2017 [6] recommend polysomnography as the diagnostic standard for all sleep-related breathing disorders with comorbidities that are suitable to reduce the significance of unattended polygraphy systems. Only in clinically clear cases with suspected SRBD without relevant comorbidities may the diagnosis be performed by means of polygraphy. Follow-up assessments are generally based on medical consultation with device-related examinations by means of polygraphy. Polysomnographic follow-up may be indicated in patients with relevant comorbidities (▶ Sect. 2.6). If an unattended polygraphic examination has already been performed with unclear results or technical problems, polysomnography is recommended.

Based on the recommendations of the AASM, oronasal thermistors may be applied to detect apneas. Regarding hypopneas, the application of nasal pressure transducer sensors is required. More recently, combination electrodes have been developed allowing the simultaneous application of dynamic pressure and thermistor measurements.

Assessment of the respiratory effort should be performed by means of esophageal pressure sensors or induction plethysmography. Elastic belts with piezoceramic sensors are not recommended because measurements are only punctual (missing circumference measurement) (▶ Sect. 2.7.1). Because in practice two different sensors cannot always be applied for the assessment of apneas and hypopneas, nasal pressure transducer is also accepted to evaluate apneas. The registration of hypopneas can also be performed by means of oronasal thermistors. If these methods are not successful or no reliable signal can be registered, the AASM criteria alternatively allow assessing apneas by means of the sum signal of thoracic and abdominal induction plethysmography (estimation of the breathing volume) or the time-related sum signal of thoracic and abdominal induction plethysmography (estimation of the airflow). As an alternative for nasal pressure transducers or oronasal thermistors, the sum signal of thoracic and abdominal induction plethysmography, the time-related sum signal of thoracic and abdominal induction plethysmography, or the separate registration of induction plethysmography of thorax and abdomen is recommended for identification of hypopneas. It is also accepted to refer to the sum signal of thoracic and abdominal polyvinylidene fluoride sensors (belts) for identification of apneas or hypopneas. In nights when positive pressure ventilation should be titrated, the use of the flow signal of the ventilation device is recommended to identify apneas or hypopneas.

According to the AASM criteria, an event is considered as *apnea* when:

- The reduction of the thermistor signal (or the dynamic pressure measurement) is ≥90%.
- The amplitude criterion (reduction ≥90%) applies for at least 10 s of the duration of the event.

An apnea is considered as being:

- Obstructive when the respiratory effort persists unrelievedly
- Central when the respiratory effort is absent
- Mixed when the respiratory effort is first absent and in a second part of the event restarts with still absent airflow (◘ Figs. 2.18, 2.19, 2.20)

After revision of the AASM criteria from 2007, the version of 2020 summarizes the alternative hypopnea aspects to one single definition:

Hypopnea is confirmed when:

- The flow signal (dynamic pressure measurement, thermistor) decreases by at least 30% compared to the original value.
- This reduction lasts for at least 10 s.
- The oxygen saturation decreases by at least 3% compared to the original value or the result is arousal correlated (see ◘ Fig. 2.21).

An event is considered as apnea when the criterion of apnea is temporarily fulfilled in the course of hypopnea.

Following the AASM again obstructive and central types of hypopneas may be differentiated.

The advantage of the new AASM criteria is, among others, the exact definition of the beginning and the end of a respiratory event.

- The beginning of an apnea or hypopnea is defined from the nadir preceding the first breath that is clearly reduced.
- The end of a respiratory event is defined as the beginning of the first breath whose amplitude approaches the baseline amplitude. In cases of unclear original amplitude, such as when breathing is highly variable, the end is set at the point where a clear increase of the oronasal breathing amplitude is observed.

  Alternatively, it is recommended in cases of accompanying desaturation to define the end at that point where resaturation of 2% or more occurs.

However, this last-mentioned criterion is supposed to be a relevant prolongation of the respiratory event because of the time shift between apnea and associated desaturation from the cardiovascular time and thus it should be declined.

Also, the consideration of respiratory events that do not meet the criterion of apnea or hypopnea but that nonetheless impair the quality of sleep and have to be rated as pathological is a merit of the AASM. The respiratory effort-related arousals (RERAs) are defined by an increase of the respiratory effort or a flattening of the dynamic

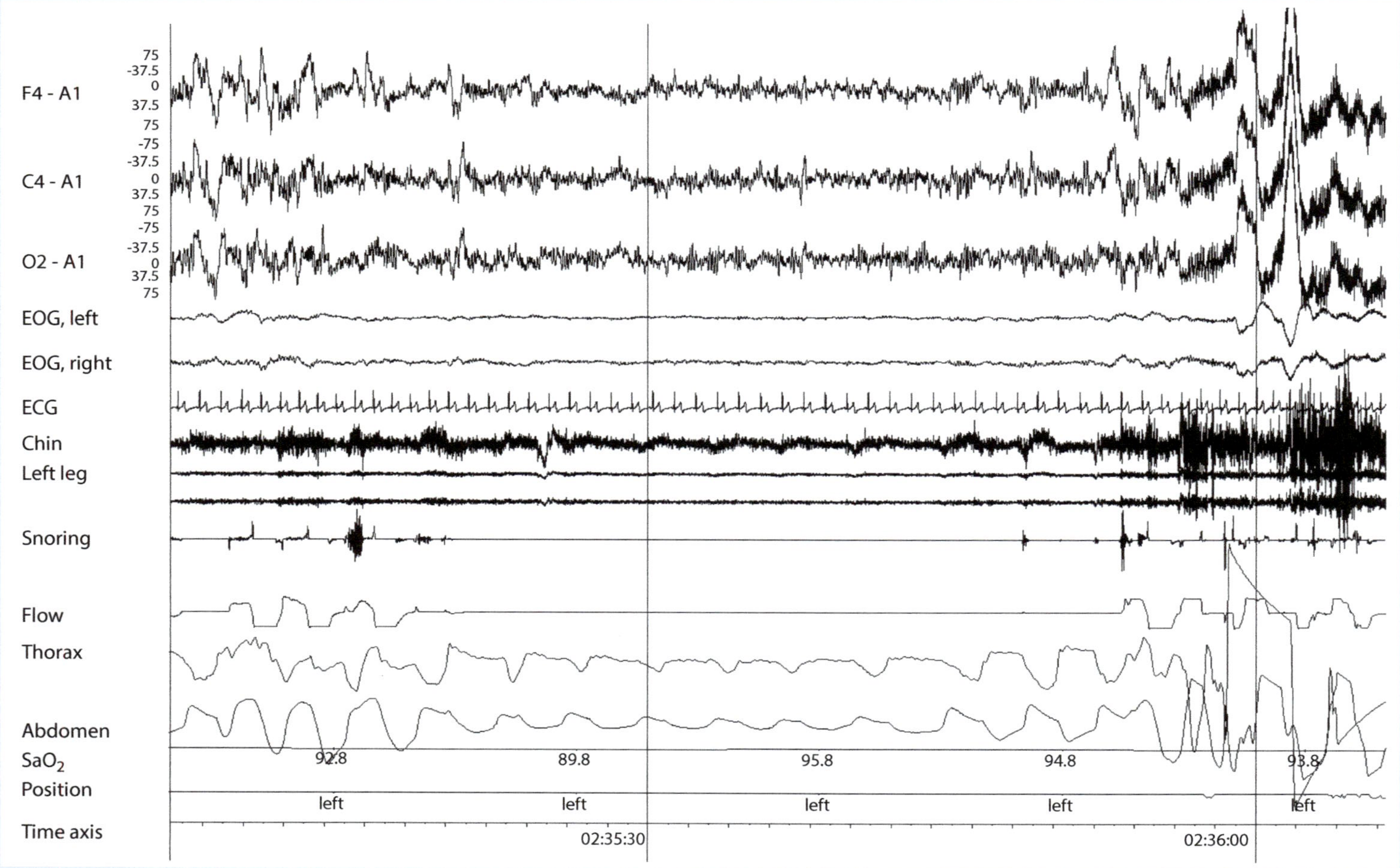

Fig. 2.18 Obstructive apnea of about 20 s with paradox thoracic and abdominal respiratory excursions. At the end of the apnea, an apnea-terminating arousal is found (increased frequency in the EEG and movement artifacts) and gradual HbO_2 decrease that continues in the consecutive epoch (not visible). The HbO_2 decrease at the beginning of the apnea as well as the previous arousal is the result of a previous apnea

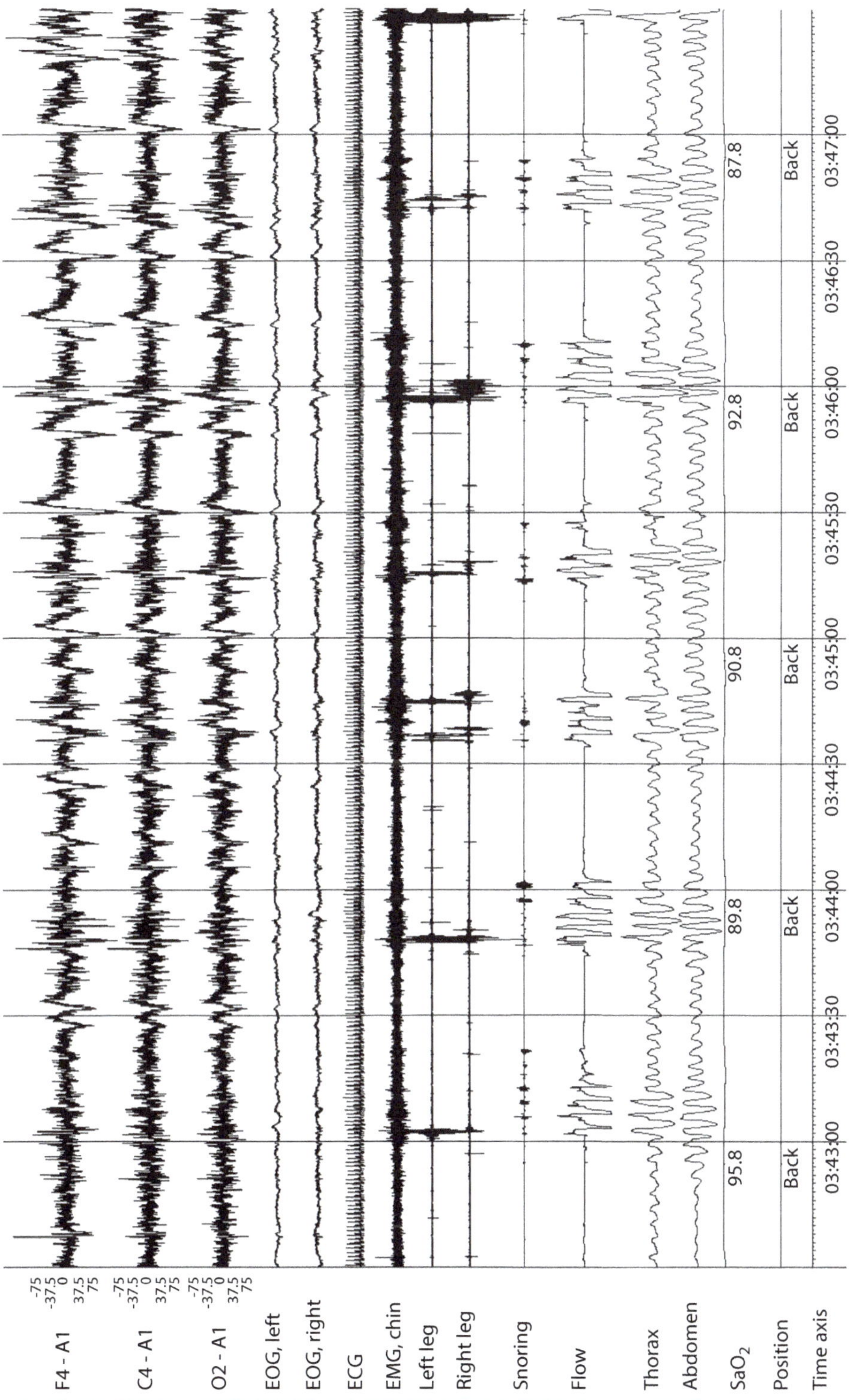

Fig. 2.19 Repeated obstructive apnea on the 5-min scale. Because of the concise presentation, the apnea-terminating arousals in the EEG can only be recognized based on the intermittent amplitude increases at the respective end of the apnea

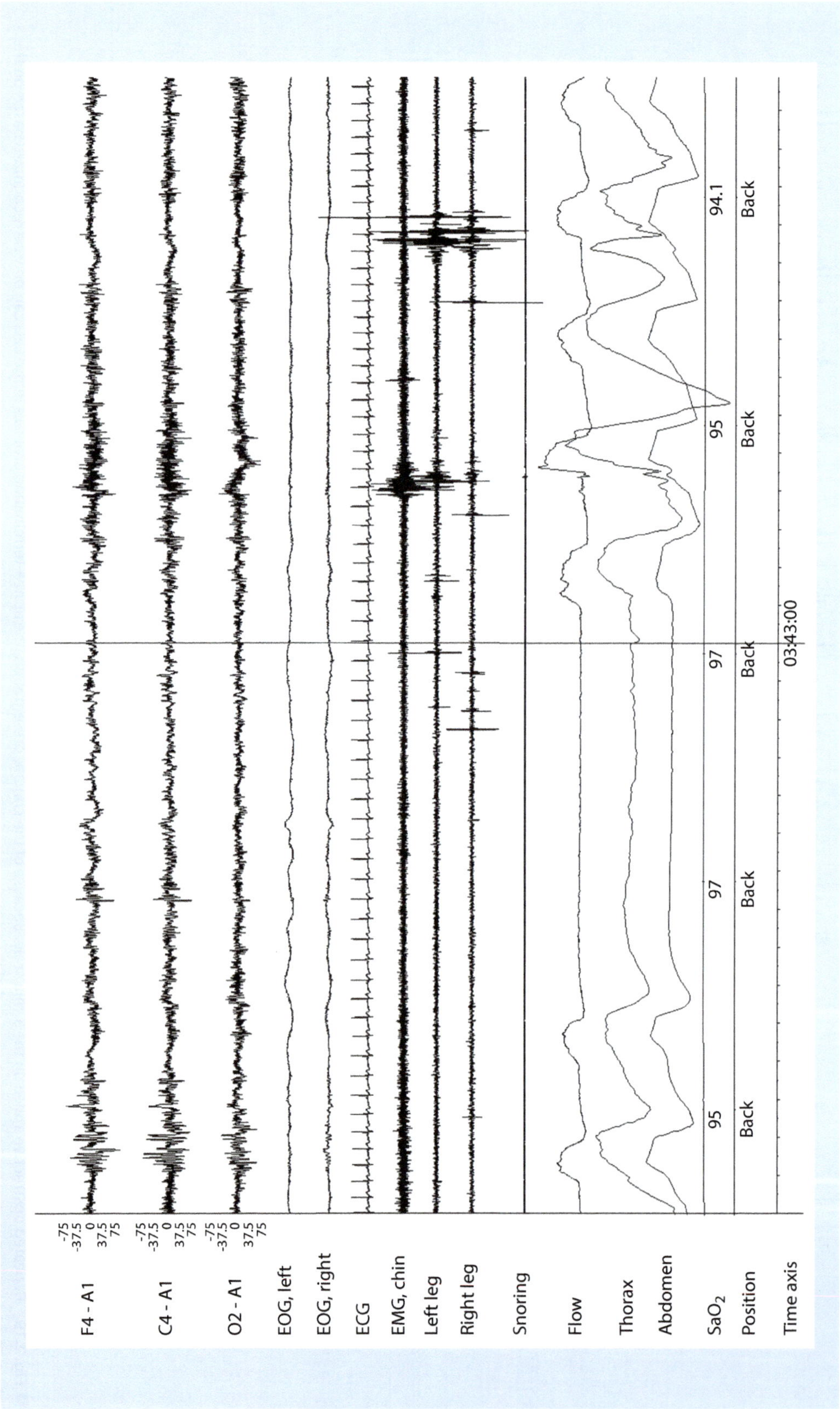

Fig. 2.20 Central apnea of 10 s with subsequent arousal reaction (accelerated frequency in the EEG and movement artifacts)

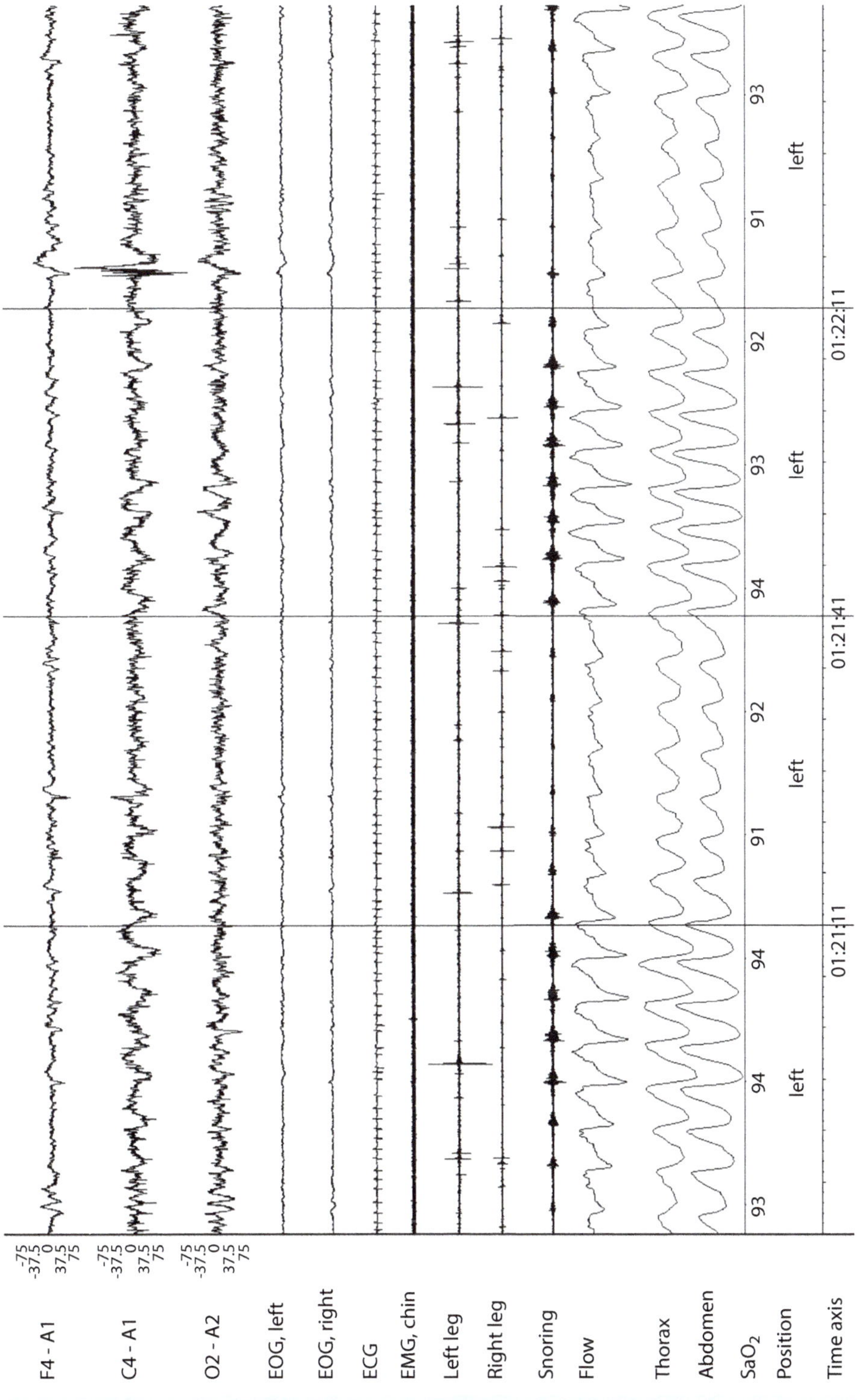

Fig. 2.21 Hypopneas in 2-min depiction. Reduction of the amplitude in the oronasal thermistor >30% and in the thoracic and abdominal respiratory excursions. Further, decrease of the HbO_2 saturation >4%

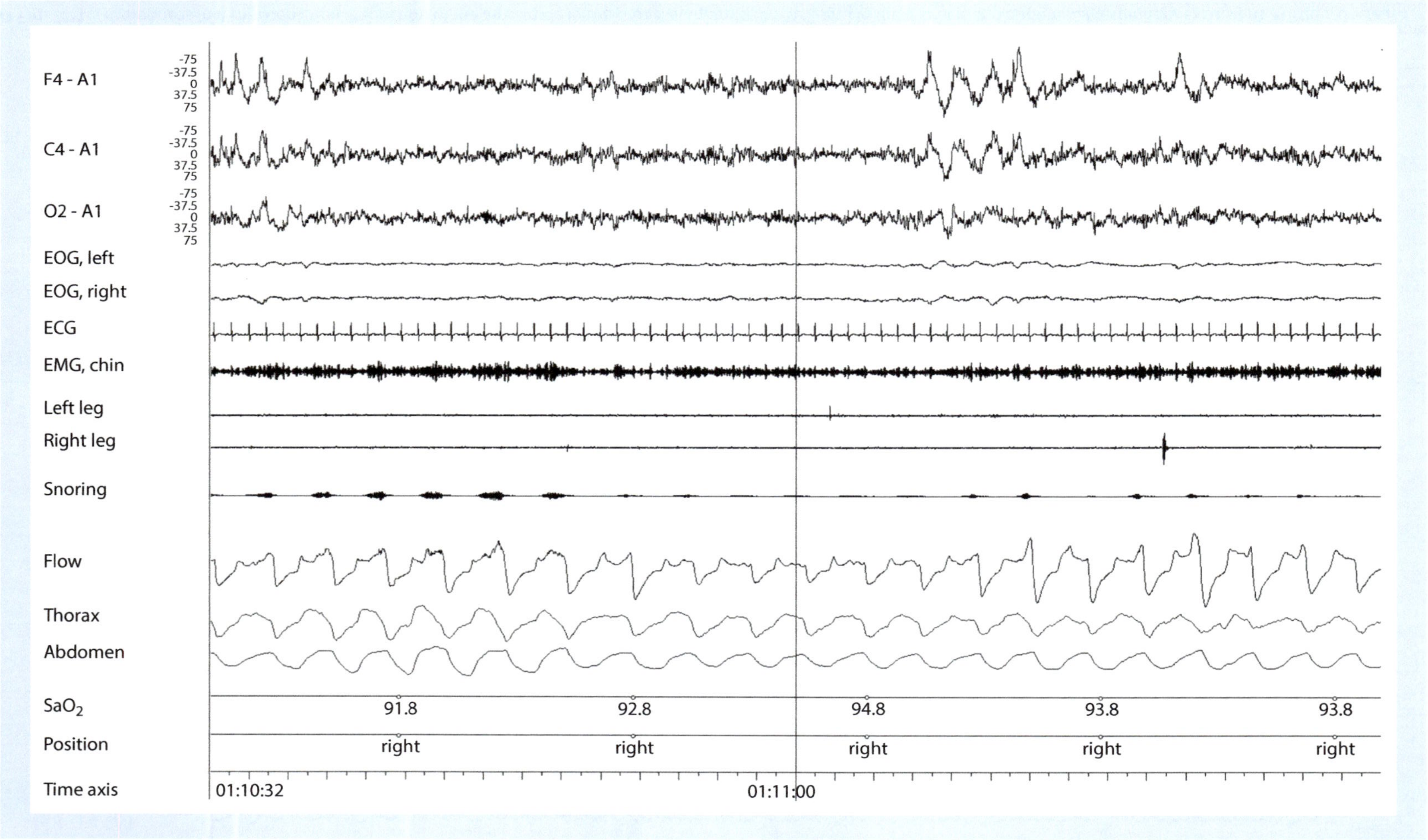

Fig. 2.22 RERA (respiratory effort-related arousal). Flattening of the curve and amplitude reduction in the oronasal thermistor by less than 30% with accompanying EEG frequency acceleration is introduced by waves with higher amplitudes (delta waves) including a K complex

pressure signal over an interval of 10 s or more. It is required that the respective event leads to arousal and the criteria of apnea or hypopnea are not met (◘ Fig. 2.22).

In cases of primary or secondary alveolar hypoventilation and central apnea, a gradual or complete loss of the airflow can be observed with open airways and reduced or absent thoracic and abdominal respiratory efforts.

The event is confirmed as *hypoventilation* when:
- The $PaCO_2$ value is at least 55 mmHg for a duration of at least 10 min.
- An increase of at least 10 mmHg of $PaCO_2$ is observed for at least 10 min over a value of 50 mmHg.

Persisting O_2 desaturation does not suffice for documenting hypoventilation (▸ Sect. 4.1.1). An increased $PaCO_2$ immediately after awakening is a clear hint to the presence of sleep-related hypoventilation. Transcutaneous as well as end-tidal (end-expiratory) measurements may be used to determine $PaCO_2$.

In the context of central sleep apnea syndromes (▸ Chap. 4), often typical airflow patterns occur that are identified as Cheyne-Stokes respiration. The AASM criteria define Cheyne-Stokes respiration as follows:
- At least three consecutive apneas and/or hypopneas emerge, in between crescendo–decrescendo breathing is observed, and the cycle length of this breathing pattern is at least 40 s.
- At least five or more central apneas or hypopneas per hour are observed within a measurement period of at least 2 h that are associated with Cheyne-Stokes respiration (◘ Fig. 2.23).

An overview of respiratory events in sleep is given in ◘ Table 2.5.

Depending on the severity of the disease, a fragmentary sleep profile with deep and REM sleep suppression is found based on apnea-terminating arousals with simultaneous increase of the superficial sleep stages. Coinciding with the apnea or hypoventilation phases, phasic HbO_2 desaturations occur that appear phase shifted because of the physiological HbO_2 saturation curve (◘ Fig. 2.24).

The AASM suggests statistically descriptive parameters for description of sleep-related breathing disorders (◘ Table 2.6). For identification of severity, the following parameters are typically measured:
- The apnea-hypopnea index (AHI)
- The desaturation index (number of HbO2 desaturations >3% per hour of night sleep)
- The respiratory effort-related arousal index (RERA-I)
- Respiratory disturbances iIndex (RDI): Number of apneas, hypopneas and RERAs per hour of night sleep.

In cases of unattended polygraphy, the assessment of sleep and RERAs is not possible because of the missing EEG. Thus, alternative calculation formulas and reference parameters are identified for description of the respiratory severity, and another classification of the severity is used compared to PSG. The respiratory event index (REI) is used instead of the RDI that considers apneas, hypopneas, and RERAs. The ODI replaces the EI.
- The REI describes the number of apneas and hypopneas with reference to the measurement time.
- The ODI describes the number of all O_2 desaturations (typically >3%) with reference to the measurement time.

For further details, see ◘ Tables 2.3 and 2.6.

In the past, the classification of the severity of sleep-related breathing disorders was only based on the extent of occurring nocturnal apneas and hypopneas. Currently, the occurrence of respiratory arousals and the daytime condition, in particular daytime sleepiness, are also considered (◘ Table 2.7).

Based on this classification of the severity, also cases with a low RDI (respiratory events per hour of sleep) and relevant daytime sleepiness with severe attentiveness disorders and proneness to fall asleep are considered as cases of severe sleep apnea.

The main criticism of the classification of the severity is that age effects and also methodical effects are not taken into account. For example, in older healthy subjects, often an RDI of more than 5/h is found. It would be desirable that the severity also includes the individual cardiopulmonary risk. Furthermore, the sensitivity of the measurement methods of the oronasal airflow is very different. Numerous studies could reveal that oronasal thermistors lead to a lower RDI compared to nocturnal pressure transducers.

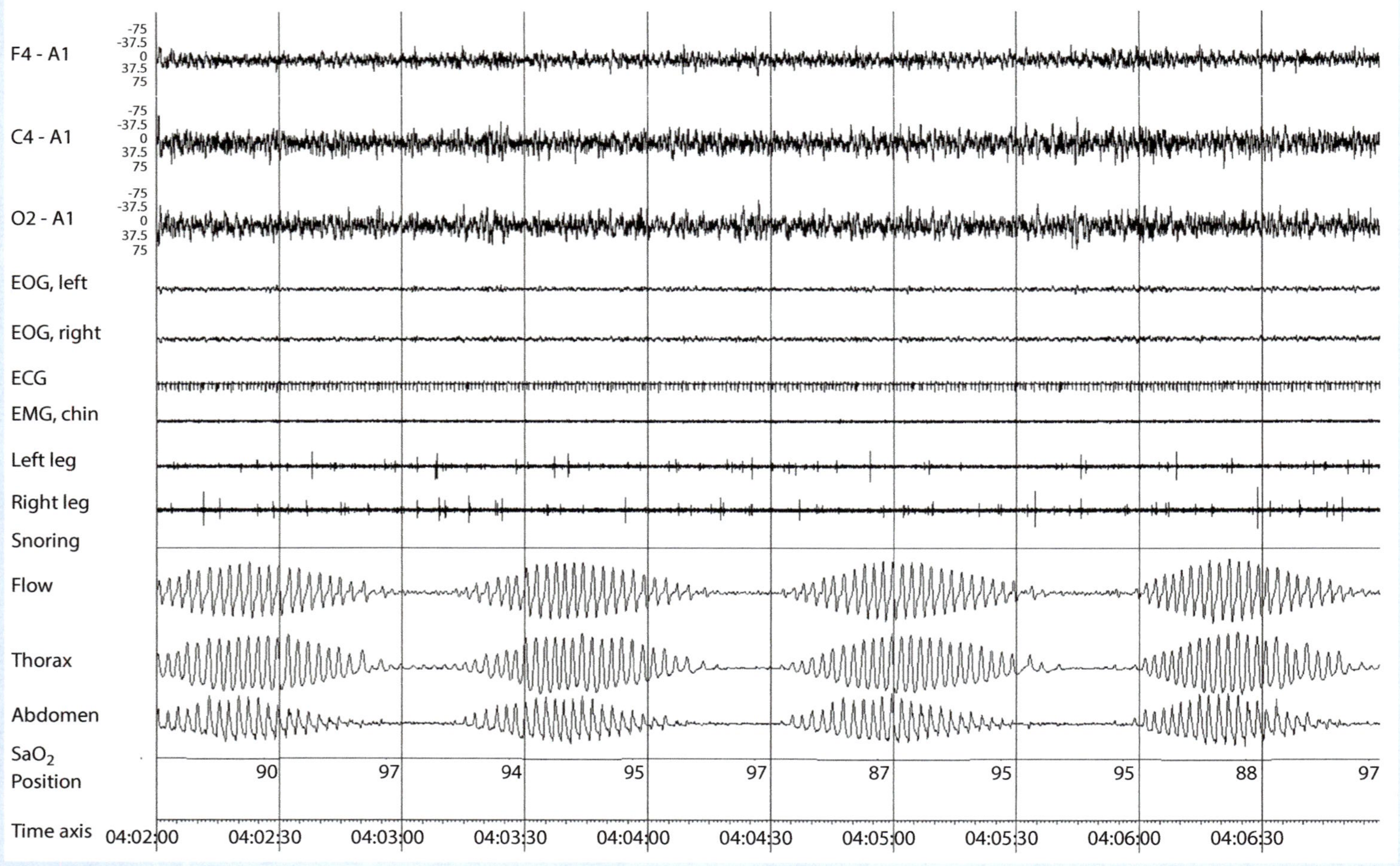

Fig. 2.23 Cheyne-Stokes respiration in the 5-min depiction of polysomnography. Crescendo–decrescendo phases of breathing follow each other. Central apneas between the events and arousals at the time of amplitude maximum. The arousal reactions are only seen because of the increased amplitude of the EEG (occipital)

Table 2.5 Systematic overview of respiratory events in sleep

Respiratory event	Oronasal airflow	Respiratory effort
Obstructive apnea	None (≥90%)	Maintained
Central apnea	None (≥90%)	None
Mixed apnea	None (≥90%)	First none, then onset
Hypopnea	≥30% (and 3% HbO_2 desaturation or arousal)	Maintained
Respiratory effort-related arousal (RERA)	Discrete reduction (<30%), not obligatory	Maintained
Cheyne-Stokes respiration	Crescendo–decrescendo-like course	Crescendo–decrescendo-like course

2.8 Examination of Sleepiness- and Fatigue-Related Daytime Impairments

Daytime sleepiness and resulting impairments at work, when driving a car, or in other socially demanding situations are a significant symptom of many diseases and in particular of many sleep disorders. A relevant percentage of 31% of the population older than 16 years report nonspecifically to suffer sometimes or frequently from sleepiness (Falkenstetter et al. 2011). A well-known, nearly legendary study of an important insurance company in Germany (HUK) reveals that about 25% of all accidents with fatal outcome on Bavarian highways are caused by driver weariness. Traffic statistics confirm that on German streets, about twice as many fatal accidents occur because of microsleeps rather than drinking/driving. About 20% of all critical events in aviation are explained by sleepiness of the safety staff, pilots, and tower staff. Numerous catastrophes, for example, the sinking of the tanker *Exxon Valdez*, the crash of the shuttle *Challenger*, or industrial accidents such as Chernobyl, Three Mile Island, and Bhopal, are supposed to be caused by, among other factors, faults because of daytime sleepiness.

The scientific interest in daytime sleepiness has been increasing in past years; however, daytime sleepiness is a young research field still with little small knowledge. A standardized scientific definition of the term is currently not available. Furthermore, a differentiation to related phenomena of fatigue has not yet been established.

Considering the current scientific knowledge, daytime sleepiness may be understood as reduced wakefulness and a reduction of the central nervous system alertness. Variations of the central nervous system activation are a universal human experience and physiological in the circadian rhythm.

Characteristics of a reduced central nervous system activation or an increased daytime sleepiness include these:

- Attention deficits
- Monotony intolerance
- Tendency to fall asleep
- Micro-sleep
- Imperative sleep attacks

These events are directly correlated with the performance in socially demanding situations as seen, for example, at work or in traffic.

In sleep medicine, nonrestorative sleep as the origin of daytime sleepiness is in the focus of diagnostic and therapeutic efforts. From a differential diagnostic point of view, it is essential to identify sleep disorders, physical diseases, and situational factors as well as the circadian phase situation as potential origins of daytime sleepiness and to include these aspects in the diagnostic and therapeutic efforts.

A theoretical model regarding the correlation between nonrestorative sleep and attention-related processes based on performance ability is described next. This neuropsychological model is based on Posner and Rafal, regarding its attention-related

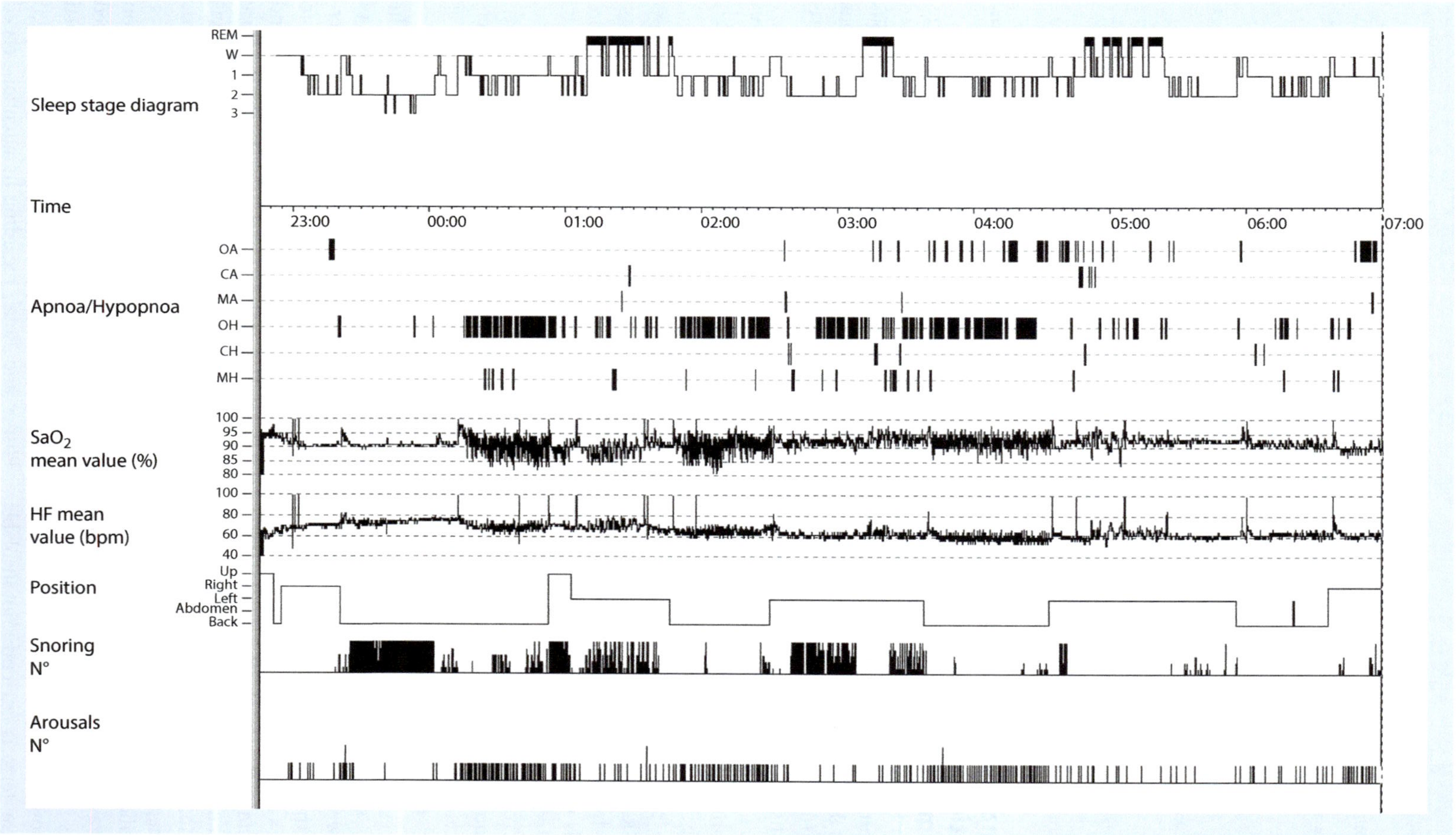

Fig. 2.24 Characteristic hypnogram of severe obstructive sleep apnea. The hypnogram shows the characteristic deep sleep suppression (Stage 3 is missing) and the increased change of sleep stages from repetitive apnea-terminating arousal reactions (*arousal N0* = *number of arousals*). The increased number of arousals (*arousal N0*) is also expressed in the higher heart frequency variation (HF mean value, bpm). Predominantly obstructive hypoventilation phases (*OH*) and obstructive apneas (*OA*) emerge independently from the body position. As a consequence of respiratory disorders, intermittent HbO_2 decreases (*SaO_2 mean value, %*) as great as 80% may be measured. The channel entitled *Snoring* reflects the increased snoring activity

Table 2.6 Statistically descriptive parameters for description of sleep-related breathing disorders

Severity	Definition
Apneas	Total number of all apneas during TST
Apnea index (AI)	Average number of apneas per hour relating to the TST
Hypopneas	Total number of all hypopneas during TST
Hypopnea index (HI)	Average number of hypopneas per hour relating to the TST
Apneas + hypopneas	Total number of all apneas and hypopneas during TST
Apnea-hypopnea index (AHI)	Average number of apneas and hypopneas per hour relating to the TST
Respiratory effort-related arousal (RERA)	Total number of all events during TST
Respiratory effort-related arousal index (RERA-I)	Average number of events per hour of sleep relating to the TST
Respiratory disturbances index (RDI)	Average number of apneas and hypopneas and RERA per hour relating to the TST
For outpatient polygraphy: Respiratory events index (REI)	Number of all apneas and hypopneas relating to the measurement time
Oxygen desaturations >3%	Total number of all events
Oxygen desaturation index >3%	Total number of all events per hour relating to the TST
For outpatient polygraphies: Oxygen desaturation index	Number of all O_2 desaturations relating to the measurement time
Mean O_2 saturation	Mean value of the O_2 concentration without desaturations in percent during TST
Occurrence of hypoventilation	Yes/no
Occurrence of Cheyne-Stokes respiration	Yes/no

TST total sleep time including N1

Table 2.7 Severity of obstructive types of sleep-related breathing disorders (this classification of the severity includes the RERAs in the RDI)

Dimension	Mild	Moderate	Severe
Sleepiness or unintended sleep episodes during the day	During activities that do not require much attention, e.g., watching TV	During activities that require attention, e.g., meetings, conferences	During activities that require active attention, e.g., driving a car
Respiratory events per hour of sleep (RDI)	5–15	15–30	>30

RERA respiratory effort-related arousal

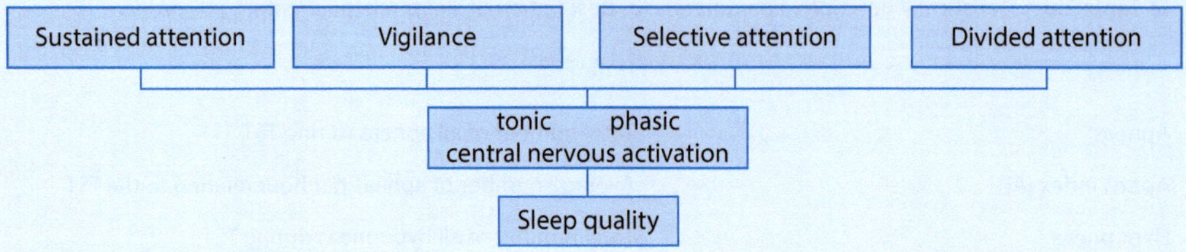

Fig. 2.25 Correlation between quality of sleep and sleepiness-related daytime impairment. The reduced quality of sleep seen in sleep disorders, for example, caused by slow-wave sleep (SWS) or REM suppression, leads to a reduction of the tonic and phasic central nervous system alertness (daytime sleepiness) that is not voluntarily controlled. In this way, also the voluntarily controlled vigilance, sustained attention, and divided and selective attention are reduced

elements, and it was confirmed in the context of numerous scientific investigations. The model differentiates five attention- and sleepiness-related aspects on which performance is based. More elaborate models are reserved for more scientific issues and are considered as too complex for the patient-oriented questions of sleep medicine.

For schematic depiction of the correlation between quality of sleep and sleepiness-related daytime impairment, see Fig. 2.25.

The model contains the tonic and phasic central nervous system alertness that is not under voluntary control.

- The tonic component is defined as the general degree of wakefulness that is influenced by circadian variations.
- The phasic component contains the ability to increase the tonic activity level triggered by requirements or a critical stimulus.

The neuronal substrate of wakefulness or also of the central nervous system arousal level is supposed to be located in the reticular formation of the brainstem. Its activity level is reflected, among others, in the frequency band of electric brain activity, heart rate, skin resistance, and pupil width (Table 2.8).

Alertness precedes the parts of attention, which are under voluntary control: vigilance, sustained attention, divided and selective attention.

In neuropsychology, *vigilance* is the ability to maintain the attention over a longer time on an increased or high level. An adequate reaction is required on rare or incidentally emerging stimuli. High requirements to vigilance are, for example, control and supervision tasks in power plants or

Table 2.8 Definition of sleepiness and associated attention processes

Attention component	Characteristics
Tonic alertness	Circadian aspect of the general arousal level, of wakefulness
	Independent of voluntary control
	Preceding vigilance, selective and divided attention
Phasic alertness	Capacity to increase the tonic activation level triggered by a critical stimulus
Selective attention	Ability to maintain the attentiveness over longer periods of time for a certain task
	Ability to suppress disturbing stimuli, interferences, and distractions
Divided attention	Speed of information processing
	Ability of divided and parallel information processing
	Ability of automated and controlled processing
Vigilance	Unspecific orgasmic readiness to react on rare and incidentally emerging stimuli over a longer time
	Under voluntary control
Sustained attention	Ability to react on incidentally emerging stimuli over a long time
	Under voluntary control

driving on a highway for a longer time. It is important to know that this definition of vigilance is not congruent with physiological definitions. In the physiological context, vigilance is used in the sense of central nervous system activation (degree of wakefulness) (▫ Table 2.8).

As a neuropsychological term, *divided attention* describes the ability to process information in a rapid, automated, and controlled way including the ability to serial and parallel actions such as driving a car in confusing, busy situations. Hence, when approaching an intersection, the driver has to pay attention to moving and standing cars, has to observe indications, traffic lights, pedestrians, etc., and at the same time has to perform coordinated motor activities such as steering, setting signals, and pressing the clutch and brakes (▫ Table 2.8).

Selective attention describes the ability of an individual to select relevant stimuli from the sum of all incoming stimuli. One classic example is a teacher who has to focus on his lesson despite a turbulent class and much disturbing noise. He has to focus (selectively) on his task to transmit knowledge and to suppress interferences that emerge because of discussions within the class (▫ Table 2.8).

Sustained attention describes the ability to correctly react on incidentally emerging stimuli of high timely density over longer periods. The difference regarding vigilance is the significantly higher density of stimuli of the critical events.

Daytime sleepiness is influenced by numerous intrinsic and extrinsic conditions such as noise, temperature, activity, body position, time of the day, motivation, ability to fall asleep, psychophysiological arousal, or intake of sedating or activity-enhancing substances. All this has to be taken into account and controlled in the examination situation.

For better understanding, the preceding paragraphs depicted the basic definitions for the assessment of daytime sleepiness. In the following chapters, single diagnostic methods will be explained in detail. In Germany, some sleep centers and other healthcare institutions have specialized on exhaustive diagnostics of daytime sleepiness, ability to work, and fitness to drive in the context of sleep disorders. In cases of such questions, patients may be referred to these institutions.

However, from a legal point of view, also physicians or therapists who are not specialized in daytime sleepiness are required to estimate the risk of pathological daytime sleepiness and its negative impact on the patient's social life by taking adequate measures. They are supposed to inform the patients about the increased potential of endangerment of self and others, for example, in traffic. In cases of positive findings, it might be recommended to transfer the patient to a specialized sleep center or a physician specialized in occupational medicine for further diagnostics.

For assessment of the fitness to drive of driving license applicants or driving licensees with SRBD and daytime sleepiness, the EU published guidelines (2015) that had to be implemented in the national legislation of the member countries until December 31, 2016. The criteria developed for each member country of the EU are available from the respective national sleep societies.

2.8.1 Diagnostics of Daytime Sleepiness

If the data of a questionnaire or history taking (▸ Sects. 2.1 and 2.3) allow suspecting pathological daytime sleepiness, in particular high-risk patients have to undergo objective examination procedures (▫ Table 2.9). In this context, sleepiness-related functions are checked:

- Central nervous system alertness
- Selective attention
- Divided attention
- Vigilance
- Sustained attention

If history taking justifies the suspicion of fatigue, no objective procedures are available (▸ Sects. 2.1 and 2.8). Moreover, the diagnosis of fatigue may be confirmed by applying respective standardized psychological questionnaires such as the Karolinska Exhaustion Disorder Scale, the Tiredness Symptoms Scale, the Fatigue Questionnaire, the Fatigue Severity Scale, and others.

For assessment of sleepiness-related impairments, numerous diagnostic methods are available (▫ Table 2.9). The examination procedures register partial aspects of daytime sleepiness on different physiological, cognitive, and subjective levels of functioning. The extent of voluntary control is highly variable. It is characteristic that the results

2

Table 2.9 Diagnostic procedures for assessment of sleepiness-related impairments

Attention component	Suitable test procedures
Tonic activation	Tendency to fall asleep, e.g., multiple sleep latency test (MSLT)
	Ability to stay awake, e.g., maintenance of wakefulness test (MWT)
	Long-term EEG (with and without behavioral observations)
	Variations of the pupil diameter in darkness; pupillographic sleepiness test (PST)
	Measurement of the reaction time with omissions, e.g., psychomotor vigilance test (PVT), OSLER test (OT)
	EEG examinations, e.g., alpha attenuation test (ATT)
	Other measurements of the reaction time, e.g., test batteries for attentional performance (TAP), Vienna Test System (VTS)
Phasic activation	Measurements of the reaction time with cues, e.g., TAP
	ERP (event-related potentials), e.g., CNV, SN
Selective attention	For example, performance sequence, test of selective attention of TAP
Divided attention	Vienna determination unit
	Test of divided attention of TAP
Vigilance	For example, vigilance test of VTS or of TAP, Vigimar
Sustained attention	Tasks with high stimulus density over longer periods
	For example, permanent attention test of VTS, test set sleep of VTS
Self-assessment questionnaires	Epworth Sleepiness Scale (ESS)
	Stanford Sleepiness Scale (SSS)
	Pittsburgh Sleep Quality Index (PSQI)

ERP event-related potentials, *CNV* contingent negative variation, *SN* sharp negative variation, *FCRT* four-choice reaction time task, *TAP* test battery for attentional performance, *VTS* Vienna Test System

of the single examination methods have only few correlations when they assess different areas of functioning or performance. Because of these mentioned differences, it was not possible previously to establish one single procedure that could serve as standard for validation of other methods.

With regard to scientific standards, PC-supported neuropsychological procedures such as these applied, for example, in the Vienna Test System (test set sleep) seem to be generally superior to electrophysiological methods such as the multiple sleep latency test (MSLT) or the maintenance of wakefulness test (MWT). In single cases, even age- and intelligence-adjusted standard values are available. Furthermore, the ecological validity of these procedures is estimated higher compared to MSLT and MWT. Nonetheless, they are still laboratory testing procedures, and their transferability to specific everyday situations, such as checking the fitness to drive, seems to be limited.

The single aspects of daytime sleepiness (central nervous system alertness, selective and divided attention, vigilance, sustained attention) depend on numerous factors that have to be considered and controlled in the diagnostic procedure.

Preconditions for Examination with Regard to Diagnostics of Daytime Sleepiness

- The examination day should be preceded by an undisturbed and regular night's sleep of at least six hours (polysomnographic control). Irregular bedtimes and shift work should be avoided on the days before examination.
- The examination should not be performed on the day immediately after the adaptation night (first night effect) in the sleep lab.
- Medication and substance anamnesis should assess drugs and substances enhancing or reducing sleepiness. In particular, in the context of medical expert reports, urine screening may be indicated.
- It is not allowed to smoke in the examination situation. Smoking should be avoided at least 30 min before the respective examination.
- Generally, patients do not consume alcohol or other stimulating substances.

In contrast to other recommendations in the literature, caffeine need not be completely omitted on the examination day but rather consumed in the usual measure in cases of habitual regular consumption.
- The examination room should have a pleasant temperature, should be soundproof, and for examinations that include the sleep-onset latency as a target parameter it should be possible to darken the room.
- Excessive physical activities or emotional stress, in particular before the respective examination, should be avoided. In this context, it must also be mentioned that information about the medical findings or the daily visits may lead to emotional stress of the patient and in this way modify the examination results.
- An important condition that has to be controlled for examination is the appointed time of day, because in the course of the day, relevant circadian and homeostatic variations of sleepiness (central nervous system activation) may occur.

2.8.1.1 Diagnostic Procedures of Central Nervous System Alertness

For most procedures of central nervous system alertness, except the pupillographic sleepiness test (PST), either only insufficient standard values are available or in healthy individuals such a broad distribution of the results is found (e.g., in the context of MSLT) that diagnostic differentiation between normal and pathological values is only possible in extreme cases. For diagnostic assessment, generally a synopsis of several procedures is required that include different measurement levels. In most procedures, the motivation of the patient has to be taken into account.

The clinically diagnostic procedures of central nervous system alertness include these:
- The multiple sleep latency test (MSLT)
- The maintenance of wakefulness test (MWT)
- The pupillographic sleepiness test (PST)
- The psychomotor vigilance test (PVT)
- The OSLER test
- Other measurements of the reaction time, such as the test battery of attentional performance (TAP) and the Vienna Test System (VTS)

Further procedures such as evoked potentials, long-term EEG, and the alpha attenuation test are mostly applied for scientific questions.

Multiple Sleep Latency Test (MSLT)

The multiple sleep latency test (MSLT) is based on the assumption that the sleep-onset latency is reduced with increasing sleepiness.

In 1977, M. Carskadon and W.C. Dement were the first who presented the MSLT as a procedure to measure daytime sleepiness. For quite a long time, average sleep-onset latencies of 5 min or less were considered as a suggestion of pathological daytime sleepiness. According to Carskadon, healthy adult sleepers show sleep-onset latencies between 10 and 20 min. Sleep-onset latencies between 5 and 10 min are conspicuous but not actually pathological.

At the beginning of the 1990s, the American Sleep Disorders Association (ASDA) defined a questionable, not evidence-based, correlation between sleep-onset latencies in the MSLT and the severity of daytime sleepiness in light of the increasing relevance of daytime sleepiness and its sociomedical risks.

Based hereon, sleep-onset latencies:
- Between 10 and 15 min correspond to mild
- Between 5 and 10 min correspond to moderate
- Between 0 and 5 min correspond to severe daytime sleepiness

The mentioned limit values are not empirically gained, but they are based on experience knowledge and do not pass empirical testing.

Since its introduction until recent times, the MSLT was established as internationally acknowledged standard procedure to assess daytime sleepiness in sleep medicine (so-called experimental MSLT). A meta-analysis published by the Atlas Task Force of the AASM in 2005, however, revealed a very limited significance and validity of the MSLT with regard to the examination of daytime sleepiness. Based on this meta-analysis, the following recommendations were given for the clearly limited indication, standardized procedure, and evaluation of the MSLT. The results of this meta-analysis have replaced it as the standard procedure for the assessment of daytime sleepiness. However, its high diagnostic validity for narcolepsy (clinical MSLT) remains undisputed.

Recommendations for the Performance and Evaluation of the MSLT According to the AASM

- The MSLT consists of five nap opportunities that are performed at 2-h intervals, starting 1.5 to 3 h after the end of nighttime PSG. Also, four nap opportunities are possible, but the MSLT is only reliable for the diagnosis of narcolepsy if in these four passes SOREM occurs twice together with nocturnal polysomnography.
- The MSLT is performed after polysomnography measurement that has occurred during the patient's major sleep period. The usefulness of the MSLT to confirm the diagnosis of narcolepsy is clearly limited if the total sleep time (TST) in the previous sleep period amounted to less than 6 h. An MSLT should not be performed after a split night sleep study (diagnostics and therapy in one night in the case of SRBD).
- A sleep diary should be kept for 1 week before the MSLT to assess the sleep–wake rhythm.
- The strict observation of the standardized conditions to perform an MSLT is crucial for obtaining valid results. The patient's sleep room has to be dark and quiet during testing; the temperature should be set at the patient's comfort level.
- Stimulants and stimulant-like medications as well as REM-suppressing medication should be ideally interrupted 2 weeks before examination. The intake of usual medications (e.g., antihypertensives, insulin) has to be critically planned before MSLT to control or minimize their stimulating and sedating side effects as well as their impact on the sleep-onset latency. Drug screening may be indicated to exclude the possibility that reduced sleep-onset latencies are not pharmacologically induced. Drug screening is typically performed in the morning before examination; sometimes it is also justified at other times. Smoking should be stopped 30 min before each nap opportunity. Vigorous physical activity should be avoided on the examination day, and the patient should end any stimulating activities at least 15 min before the MSLT. The patient should abstain from caffeine-containing beverages and avoid exposure to bright sunlight. A light breakfast 1 h before the first trial and a light lunch immediately after the second noon trial are recommended. It must be borne in mind that diagnostic-therapeutic discussions with the patient on the examination day may have a stimulating effect, such as when the patient is informed about the presence of sleep apnea or other diseases.
- The MSLT should only be performed by specifically trained and experienced specialists.
- The standard electrodes (C3-A2, C4-A1) are positioned according to the criteria of Rechtschaffen and Kales; in addition, occipital (O1-A2, O2-A1) derivations are performed for better identification of the sleep–wake transition. Furthermore, EOGs from the left and right orbita edge of the respective eye are measured as well as a mental/submental EMG and a single-channel ECG.
- Before each nap opportunity, the patients are asked if they need to use the bathroom or need other things for their comfort. The biosignal calibration before each trial comprises the following standardized instructions:
  1. Please lie quietly with your eyes open for 30 s.
  2. Close both eyes for 30 s.
  3. Without moving your head, look to the right, then to the left, then right, then left, right and left.

4. Blink eyes slowly for five times.
5. Clench your teeth tightly together.

- For each trial, the patient should be instructed as follows: "Please lie quietly, assume a comfortable position, keep your eyes closed and try to fall asleep." Immediately afterward, the lights are turned off, signaling the start of the test. Between the trials, the patient should leave the bed and be prevented from sleeping. This procedure requires continuous observation by the staff.
- Sleep onset for the clinical MSLT is determined by the time from lights out to the first epoch with sleep, including stage S1 (according to Rechtschaffen and Kales), defined as the first 30-s epoch with more than 15 s of cumulative sleep. In the so-called experimental MSLT, the sleeper is awakened after three consecutive sleep epochs. The absence of sleep during one nap opportunity is recorded as a sleep latency of 20 min. The latency is also included in the calculation of the mean sleep latency. For assessment of the REM sleep, the clinical MSLT is performed for a further 15 min after the first epoch of sleep, regardless of the occurrence of sleep. The REM latency is taken as the time of the first epoch of sleep to the beginning of the first epoch of REM sleep, regardless of the intervening stages of sleep or wakefulness.
- One MSLT trial is terminated after 20 min if sleep does not occur.
- The MSLT findings include the start and end times of each trial, the latency from lights out to the first epoch of sleep, the mean sleep latency (arithmetic mean of all naps or nap opportunities), and the number of SOREM periods. For the diagnosis of narcolepsy, at least two MSLTs with SOREM of a total of five MSLTs and two PSG are required.
- Events and conditions that require deviation from the standard protocol have to be documented thoroughly by the staff so that they may be included in the interpretation.

Table 2.10 Mean sleep-onset latencies of healthy individuals and narcolepsy patients for MSLT with four and five nap opportunities

Condition	Mean value	± SD (min)
MSLT with four nap opportunities	10.4	±4.3*
MSLT with five nap opportunities	11.6	±5.2*
MSLT for narcolepsy	3.1	±2.9

* = 4 vs. 5 nap MSL $p<0.01$

For interpretation of the mean sleep-onset latency, the mean sleep-onset latencies of healthy individuals were depicted for MSLT with four and five nap opportunities (Table 2.10).

Because the mean sleep-onset latency in MSLT is clearly age related, common age-dependent standards were determined for the clinical as well as experimental version (Table 2.11). The meta-analysis of the AASM did not reveal significant differences between the clinical and experimental version of the MSLT, except for the group of 30- to 39-year-old individuals, in contrast to the theoretical assumption. Thus, the values of both versions are pooled in Table 2.11.

Indications for MSLT According to AASM Criteria

- The MSLT is indicated in patients with suspected narcolepsy for confirmation of the diagnosis.
- The MSLT may be indicated as part of the diagnostic process to differentiate between idiopathic hypersomnia and narcolepsy.
- The MSLT is not indicated in the clinical routine for diagnosis or therapy evaluation of obstructive sleep apnea.
- The MSLT is not indicated in the clinical routine for the determination of sleepiness in cases of medical and neurological disorders (except narcolepsy), insomnia, and circadian rhythm disorders.

2

Table 2.11 Age dependency of experimental and clinical MSLT in healthy individuals

Age	Mean sleep-onset latency (min)	SD	Hours	Remarks
10–20 years	10.0	4.5	25	–
20–30 years	10.4	5.4	284	Sign diff to 50–80 years
30–40 years	10.8	3.9	192	Sign diff to 50–80 years
40–50 years	11.7	4.4	72	Sign diff to 80 years
50–60 years	12.1	1.1	11	Sign diff to 80 years
60–70 years	11.2	5.2	54	Sign diff to 80 years
70–80 years	n.i.	n.i.	n.i.	n.i.
80–90 years	15.2	6.0	22	Sign diff to all

Sign diff to significant difference to, *n.i.* no information

Practical Tip

The MSLT seems to be a procedure that assesses the ability to fall asleep. The sleep-onset ability is influenced by daytime sleepiness but also other factors such as the ability to relax and rest. The ability to fall asleep rapidly is not necessarily pathological, but it may also be an adaptive physiological behavior that allows switching quickly from activity to rest.

The MSLT should be included only as one of several procedures if daytime sleepiness has to be assessed. For statements in the context of individual cases, in particular with regard to fitness for work and driving, its significance is very limited.

For diagnostics of narcolepsy, the validity of the procedure is confirmed.

Maintenance of Wakefulness Test (MWT)

The maintenance of wakefulness test (MWT) was developed from the MSLT and represents a modification. Methodically, it is based on identical electrophysiological parameters as the MSLT: the EEG, EOG, and EMG.

The MWT is based on the assumption that it is more interesting in the field of sleep medicine to determine the ability to stay awake rather than the ability to fall asleep, especially in cases of hypersomnia. In comparison to the MSLT, the MWT has a higher face validity or ecological validity.

Thus, in modifying the MSLT, the examination is performed in a sitting position, such as in a comfortable armchair, and the patient is instructed to stay awake. Basically, the MWT has to contend with the same influencing factors as the MSLT.

The Atlas Task Force of the AASM gives the following recommendations for performing and evaluating the MWT. These recommendations are based on knowledge obtained from a trial performed by Doghramji and colleagues that was completed by expert opinions from a consensus process.

Recommendations of the Atlas Task Force of the AASM for Performance and Evaluation of the MWT

- The MWT consists of four trials of 40 min each performed at 2-h intervals, with the first trial beginning about 1.5–3 h after the patient's usual wakeup time. Thus, usually, the first trial starts at 9:00 or 10:00 in the morning.
- The examining physician decides if PSG is necessary in the night before MWT, based on the clinical conditions.

- The examination room should be maximally insulated from external light. A light source should be placed slightly behind the patient so that it is just out of the field of vision. It should deliver an illuminance of 0.10.0.13 lux at the corneal level. A 7.5 W nightlight may be used placed about 30 cm above the floor, and about 90 cm laterally removed from the patient's head. The room temperature should be set based on the patient's comfort level. During examination, the patient should be seated in a comfortable armchair or in bed with the back and head supported by a bedrest (alternatively, pillows may be used).
- Consumption of alcohol, caffeine, and other medications before and during MWT should be determined by the sleep clinician preceding the MWT. Drug screening may be indicated to clarify if the wakefulness or sleepiness is induced by other than the prescribed medication. Drug screening is usually performed on the morning of the MWT, but the timing may be modified according to the clinical conditions. A light breakfast is recommended at least 1 h before the first trial; a light lunch is recommended immediately after the termination of the second noon trial.
- The MWT should only be performed by specialized and experienced staff.
- The standard electrode montage for the MWT includes two central EEG (C3-A2, C4-A1) and occipital (O1-A1, O2-A1) derivations, left and right eye EOGs, mental/submental EMG, and a single-channel ECG.
- Preceding each trial, the patient is asked if he/she needs to use the bathroom or requires other things for comfort. Biosignal calibration before each trial encompasses the following standard instructions:
  - Please lie quietly with your eyes open for 30 s.
  - Close both eyes for 30 s.
  - Without moving your head, look to the right, then left, then right, then left, right and left.
  - Blink eyes slowly for five times.
  - Clench your teeth tightly together.
- Before each trial, the patient is instructed: "Please sit still and remain awake for as long as possible. Look directly ahead of you and do not look directly at the light." The same instructions are supposed to be given before each trial. Immediately afterward, the lights are turned off, signaling the beginning of the examination. The patient is not allowed to perform self-stimulations such as singing or slapping the face. Video surveillance during MWT may be helpful. Between the trials, the patient has to leave the bed or armchair and is prevented from sleeping. This procedure requires continuous surveillance by the staff.
- Sleep onset is defined as the first epoch of more than 15 s of cumulated sleep in the first 30-s epoch.
- Trials are terminated after 40 min if no sleep occurs or after unequivocal sleep, defined as three consecutive epochs of Stage 1 sleep or one epoch of any other stage of sleep.
- The following data are documented:
  - Start and stop times for each trial
  - Sleep-onset latency
  - Total sleep time (TST)
  - Stages of sleep achieved for each trial
  - The mean sleep latency (arithmetic mean of the four trials)
- Events and conditions that represent a deviation from the standard protocol have to be thoroughly documented by the sleep technologists so that they may be taken into account for interpretation.

Similar to the MSLT, the AASM does not present cut-offs for the presence of pathological sleep-onset latency in the MWT. Moreover, the unsatisfactory study situation regarding standard values and manifold influencing factors on the sleep-onset latency is mentioned. The mean sleep-onset latency (occurrence of the first epoch of sleep) in the MWT (40-min protocol) was 30.4 ± 11.2 min in control persons. The upper limit of the 95% confidence interval (ceiling effect) was 40.0 min and the lower limit 12.9 min.

Sleep-onset latencies below a value of 13 min are classified as pathological. This type of limit value definition is based on statistical conventions and not on standardization studies with hypersomnia patients.

Indications for the MWT According to the Atlas Task Force of the AASM

- The MWT is an objective and valid examination procedure for assessment of the ability to stay awake for a certain period of time.
- The MWT is performed in combination with clinical history taking to assess the ability to stay awake.
- The 40-min protocol of the MWT is required for objective assessment of the individual ability to stay awake.

To ensure a valid assessment of the sleepiness/wakefulness, the MWT must be performed under suitable conditions (derivation techniques, acknowledged protocols, experienced and qualified staff).

The MWT is not suitable to assess sleepiness if it is the only method applied. Moreover, it is recommended to apply other test procedures and to consider the clinical symptoms of the patient.

Practical Tip

The MWT is an important element in the diagnostics of central nervous system activation. In contrast to the MSLT, it provides higher face validity because sleep medicine is more frequently interested in the patients' ability to stay awake than their ability to fall asleep. Similar to MSLT, MWT is a staff- and time-consuming procedure.

Cut-offs based on normative data are not available. Statements made in individual cases seem to be problematic, as also for MSLT, and require at least confirmation by other test procedures on daytime sleepiness.

Pupillographic Sleepiness Test

If a healthy awake person looks into the dark, his/her pupils widen immediately. In the wake stage, the pupil width remains stable for a long time under exclusion of light.

In cases of severe daytime sleepiness, however, relevant variations of the pupil width occur after just a few minutes. This wavelike phenomenon was defined as "fatigue waves" by Löwenstein, who was the first to describe this phenomenon. The low-frequency pupil oscillations increase with the extent of sleepiness; their amplitude increases to several millimeters.

The pupillographic sleepiness test (PST) is based on the measurement of the spontaneous pupil motor activity. A stable pupil width indicates a high alertness level; however, instability of the pupil width signals sleepiness.

During examination, the patient sits on a comfortable chair at the measurement table; the head is placed on a combined chin-forehead support. The eyes are protected against light by means of soft, light-insulated goggles (infrared). The typical sleepiness-related pattern of the pupil is assessed by means of an infrared-sensitive video camera and subsequent PC-assisted evaluation.

Target variables are the pupillary unrest index (PUI) in millimeters (mm)/minute as well as the amplitude spectrum of 0.8 Hz or less as measure for the oscillations of the pupil width; these describe pupillary variations of different amplitudes of less than 0.8 Hz as measure for the reduction of the central nervous system activation.

In a normal cohort of 349 subjects between 20 and 60 years of age, a mean value for the common logarithm (ln) of the PUI was 1.50 ± 0.39 mm/min (for standard values, see ◘ Table 2.12). Thus, values as of ln PUI >1.89 are conspicuous and as of ln PUI >2.28 they are pathological. This critical definition of the limit values corresponds to statistical conventions and results less from content-related reflections.

Compared to the classic procedures of sleep medicine such as the MSLT and the MWT, the PST is clearly more economical. Taking into account the short time of developing this procedure, an extensive verification of test-theoretical quality criteria is already available.

Table 2.12 Percentiles of the norm value range for ln PUI and PUI

Value range	MV−2SD	MV−SD	MV	MV+SD	MV+2SD
ln PUI/[mm/min]	0.73	1.11	1.50	1.89	2.28
Percentiles [%]	2.3	15.9	50	84.1	97.7
PUI [mm/min]	2.07	3.05	4.50	6.64	9.80

ln common logarithm

2.8.1.2 Diagnostic Procedures to Assess Vigilance

In neuropsychology, vigilance is defined as the ability to rapidly and adequately react to rare and incidentally emerging stimuli in long-lasting and monotonous situations.

Generally, it must be mentioned that some examination procedures that are available on the market have such a high stimulus density that they test less the vigilance but rather represent a task for sustained attention. The duration of the tasks has to be strictly observed. Methods with a duration of the tasks of less than 30 min frequently cannot differentiate between healthy individuals and sleep patients, probably because of motivational influences, or they mask vigilance impairments in patients.

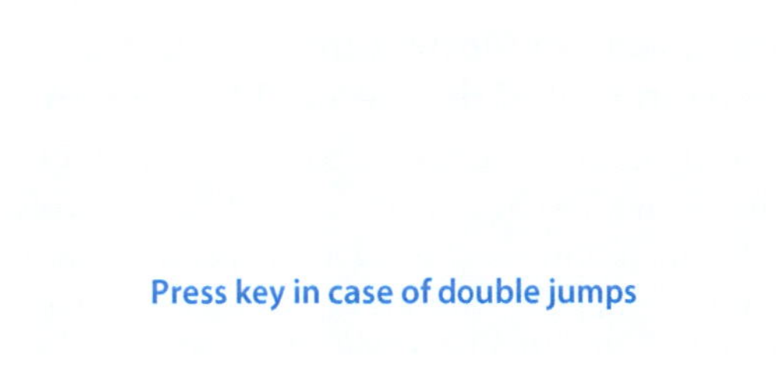

Fig. 2.26 Tasks of the vigilance test according to Quatember and Maly. Bildrechte: Stuck [Urheberrecht beim Autor]. Datei: Abb. 2.24

Vigilance Test According to Quatember and Maly

The computer-based test procedure regarding vigilance from the Vienna Test System (Fig. 2.26) is based on the clock test that had been developed in 1950 by Mackworth for measuring the vigilance of American soldiers. Based on this procedure, soldiers could be identified who showed good discovering abilities in the context of radar surveillance.

The patient is invited to follow a jumping light spot along the circumference of the circle shown on the computer screen. Each time the light spot makes jumps of double length, the patient has to rapidly press a button. Three different test versions vary with regard to the installation, the duration, the number of critical stimuli, the intervals, the number of times, and the steps and jumps.

If the vigilance is suspected to be impaired, as in cases of sleep-related breathing disorders, the test duration should be 60–90 min, at least 30 min. Test durations of less than 30 min often lead to a strong weighting of motivational effects and in this way to masking of vigilance impairments.

Standardization of the vigilance test is available; however, it is only limited in the version with a test duration of 66 minutes. One version of the vigilance test, according to Quatember and Maly, was standardized by the Siesta Group of Vienna in cooperation with the working group on vigilance of the DGSM based on the data of 200 healthy sleepers. The selected stimulus density, however, rather corresponds to a task of sustained attention.

Sub-test of Vigilance of the Test Battery for Attentional Performance

To work on a vigilance test, the patient sits in front of a computer screen. Four tasks with different stimuli (optic, acoustic, optic/acoustic) are available. All procedures can be performed with high or low stimulus density. The duration of the examination that has to be particularly taken into account when assessing the vigilance can be varied up to 60 min. A sufficient standardization with good description of the norm sample is available.

Other procedures are available to assess the vigilance.

2.8.1.3 Diagnostic Procedures to Assess Selective Attention

Selective attention includes the ability of a subject to selectively differentiate relevant stimuli from the sum of all inflowing stimuli. The stimuli may come from different modalities. In the following, two of the most frequently applied computer-based procedures are described that are used in sleep medicine. They are also used in occupational medicine and for determination of the fitness to drive.

Achievement Motivation Test Series, Version 3.00 of the Vienna Test System

During the achievement motivation test series of the Vienna Test System, the subjects have to solve different arithmetical problems depending on the level of difficulty. According to the test version, they have 10–20 min at their disposal. The test is considered as being independent from the intelligence. Sufficient standardization is ensured.

Go/NoGo of the Test Battery for Attentional Performance

The selective attention can be verified by means of the sub-test Go/NoGo of the test battery for attentional performance (TAP). Two performance variants are available, and the second variant measures especially the selective attention. On a screen, five squares with different filling patterns are shown. The patient has to react when one of the five squares corresponds to the two given squares with the critical stimuli. Sufficient standardization is ensured.

2.8.1.4 Diagnostic Procedures to Assess Divided Attention

Situations requiring divided attention are usually the rule than the exception. The divided attention may be tested by means of so-called dual tasks where the subjects have to consider two simultaneous stimuli, sometimes of different modality. In the following, the examples of two computer-based procedures are described that are frequently applied in sleep medicine as well as in occupational medicine and for assessment of the fitness to drive a car.

Test of Divided Attention of the Test Battery for Attentional Performance

The subject sits in front of a computer screen and has to react whenever a series of crosses that are rapidly changing their positions form a square. At the same time, the verification of a monotonous sound sequence is performed as acoustic task. Four different stimulus sequences may be chosen to avoid learning effects during test repetitions. Sufficient standardization is ensured.

Vienna Determination Unit

The computer-based Vienna determination unit (Vienna Test System) provides a procedure to measure sensor-motor functions in the selective reaction behavior. Optic stimuli with lamps of five different colors have to be reacted on by pressing allocated keys. Two additional white lamps require a reaction with the left and right foot pedal. Two acoustic stimuli, high and low sound, require pressing of respectively assigned keys. Up to four stimuli may be offered at the same time. Sufficient standardization is ensured.

2.8.1.5 Subjective Diagnostic Questionnaires for Assessment of Sleepiness-Related Impairments

Self-assessment questionnaires are applied for qualitative and quantitative assessment of the patient's subjective level of suffering regarding sleepiness-related disorders.

Scientific investigations often reveal only few correlations between subjective and objective measurements, which is especially true for the MSLT and the MWT but also for neuropsychological examination procedures. The background might be that subjective procedures are applied unsystematically in cases of sleepiness as well as fatigue. Furthermore, objective procedures generally assess aspects of sleepiness, whereas subjective procedures rather aim at the subjectively stressing phenomenon of sleepiness in its entirety. In general, the results of subjective questionnaire data depend on the patient's ability of introspection.

Basically, subjective statements and complaints should not be neglected even if objective findings are inconspicuous, also because some objective procedures applied in sleep medicine do not meet test-theoretical quality criteria. In the context of expert opinions, the possible falsification of the results of questionnaire data (simulation or dissimulation) must be taken into account.

In the following, questionnaire procedures for assessing the subjective sleepiness and one questionnaire for differential diagnostic assessment of sleepiness and fatigue are described. Both procedures are internationally applied in sleep medicine.

Stanford Sleepiness Scale (SSS)

The Stanford Sleepiness Scale (SSS) is applied in clinical routine and in particular in the context of scientific investigations in intra- and intergroup comparison.

In regular intervals, and also before each trial of the MSLT, patients estimate their degree of wakefulness based on a seven-step scale. To assess the circadian course of the subjective sleepiness, the evaluation of 1 h in 15-min intervals within a 3-h bloc over the day is recommended.

Investigations on the sensitivity reveal that already evaluations in 15-min intervals reflect discrete changes of the degree of wakefulness. From the scores of each time interval, a sum score is calculated.

Validity checks in the proper sense of the word are not known. The test correlates only weakly with the sleep-onset latency of the MSLT. Because of the doubtful validity of the MSLT, such low correlations must not be overstated.

Practical Tip

The SSS is a good, widely distributed questionnaire to assess the individual circadian rhythm of subjective daytime sleepiness. Because standardization is currently not performed, interindividual evaluation of the results is limited.

Regarding intraindividual comparison, such as in the context of therapy evaluations, it might be a suitable procedure.

Epworth Sleepiness Scale (ESS)

The Epworth Sleepiness Scale (ESS) is a simple procedure to quantify the tendency to fall asleep in everyday situations.

Because of behavior-related questions (items), a sufficient interindividual comparability may be assumed. The patients are interviewed with regard to the probability to fall asleep in eight typical everyday situations. The single results are summed up to a total score between 0 and 24. Based on some clinical trials, a score of more than 10 is considered as pathological.

However, the results have to be interpreted reluctantly when the patients never experience certain everyday situations that are mentioned, for example, theater visits, or passenger or driver in a car, because then the low values of the ESS mask the actual severity of the disorder. Validity checks and standardization studies are currently not available.

Practical Tip

ESS is the most frequently applied and best acknowledged procedure to assess the subjective sleepiness and tendency to fall asleep in monotonous everyday situation. It is operationalized by data on the probability to fall asleep in certain everyday situations. Sum scores greater than 10 are considered as pathological.

Practical Tip

The risk assessment of pathological daytime sleepiness includes these aspects:

- Intensive history taking regarding sleepiness with particular attention to risk factors in the past, supported by a procedure on self-assessment of daytime sleepiness, for example, ESS (▶ Sect. 11.2)
- If the patient's history and/or the questionnaire reveal an increased risk at work or in road traffic, the application of an objective procedure for examination of the central nervous system activation, such as MWT or PST, and a procedure to verify the vigilance with a test duration of at least 30 min are required.

If needed, information of the patient about potential endangerment of self and others in traffic or at work should follow. For the legal security of the treating physician, this information has to be documented in the files.

2

It must be taken into account that both procedures on central nervous system alertness and vigilance should be applied at two different times of a day, if possible (in the morning, peak performance; in the afternoon, performance slump).

2.9 Questions

? 1. Please list the rules for classification of respiratory events in sleep.

? 2. Which indications for performing an outpatient apnea screening do you know?

? 3. Which indications for polysomnography are given for RLS?

? 4. Which aspects of daytime sleepiness are differentiated?

? 5. Which types of history taking for sleep disorders are differentiated?

Further Reading

1. American Academy of Sleep Medicine. International classification of sleep disorders, vol 3. Aufl: diagnostic and coding manual. Westchester: American Academy of Sleep Medicine, 2014.
2. American Academy of Sleep Medicine. The AASM-manual for the scoring of sleep and associated events: rules, terminology and technical specifications. Version 2.3. Darien: American Academy of Sleep Medicine; 2020.
3. Carskadon MA, Dement WC. Sleep tendency: an objective measure of sleep loss. Sleep Res. 1977;6:200.
4. Falkenstetter T, Frauscher B, Anderer P, Bolitschek J, et al. Erhöhte Tagesschläfrigkeit in Österreich. Somnologie. 2010;14(1):15.
5. Hennig A, Gesche H, Fietze I, et al. Messung von apnoebezogenen Blutdruckänderungen mittels Pulstransitzeit und Penaz-Prinzip. Atemwegs Lungenkrankheiten. 2012;38:1–8.
6. Kapur VK, Auckley DH, Chowdhuri S, Kuhlmann DC, et al. Clinical practice guideline for diagnostic testing for adult obstructive sleep apnea: an American Academy of Sleep Medicine clinical practice guideline. JCSM. 2017;13(3):479–504.
7. Kryger M, Roth T, Dement WC. Principles and practice of sleep medicine. Philadelphia: Elsevier; 2017.
8. Küchler G. Non-invasive blood pressure determination method and apparatus. 2006, 2008, 2010, 2012. Patent Numbers US 11/364 174, US 2006/0217616 A1, 7374542, DE 102005014048.3-35, EP 20060001181.4-1526.
9. Kushida CA, Littner MR, Morgenthaler TM, et al. Practice parameters for the indications for polysomnography and related procedures: an update for 2005. Sleep. 2005;28:499–519.
10. Kushida CA, Nichols DA, Holmes DA, et al. SMART DOCS: a new patient-centered outcomes and coordinated-care management approach for the future practice of sleep medicine. Sleep. 2015;38(2):315–26.
11. Park CY, Hong JH, Lee JH, Lee KE, Cho HS, Lim SL, Kwak JW, Kim KS, Kim HJ. Clinical usefulness of watch-PAT for assessing the surgical results of obstructive sleep apnea syndrome. J Clin Sleep Med. 2014;10(1):43–7.
12. Portable Monitoring Task Force of the American Academy of Sleep Medicine: Collop NA, McDowell Anderson A, Boehlecke B, et al. Clinical guidelines for the use of unattended portable monitors in the diagnosis of obstructive sleep apnea in adult patients. J Clin Sleep Med (JCSM). 2007;3(7):737–74.
13. Rechtschaffen A, Kales A. A manual of standardized terminology, techniques and scoring system for sleep stages in human subjects. Washington, DC: National Institutes of Health, Publication; 1968.
14. Redline S, Kirchner HL, Quan SF, et al. The effect of age, sex, ethnicity and sleep disordered breathing on sleep architecture. Arch Intern Med. 2004;164:406–18.
15. Weeß H-G, editor. Update Schlafmedizin. Bremen: UniMed Verlag; 2015.
16. Weeß H-G, Sauter C, Geisler P, et al. Vigilanz, Einschlafneigung, Daueraufmerksamkeit, Müdigkeit, Schläfrigkeit – Diagnostische Instrumentarien zur Messung müdigkeits- und schläfrigkeitsbezogener Prozesse und deren Gütekriterien. Somnologie. 2000;4:20–38.

Insomnia

H.-G. Weeß

B. A. Stuck et al., *Practice of Sleep Medicine*, https://doi.org/10.1007/978-3-030-17412-5_3

Insomnia is the most frequent sleep disorder and is characterized by a discrepancy between the need and the ability to sleep. Increased sleep latencies are typically observed, as well as frequent awakenings after sleep onset and waking up very early in the morning. It is essential for diagnosting insomnia that the sleep problems cause complaints to occur during the daytime, for example, impairments in performance and motivation and mood disturbances. Chronic insomnia is associated with increased absenteeism from work, reduced productivity, and an increased risk of accidents. Furthermore, health risk is increased, i.e., the likelihood of developing cardiovascular diseases, metabolic diseases, and mental disorders like depression is increased in chronic insomnia, and thus life expectancy might be reduced.

Insomnia is one of the most prevalent sleep disorders. In epidemiological studies, more than 30% of the population reported insomnia complaints. Ohayon [14] summarized the epidemiological data regarding insomnia disorders and concluded that about 10% of the adult population in industrialized countries suffers from chronic insomnia and about 3% require treatment. For Germany, the Robert Koch Institute [18] showed that in the age group of 18 to 79 years, 69.7% of individuals had insomnia symptoms at least once during the previous year. In 30.3% of the participants, the symptoms occurred at least three times per week. Adding the complaint of poor sleep quality, the percentage of affected individuals was reduced to 21.9%. Further clinically relevant impairments during daytime such as sleepiness or fatique were observed in 5.7% of the individuals who thus would fulfill the diagnostic criteria of insomnia.

Insomnia is very likely to chronify. A study performed by Morin et al. [13] showed that about 70% of all patients with insomnia had persisting complaints over at least 1 year. Forty-six percent of all patients enrolled in this trial reported complaints that occurred since more than 3 years.

Depending on the study, the gender ratio ranges from 2:1 to 4:1, with females reporting insomnia more often than males. Older people complain more frequently about insomnia than younger people. In individuals older than 60 years, incidences of insomnia up to 50% and more have been observed. It is notable that older people are more likely to be treated with classic hypnotics like benzodiazepines or benzodiazepin receptor agonists over very long time periods. Even other psychotropic drugs such as sedating antidepressants are more frequently applied in the treatment of insomnia in this age group.

Chronic insomnias represent a risk factor for somatic and mental disorders. For cardiovascular diseases, it was shown that insomnia as an independent risk factor increases the risk of heart attack, heart failure, and hypertension in the long run. Meta-analyses suggest that short sleep is associated with weight gain and may thus be a risk factor for metabolic syndrome. Insomnia is also a risk factor for diabetes. In addition, neurological disorders are often accompanied by insomnia. An increased risk for developing neurodegenerative diseases such as dementia and Parkinson's disease in insomnia has been reported. A cross-sectional study showed a correlation between poor sleep quality and cortical atrophy in older individuals.

Clear-cut findings reporting an association between insomnia and mental disorders have been published. In a meta-analysis, Baglioni et al. [4] included more than 20 primary studies and could show that patients with insomnia had a higher risk of developing depressive episodes compared to healthy individuals at a later time point (odds ratio: 2.1). Epidemiological surveys further confirm that insomnia is a risk factor for the development of anxiety disorders and substance addiction. In addition, correlations could also be shown for insomnia complaints are independent predictors of suicidality, suicide attempts, or committed suicides.

Finally, insomnia disorders cause high expenses for the healthcare system; on the one hand, there are direct costs, such as sleep medication and/or psychotherapy, but on the other hand indirect expenses also must be considered, such as those caused by absences from work, accidents in the workplace or traffic accidents, and reduced productivity at work or early retirement. It is estimated that costs related to insomnia disorders, especially the chronic type, add up to 1.7% of the gross national income. However, more data have to be collected to verify this assessment.

In clinical practice, the treatment of insomnia is mainly based on drugs even if the effectiveness of the compounds is not or not sufficiently well documented and often does not address the causes underlying the insomnia disorder. Drug-related therapies usually are symptom-oriented. A decrease in prescription hypnotics has been observed, but the overall sales of the pharmaceutical industry regarding hypnotic drugs was increased, implying that hypnotics are being increasingly prescribed on a private basis and an increase in over-the-counter sleep aids. The percentage of sedating antidepressants has increased because of the widespread knowledge about tolerance and addiction to benzodiazepines (BZD) and, with lower probability, of the benzodiazepine receptor agonists (BRZA) (▶ Sect. 3.7.3). New-generation hypnotics are currently being developed or tested in clinical trials and one of them, suvorexant, is approved in the US.

Meta-analyses indicate the long-term effectiveness of psychoeducation combined with cognitive behavioral therapeutic methods in insomnia. In particular, cognitive behavioral therapy for insomnia (CBT-I) is considered the method of choice for the treatment of insomnia. Thus, the guidelines of the European Sleep Research Society, the Germany Sleep Research Society, and the American Academy of Family Physicians require application of behavior therapeutic techniques as first-line therapy before prescribing hypnotics. In addition, CBT-I is also effective in patients with a variety of diseases (somatic or mental disorders) and comorbid insomnia. Often CTB-I not only can improve the sleep complaints but also lessen the symptoms of the somatic disorder, e.g., in chronic pain syndromes, or depression. Many studies confirm that the effectiveness of cognitive behavioral therapy is comparable to that of hypnotics and that it is superior regarding its long-term effects (see ▶ Sect. 3.7.3).

Specifically, a multimodal procedure integrating pharmacological, behavioral-medical, and cognitive-behavioral therapy elements into the treatment program seems to be superior to monotherapeutic efforts that are often limited to the application of hypnotics.

The enormous time- and staff-consuming efforts of applying CBT-I have led to the development of a stepped-care approach in order to treat the large number of patients suffering from insomnia. In a first step, self-help manuals or Internet-based programs are recommended. If this method does not show the expected results, psychoeducative measures (sleep hygiene) are taught by healthcare professionals (e.g., trained nurses or family physicians). Only if these methods are not successful and the insomnia tends to chronify, should psychotherapists and in a last step psychotherapists certified in sleep medicine carry out a state-of-the-art CBT-I in a small group setting or as individual therapy.

3.1 Classification of Insomnia Disorders

In 2014, the third edition of the *International Classification of Sleep Disorders* (ICSD-3) was published, which led to a fundamental change in the assessment of insomnia disorders. Hence, the diagnostic criteria of insomnia were completely revised regarding their formal aspects as well as their content compared to the ICSD-2.

One of the most important innovations is the introduction of the concept of "insomnia disorders," which includes all causes and symptoms of insomnia. The differentiation between primary and secondary insomnia comorbid to somatic and mental disorders and also as a consequence of substance or drug abuse is no longer applied. In the ICSD-3, insomnia disorders might be the trigger or the consequence of comorbid disorders, i.e., the causal relationship cannot always be clarified. This conceptually new assessment of insomnia takes into account that insomnia disorders often have a multifactorial etiology and manifold symptoms, which does not allow a simple causal classification. In the ICSD-3, additional disorders can be coded as comorbidities of insomnia. The implementation of this approach in the DSM-5 has already taken place. Currently, the DSM-5 describes insomnia disorders as independent disorders, comparable to the ICSD-3: it is coded independently of the fact of whether a patient also has a mental disorder or somatic disease. The classification into primary and secondary sleep disorders was also discarded.

3

In the ICSD-3, complaints during daytime like impairment of social and/or academic performance and the mood disturbances are still required for diagnosis of "insomnia," comparable to the ICSD-2 or the DSM-5. However, nonspecific daytime complaints, for example, tension headaches, are no longer among the diagnostic criteria. As daytime impairment is important, merely age-related physiological changes in sleep do not implicate an insomnia diagnosis. Older people show, without necessarily having a pathology, higher sleep fragmentation, longer sleep-onset latencies, and an increased number of nocturnal awakenings. By definition, all diagnostic manuals only assess those age-related changes of sleep as relevant if they are accompanied by impairment of daytime performance.

In the ICSD-2, a total of 11 types of insomnia were distinguished. The ICSD-3 classifies only 2 types: *chronic insomnia disorders* and *short-term insomnia disorders*. The main categories that had been differentiated in the ICSD-2 are now mentioned as subtypes of chronic insomnia disorders. Furthermore, the ICSD-3 describes *other insomnia disorders* and *excessive time in bed* as well as *short sleep* duration as isolated symptoms and normal variants.

The complaint about nonrestorative sleep was excluded as a diagnostic criterion for *short sleeper time* as well as *chronic insomnia* as this symptom is not specific to insomnia. Because the symptom of nonrestorative sleep occurs in many sleep disorders, for example, sleep-related breathing disorders or periodic movement disorders during sleep, its removal from the ICSD-3 insomnia criteria was overdue, and thus it has also been excluded in the DSM-5.

The key symptoms of short-term sleep and chronic insomnia are a difficulty initiating and maintaining sleep or waking up very early in the morning. For diagnosis, daytime impairment due to sleep problems is indispensable.

Diagnostic Criteria of the American Academy of Sleep Medicine (AASM) for Insomnia in Adults

- Complaints about difficulties initiating sleep, maintaining sleep, and/or waking up earlier as desired.
- At least one of the symptoms occur in relation to insomnia complaints.
  - Fatigue or general discomfort
  - Attention, concentration, and memory impairment
  - Impaired social, family, occupational, or academic performance
  - Mood disturbances or irritability
  - Daytime sleepiness
  - Behavioral problems (hyperactivity, aggression, impulsivity)
  - Increased proneness for errors or accidents
  - Reduced motivation, energy, initiative
  - Dissatisfaction or worries with regard to the sleep disorder
  - In the context of chronic insomnia, the sleep complaints and at least one of the above-mentioned associated daytime symptoms occur at least three times per week over a period of more than 3 months. In cases of *short-term insomnia*, no time criterion exists
  - The impairments are not explained by chronic sleep deprivation or inadequate sleep conditions

According to the ICSD-3, a frequency of complaints of at least three times per week over a period of at least 3 months is required for chronic insomnia. This time criterion takes into account the clinical experience that insomnia disorders are characterized by a high probability to chronify but that, on the other hand, they can also be a reaction to acute stressors and subside very quickly. The diagnosis of *chronic insomnia disorder* is also possible if brief periods of insomnia complaints occur intermittently over several years even though these single phases do not meet the 3-month criterion. In this way, insomnia disorders that may appear intermittently over several years with short-term remissions in the interval can also be diagnosed and treated. For adults, a subjective sleep latency of more than 30 min is considered clinically relevant. Subjective awake time after sleep-onset and waking up very early in the morning before the selected time of arising should exceed 60 min. Insomnia disorders that do not meet the criterion of a duration of 3 months are classified as *short-term insomnia*.

Thus, it is not required that the nighttime and daytime complaints occur at least three times per week.

The previous diagnostic categories of so-called primary insomnia (psychophysiological insomnia, idiopathic insomnia, sleep-state misperception, and inadequate sleep hygiene) are included as subtypes of chronic insomnia in adults. Secondary insomnia comorbid to mental disorders, medical conditions, or drug or substance consumption are also included in the diagnosis of *chronic insomnia* because the differentiation between primary and secondary is no longer made. Nonetheless, they are still taken into consideration as subtypes of chronic insomnia as this allows the correct diagnosis and indication for sleep-specific therapeutic interventions. The adjustment insomnia is included in short-term insomnia.

The classification of insomnia disorders into different main categories previously found in the ICSD-2 was based on theoretical considerations and did not reflect the clinical practice as most insomnia types showed a clear overlapping of symptoms. Moreover, many of the criteria of the previous main types (ICSD-2) were very unspecific and could not be associated with one main category of insomnia. However, the new classification of chronic insomnia will yield a heterogenic group of patients with manifold and different origins of their sleep complaints. Especially in the context of empirical research, scientists will face great difficulties regarding defining specific patient groups. Hence, specification and classification into subtypes, if applicable, are always recommended.

Subtypes of Chronic Insomnia in Adults, Adapted from ICSD-3

- Psychophysiological insomnia
- Idiopathic insomnia
- Paradoxical insomnia
- Insomnia caused by inadequate sleep hygiene
- Insomnia caused by a mental disorder
- Insomnia caused by a medical condition
- Insomnia caused by drugs and substance use

Short-term insomnia is distinct from chronic insomnia with regard to the aspect that the complaints occur less often than three times per week and/or less than 3 months. Short-term insomnia is often triggered by a specific stressor and generally lasts only for a brief period or intermittently when the patient is exposed to this stressor. The insomnia vanishes if the stressor is no longer present or the individual copes with the stressor. The stressor may be psychological, psychosocial, physical, somatic, or environment based e.g., work-related stress, family conflicts, moving to another place, hospitalizations, untreated dysfunction of the thyroid, and other medical diagnoses. Also, positive events, for example, being in love or winning the lottery may temporarily disturb sleep. However, those events are rarely perceived as disstressing.

The group of *other insomnia disorders* as a further diagnostic category is reserved to those disorders that cannot be classified as short-term insomnia or chronic insomnia. In the course of the diagnostic process, this term is used as a "working hypothesis" until it is possible to make a clear decision in one direction or another.

In the new category of isolated symptoms and normal variants, *excessive time in bed* and *short sleeper* are listed. Both phenomena have in common that they are not associated with daytime impairments and that they do not meet the criteria of being a disorder. In the ICSD-3, both phenomena are defined more precisely.

Excessive time in bed is understood as an isolated symptom that is characterized by prolonged time of sleep onset or long periods of wakefulness during the night. However, neither daytime impairment nor insomnia complaints are reported. A lack of social zeitgebers, e.g., in unemployed people or retired persons, may contribute to longer times in bed. In children, longer times in bed may be observed when parents have unrealistic ideas of their children's sleep need.

The phenomenon of *short sleeper* is characterized by the fact that sleep duration is less than 6 h without experiencing daytime impairments like tiredness. That is, the short sleep duration is not caused by a reduced ability to sleep but rather attributed to a naturally occurring reduced sleep need. Even if criteria of insomnia regarding sleep continuity may be present, it is recommended not to diagnose insomnia. The concept of short sleepers is in line with the data that individual sleep duration is highly variables, likely due to genetically determined differences in sleep need.

3.2 Chronic Insomnia Disorder

In the following, the clinical symptoms, polysomnographic findings, differential diagnoses, etiology, pathogenesis, risk factors, and sleep diagnostics of *chronic insomnia* in adults are reviewed. In addition, subtypes are discussed (for insomnia in children, see ▶ Chap. 11). The treatment of chronic insomnia is presented in ▶ Sect. 3.7.

3.2.1 Definitions

Insomnia is characterized by reduced ability to initiate or maintain sleep or waking up very early in the morning. Frequently, these characteristics co-occur and intensity of each symptom may vary in the further course of the disorder. In addition, complaints about poor and nonrestorative sleep with low awakening threshold are reported, however, as already mentioned, this is no longer a diagnostic criterion according to the ICSD-3 (only daytime complaints). Patients often report that they sleep deeper in the early morning hours, at the nadir time of the body temperature, and shortly before the alarm clock ends the night. Prolonged sleep episodes until noon can be the consequence, especially in individuals who do not have social zeitgebers. It is characteristic that patients with insomnia tend to underestimate their actual sleep duration, which is explained among other factors by frequency changes in sleep electroencephalogram (EEG) and frequent arousals during sleep.

People typically complain about daytime impairment regarding their psychosocial performance. Complaints and symptoms that are frequently reported are daytime tiredness, attention and memory problems, reduced energy and motivation, mood disturbance, and social withdrawal in the evening. Patients complain about being tired, but in contrast to patients with hypersomnia disorders, they are often not able to sleep during the daytime. Reports about reduced performance at work or when studying are characteristic, as well as complaints about more errors because of fatigue and micro-sleep at work or in road traffic. Additional symptoms are described in the following sections about the subtypes of chronic insomnia.

3.2.1.1 Subtype of Psychophysiological Insomnia

The subtype of psychophysiological insomnia is a frequently observed type of insomnia caused by increased psychophysiological arousal (see ▶ Sect. 3.2.2 on Etiology and Pathogenesis) that is related to sleep-related negative thoughts. The core symptomatology is an increased cognitive, emotional, and physiological arousal in the sleep situation.

Patients frequently report deliberate efforts to fall asleep. The fear regarding the effects of sleep loss and inadequate sleep hygiene (e.g., irregular bedtimes, working at nighttime, or watching TV) are as characteristic as the inability to relax and an increased cognitive activity during sleep onset, e.g., rumination. Often the individual is able to fall asleep in the early morning hours after stopping excessive efforts of initiating sleep. Patients of this group commonly sleep in front of the TV, because in this situation, thoughts are not focused on sleep.

3.2.1.2 Subtype of Paradoxical Insomnia

Paradoxical insomnia as a subtype of chronic insomnia is mainly characterized by complaints about the reduced ability to sleep without objective markers for this complaint. The modern view is that these patients have problems perceiving their current state as sleep. There is a high discrepancy between the perception of sleep by an individual and objective findings regarding the quantity of sleep. Some studies allow the assumption that there is a correlation between an increased level of psychophysiological arousal, changes of the power spectrum of the sleep EEG, and the misperception of sleep (see ▶ Sect. 3.2.2).

3.2.1.3 Subtype of Idiopathic Insomnia

Idiopathic insomnia describes a type of chronic insomnia that begins in childhood without apparent triggers. Idiopathic insomnia cannot be explained by any other sleep disorder, somatic or mental disorder, drug effects, or any other substance consumption. Generally, no triggering factor can be identified for the sleep disorder; at the same time, longer symptome-free phases are not reported.

3.2.1.4 Subtype of Insomnia Caused by a Mental Disorder

As a subtype of chronic insomnia, insomnia comorbid to a mental disorder is a sleep disturbance that is conceptualized as a symptom of the mental disorder. Insomnia symptoms are commonly the major complaint and may require separate and/or specific therapy. Sometimes, patients report the sleep disorder as the main cause of their psychopathological symptoms. In these cases the underlying mental disorder only becomes evident after focused and intense psychiatric exploration. The pathophysiology of the sleep disorder is part of the etiology of the underlying mental disorder and the resulting increased psychophysiological arousal due to the mental disorder, e.g., in mood disorders. Especially anxiety disorders with the fear of not being able to fall asleep as a single symptom are easy to differentiate from chronic insomnia that also include sleep-related worries.

3.2.1.5 Subtype of Insomnia Resulting from Inadequate Sleep Hygiene

In the context of the subtype of insomnia caused by inadequate sleep hygiene, the origins of chronic insomnia are assumed to be based on sleep-incompatible behavior.

Those behavioral patterns may be classified into two categories: those that trigger an increased cognitive, emotional, or somatic arousal before going to bed and those that are not compatible with the sleep–wake rhythm. The latter might show up in irregular sleep times, excessively long phases in bed, using the bed for activities other than sleep (e.g., TV, smartphone use), naps during daytime, stimulating activities before going to bed, nighttime activities such as watching TV, and getting up and doing some work as well as consumption of stimulating or sleep-disturbing substances (caffeine, nicotine, alcohol). The origin of such behavior is assumed to be mainly the incorrect assessment of the consequences of irregular periods of staying awake at different times over the course of a 24-h period. Stress, ambition, and work overload may cause behavioral patterns that lead to insomnia complaints or sleep–wake rhythm disorders. These behaviors that might be incompatible with sleep, however, do not automatically lead to sleep disorders in every individual.

In view of recent developments, the use of new media such as smartphones and tablet PCs used while in bed might be a sleep-disturbing factor. Further studies could demonstrate that increased use of these devices during time in bed reduces sleep and causes sleep disorders and daytime sleepiness as a consequence. This behavior is frequent in adolescents. In some studies, poorer performance at school was a consequence of excessive media use. Two factors are likely responsible for the negative effect of these devices on sleep. First, the color spectrum of the LED screens containing blue light suppresses melatonin production. However, findings indicate that sleep onset is only marginally prolonged despite reduced melatonin concentration. Second, the type of activity, such as surfing the Internet, chatting with friends, reading e-mails, etc., increases the cognitive-emotional arousal level, and might interfere with falling asleep.

According to epidemiological studies, about 1–2% of adolescents and young adults show sleep-incompatible behaviors; probably a similar percentage of older adults is affected. In sleep centers, up to 10% of the patients report inadequate sleep hygiene that might be the origin of their insomnia. As a broad variety of sleep-impairing behaviors is often seen in insomnia patients, the actual prevalence of inadequate sleep hygiene in this group might be higher.

3.2.1.6 Subtype of Insomnia due to Psychiatric Disease, Medical Condition, or Drug and Substance Consumption

In this context, insomnia is the characteristic symptom of a psychiatric, neurological, or internal disease, or it is sometimes even caused by chronic drug intake. Also, insomnia disorders based on withdrawal effects are grouped into this diagnostic category. The distinction is made regarding excessive use and addiction to drugs or other substances.

3

3.2.2 Etiology and Pathogenesis

Chronic insomnia is caused by a multifactorial complex of triggering and maintaining factors. Often the interrelations and the cause–effect relationship of single factors cannot be clearly determined. Psychological and psychodynamic factors also play a role for the subtypes of *psychophysiological*, *idiopathic*, and *paradoxical insomnia*. Situational factors are described for the subtype of insomnia due to inadequate sleep hygiene. Furthermore, mental disorders, medical conditions, and (side) effects of drugs and substances may cause and maintain insomnia: these are considered in the description of the subtypes of *insomnia caused by psychiatric disorder*, *insomnia caused by a medical condition*, and *insomnia caused by drug and substance consumption* (see ▶ Sect. 3.2.1.6).

Many studies investigating the pathophysiology of chronic insomnia focus on the increased psychophysiological arousal in connection with sleep but also on the wake-sleep schedules of patients. The increased arousal is on the subjective level experienced as increased cognitive and emotional activity. These patients generally show an increased proneness to rumination. Patients often have difficulties relaxing, physically and mentally. Furthermore, if emotions are processed they are frequently negative. Positive experiences such as lottery winnings or being in love may lead to sleep disorders via activation due to positive emotions. If patients focus on their sleep problems, often associated with anticipatory anxiety regarding the negative effects of sleep deprivation, increase cognitve arousal even more and that may exacerbate and stabilize the sleep complaints.

Regarding pathophysiology, increased activity on the hypothalamus-pituitary-adrenal axis has been found. Studies indicate an increased heart rate, an altered heart rate variability, increased metabolism, increased cortisol release, as well as increased corticotropin-releasing factor (CRF) values in insomnia patients. In addition, increased beta and gamma activities in the sleep EEG can be seen in insomnia patients compared with healthy control groups.

Functional MRI (fMRI) of insomnia patients showed increased regional glucose metabolism in sleep-regulating centers such as the thalamus, upper brainstem, and the anterior cingulate and limbic cortex compared to healthy controls. Furthermore, regionally reduced GABA activity is described in sleep-regulating brain areas.

Personality factors are considered as predisposing aspects for increased rumination about everyday experiences and the lack of ability to relax while lying in bed. Some of those factors are, for example, increased perfectionism, hypochondriac personality, reduced self-esteem, social introversion, and increased neuroticism scores.

Mental disorders, in particular affective disorders such as depression or anxiety disorders, may be accompanied by insomnia complaints. Somatic disorders such as chronic pain and metabolic syndrome, and pulmonary diseases are also accompanied by a higher risk of developing insomnia. Numerous drugs and substances may trigger sleep problems via, for example, activation of central nervous systems.

Situational factors that are summarized under the misleading term of "sleep hygiene" may negatively influence sleep and cause sleep problems. The term "*observing adequate rules for healthy sleep*" would be more appropriate. Environmental factors are noise, light pollution, and inadequate temperatures, but also inappropriate behavior such as irregular wake-sleep schedules, and heavy meals and sports directly prior to sleep onset. Also, alcohol and tobacco consumption in the evening may lead to sleep problems.

3.2.2.1 Developmental Model of Chronic Insomnia

Chronic insomnia develops from *short-term insomnia*. Triggering factors of physical or mental nature and inappropriate behavior may perpetuate the condition, even if these factors can also disappear after some time. For chronification, processes that are characterized by establishing inadequate sleep hygiene and misconceptions about sleep are often the driving force, independent from the triggering factors. On the physical level, habituation to the problematic sleep–wake rhythm occurs. Even if the original reasons for nocturnal awakenings are no longer present at night, this habituation may still cause sleep fragmentation. Furthermore, misconceptions and inappropriate behaviors can stabilize themselves without being consciously reflected by the individual. Increased cognitive and emotional arousal, e.g., an increased likeliness to ruminate about positive as well as negative everyday situations that is accompanied by emotional activation, develops in bed and hampers falling asleep. Thus, the sleep disorder may persist even after the original trigger(s) are long gone. Furthermore, the individual often develops sleep-incompatible behavior in the acute phase of insomnia that chronifies the sleep disorder; for example, household activities or home office work at night, TV watching, or other stimulating activities done during the night.

The distress during the day due to sleep deprivation can result in increased self-observation with focus on one's own sleep disorder and the in ability to sleep. This often results in stronger efforts to fall asleep and, in turn, to the frustrating experience of nocturnal sleeplessness. Both factors increase psychophysiological arousal at night and enhance sleep fragmentation. The vicious circle can be described as: "Who desperately wants to fall asleep, stays awake!"

◘ Figure 3.1 summarizes the outlined model.

3.2.2.2 Risk Factors for the Development of Chronic Insomnia

Women showed a higher risk compared to men for developing insomnia. Also, education level and income (socioeconomic status) had an impact on the incidence of problems of initiating and maintaining sleep. Individuals with a lower level of education and lower income are more prone to develop insomnia. Another risk factor is unemployment. Individuals who live alone, widowed or divorced individuals, or single persons often suffer from difficulties of initiating and maintaining sleep. Even an increased incidence within families was observed. It is not yet determined whether genetic factors, traditional family values, or both these factors may be responsible. Older individuals are more likely to develop insomnia. Age itself seems not to be the basic factor but rather the somatic and psychological changes accompanying aging, including the higher incidence of somatic diseases. Personality is associated with a higher

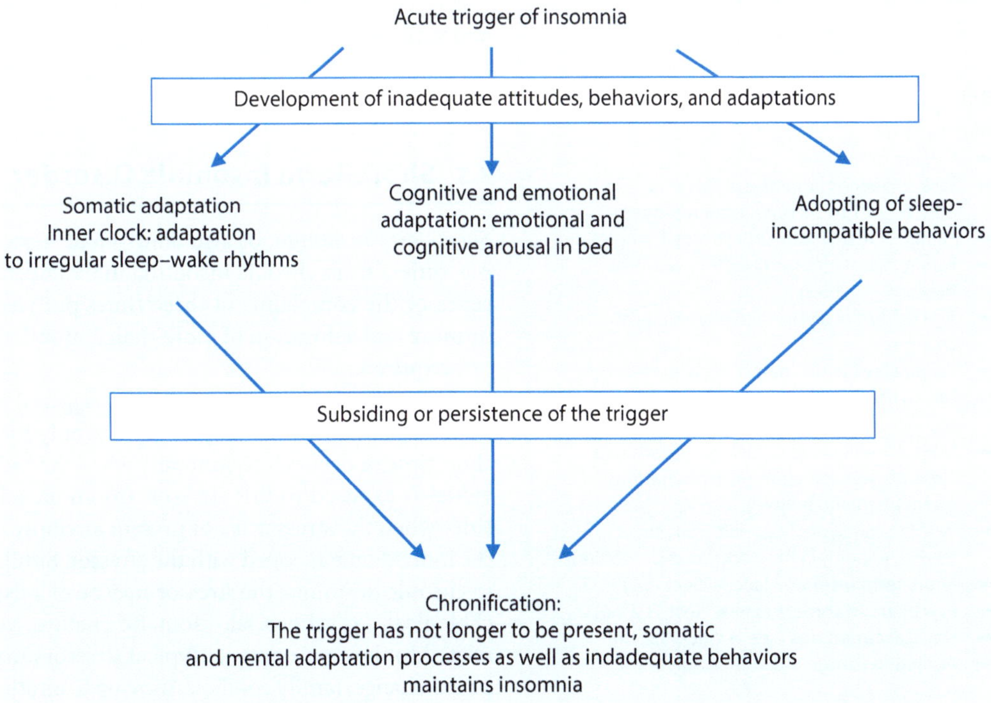

◘ **Fig. 3.1** Model of chronification of insomnia

probability for developing insomnia complaints, in particular neuroticism, perfectionism, hypochondriac personality, reduced self-esteem, social introversion, and internalization. The increased psychophysiological arousal and/or increased stress levels are often responsible for developing insomnia. Major life events such as divorce, the death of a close person, job change, or examinations (academia) can also increase problems of initiating and maintaining sleep. Recent studies also showed a higher prevalence of insomnia disorders in shift workers. Furthermore, employment with high workloads (executive tasks, self-employment) or jobs with low autonomy can foster insomnia. Individuals who frequently suffer from short-term insomnia have a higher risk of developing chronic insomnia. Finally, mental disorders also show a significantly increased risk for insomnia: mood disorders, anxiety disorders, posttraumatic stress disorders, addiction, and drug or substance consumption may cause problems with initiating and maintaining sleep. Medical conditions, for example, endocrine diseases, neurodegenerative diseases, chronic pain symptoms, and other factors, may also be associated with a higher risk of insomnia (see ▶ Box 3.1).

Box 3.1 Risk Factors for the Development of Insomnia

- Female gender
- Low socioeconomic status (level of education, low income, not employed)
- Family status (widowed, divorced, single)
- Family history (genetic factors, learned behaviors, values)
- Age-related cognitive and physiological changes
- Personality factors (neuroticism, perfectionism, hypochondriac personality, reduced self-esteem, introversion, internalization)
- Major life events (e.g., divorce, death of a close person, job change, examinations, marriage, being in love)
- Working conditions (e.g., shift work, stress levels, autonomy in the work process, mobbing)
- Short-term insomnia (see ▶ Sect. 3.3)
- Psychiatric disorders (see ▶ Sect. 3.2.1.6)
- Medical conditions (see ▶ Sect. 3.2.1.6)
- Addiction (drugs, substances, alcohol)

3.2.3 Polysomnographic Findings

Polysomnographic findings often show a sleep-onset latency longer than 30 min. Wake phases after sleep onset of 1 or 2 h duration are often observed. Some patients report a reduced sleep duration of less than 6 h. An increase of the sleep stage N1 and a reduction of slow wave sleep, stage N3, are characteristic. In the sleep lab, some patients show an inverse first-night effect, meaning that they sleep better in the lab compared to sleeping at home despite the unfamiliar environment and the stress caused by electrodes, video, etc. A few patients show a change in the power spectrum of the sleep EEG: the power of the beta and gamma band may be increased. Some studies reported a correlation of these frequency band changes and sleep misperception. In comparison to healthy individuals, insomnia patients tend to overestimate their sleep latency and to underestimate their real overall sleep period.

Despite complaints about sleep loss and tiredness, patients with insomnia often show normal sleep latencies in the MSLT and performances within normal ranges in psychometric tests measuring sleepiness-related aspects such as attention and vigilance.

3.3 Short-Term Insomnia Disorder

Short-term insomnia, or also adjustment insomnia, differs from chronic insomnia in that occurrence of the complaints of three times per week or more and a duration of more than 3 months is not required.

Short-term insomnia is typically triggered by a specific stressor. Generally, it persists only for a short time or occurs intermittently when the individual is exposed to this stressor. Insomnia subsides when the stressor is not present anymore or the individual has coped with the stressor. Similar to chronic insomnia, the stressor may be of a psychological, psychosocial, somatic nature, or related to the environment. Typical stressors may be job change, family conflicts, moving to another city, hospitalizations, and major medical diagnoses. Also, positive experiences, for example, being in love or winning a lottery, can meet the criterion of a stressor and temporarily disturb sleep; however, these sleep disturbances are rarely perceived as disstressing.

The complaints regarding sleep and daytime impairments in *short-term insomnia* are similar to those reported by patients with *chronic insomnia*.

Especially with psychological and somatic predispositions, *short-term insomnia* may become chronic. Thus, special care should be given to these patients preventing chronification with all the associated risk factors of chronic insomnia.

With regard to the diagnostic and therapeutic procedure, the same strategies and interventions should be applied in short-term insomnia as in chronic insomnia.

3.4 Other Insomnia Disorders

The diagnosis of "other insomnia disorder" represents a category for nonspecific insomnias that do not meet the criteria of *chronic* or *short-term insomnia*. This diagnosis is often made in the course of the diagnostic process as preliminary diagnosis or "working diagnosis" until further examinations allow specification of the insomnia disorder into *chronic* or *short-term insomnia*.

3.5 Isolated Symptoms and Normal Variants

In the category of *isolated symptoms and normal variants*, *excessive time in bed* and *short sleeper* are listed. Both phenomena have in common that they are not associated with daytime impairments and are not considered as a disorder. Both phenomena are outlined more precisely in the ICSD-3.

3.5.1 Excessive Time in Bed

Excessive time in bed is understood as an isolated symptom that is characterized by a prolonged sleep latency and/or long times being awake after sleep onset. However, no daytime impairment is observed, nor is subjective suffering reported. Lack of social contacts, e.g., in unemployed or retired individuals, may partly explain these long bed times. Longer times in bed may also be observed in children whose parents have unrealistic ideas of their children's need to sleep, i.e., overestimating the sleep duration.

3.5.2 Short Sleeper

Short sleepers are characterized by sleep durations of less than 6 h without experiencing daytime impairment. Mainly, the short sleep duration is not caused by an inability to sleep but rather due to a reduced need of sleep. Even if the criteria of insomnia (long sleep latency, time awake after sleep onset) are fulfilled, it is recommended not to diagnose insomnia in those cases as they do not report daytime complaints. The concept of short sleepers is congruent with the finding that sleep duration is highly variable between individuals, genetically determined.

3.6 Diagnostics of Insomnia

Insomnia etiology is multifactoral, therefore an interdisciplinary approach is recommended to successfully diagnose and treat the disorder. Knowledge of internal medicine, neurology, psychiatry, otolaryngology, psychology, and psychotherapy is essential for the diagnosis and therapy of insomnia. Treatment and assessment approaches of one speciality only are generally not beneficial for patients.

The diagnostic procedures should include general, drug-related, and substance consumption history and a physical examination together with laboratory parameters (see ▶ Chap. 2).

The general history taking serves as assessment of the general health status, which refers to somatic diseases, psychiatric stress, drug and substance consumption, psychosocial impairments, and other aspects of the patient's wellbeing. Based on this general history, subsequent detailed history taking completes the anamnesis.

In the diagnostic process, triggering and maintaining factors have to be assessed. For example, endocrine, chronic renal, gastrointestinal, cardiopulmonary, and neurological diseases and chronic pain syndromes, may cause or maintain sleep disorders (see ▶ Chap. 10). ▶ Box 3.2 gives an overview of medical conditions that have to be considered in the diagnostic process. Performing brain imaging to exclude organic brain origins may be indicated in insomnia with sudden onset and in chronic courses if persisting somnolence is one of the key symptoms.

Box 3.2 Medical Conditions That May Lead to Chronic Insomnia

- Chronic renal disease
- Gastrointestinal diseases
- Endocrine diseases
- Cardiopulmonary diseases
- Headaches
- Malignant diseases
- Polyneuropathy
- Stroke
- Multiple sclerosis
- Severe itching as symptom of dermatological diseases and allergies

It is important to bear in mind that the typical vicious circle with anticipatory anxieties, and increased cognitive-emotional and psychophysiological arousal can also develop in insomnia disorders due to medical conditions, and thus treatment of the underlying disease does not always alleviate the sleep problems, especially in cases where chronic insomnia is fully developed.

History taking with regard to drug and substance consumption includes not only medication available on prescription but also those obtainable over-the-counter. Furthermore, the consumption of stimulants and related substances is assessed. The objective is to assess all substances that might have potentially negative effects on sleep, and, thus, may have caused or maintained the sleep disorder (▶ Sect. 2.1.4).

The long-term use of BZD and BZRA should be elicited. Alcohol consumption might be a maladaptive self-treatment of sleep problems and may even worsen sleep problems over time. Many addictions might be explained by the attempt to treat evening arousal levels and corresponding sleep problems.

Sleep diagnostics include sleep history, sleep diary, and if needed a sleep questionnaire and actigraphy (▶ Chap. 2). The identification of triggers and maintaining factors is one focus within the diagnostic process. Furthermore, the behavior and well-being in the sleep environment and directly in the pre-sleep situation are also in the center of interest.

Eliciting sleep-incompatible behaviors and inner attitudes via sleep diaries may support diagnostic as well as therapeutic efforts. Furthermore, it can provide important clues regarding the current sleep duration, awake periods after sleep onset, sleep latency, and the feeling of being refreshed in the morning. The sleep diary should be kept during the diagnostic processes for at least 2 weeks, although focusing on the sleep–wake behavior may impair sleep in this patient group. Additional sleep questionnaires, for example, FEPS I and II (▶ Chap. 2), serve for the assessment of psychodynamic aspects of insomnia.

Actigraphy might help objectify the irregular sleep–wake schedules, especially in patients with sleep misperception (▶ Sect. 2.4). Regarding differential diagnosis, actigraphy may also be suitable to assess possible phase delays or advances as well as the identification of the circadian rhythm.

Asking about tiredness and fatigue during daytime helps to assess the psychosocial impairment of performance and classify severity (▶ Sect. 2.1.3). These measures can help to identify risk factors at work or in road traffic due to disturbed sleep. Sometimes the results may justify sick leave certificates or the withdrawal of the driver's licence. In these cases, objective measures of the impairments should be performed by using neuropsychological tests (▶ Sect. 2.7).

A substantial number of patients with chronic insomnia suffers from a co-morbid mental disease. It is not always clear whether the insomnia complaints are a symptom of the mental disorder or if the insomnia complaints are responsible for the mental disorder due to their severity and duration. One must bear in mind that some patients might feel ashamed mentioning emotional problems to their therapists, and it is easier for them to complain about a sleep disorder rather than report depressive complaints. Other possible psychiatric symptoms should be assessed within the diagnostic process, even if the patient focuses only on sleep-related problems. ◘ Table 3.1 summarizes mental disorders that are typically associated with insomnia disorders according to [5].

Table 3.1 Sleep disorders associated with associated with mental disorders

Disease	Disorder in initiating or maintaining sleep	Reduction of slow wave sleep	REM sleep disinhibition	Hypersomnia
Mood disorders	+++	++	+++	+
Anxiety disorders	+	/	/	/
Alcoholism	+	+++	+	/
Borderline personality disorder	+	/	+	/
Dementia	+++	+++	/	+
Eating disorders	+	/	/	/
Schizophrenia	+++	+	+	+

Adapted from [5]
+++ found in nearly all patients, ++ found in about 50% of patients, + found in 10–20% of all patients, / not previously described

Not every patient suffering from disorders of initiating and maintaining sleep requires diagnostic assessment via polysomnography. Generally, extensive history taking and physical examination are sufficient for a valid diagnosis. Many studies and meta-analyses showed that there is a significant discrepancy between objective polysomnographic findings and subjective perception of sleep by patients with insomnia. Sometimes, patients overestimate their times awake dramatically, but a few tend to underestimate the time being awake during the night. These findings indicate that polysomnography in insomnia might not be useful as these parameters rarely correspond with the subjective complaints. On the other hand, polysomnography is indicated in patients with chronic insomnia who did not respond classic outpatient treatment procedures like CBT-I. Another important aspect of performing polysomnography is that some insomnia patients may have sleep apnea syndrome and/or periodic leg movements syndrome even when the diagnosis based on the anamnesis was clearly a primary insomnia.

Thus, diagnostic polysomnography should be performed if insomnia might be caused by medical conditions, in particular if the presence of a sleep apnea syndrome, or periodic leg movements are probable. In therapy-nonresponders, polysomnography may provide additional diagnostic and therapeutic information, especially for risk groups such as professional drivers or patients who work with dangerous machines. Polysomnography may also provide further diagnostic as well as therapeutic information in cases in which there is a significant discrepancy between the subjectively perceived severity of the insomnia and the polysomnographic findings (Table 3.2).

Table 3.2 Main indications for polysomnography in the sleep laboratory in cases of insomnia, based on the AWMF guideline on insomnia, 2017

Indication	Recommendation level
Therapy-resistant insomnia	B
After exhaustion of other diagnostic measures and suspected insomnia caused by a medical condition	A
Insomnia in risk groups in relationship to endangerment of self or others, e.g., professional drivers or patients working with dangerous machines	B
Expected significant discrepancy between subjectively perceived severity of the insomnia and polysomnographic findings	B

3

3.7 Therapy of Insomnia

Insomnia disorders may be explained by psychiatric, somatic, behavioral, and substance-induced origins. In the course of the disorder patients often develop dysfunctional attitudes and behaviors that are not compatible with sleep and exhibit an enhancing effect on the insomnia complaints. Those behavioral patterns are summarized with the term of "inadequate sleep hygiene."

The multifactorial conditions of insomnia requires a multimodal treatment approach. The treatment of triggers and maintaining factors and conditions is the main focus. In insomnia, psychological factors play a major role in the etiology and especially in maintaining insomnia. Thus, cognitive-behavioral and other psychotherapeutic interventions are the key elements in the treatment regime-even if sleep medication is prescribed. In 2016, the American Academy of Family Physicians considered cognitive behavioral therapy of insomnia as first line treatment and not pharmaceutical therapy.

Without extensive diagnostics, a symptomatic approach applying hypnotics is not very promising. Especially the long-term treatment is problematic due to the high risk of addiction and habituation. The following paragraphs review the major elements of insomnia therapy.

Psychoeducation regarding the basics of sleep hygiene helps to reduce sleep-incompatible behaviors and increase sleep-promoting behavior. This is the basic element of each insomnia therapy. However, one must bear in mind that information and counselling about sleep hygiene are often not sufficient as single therapeutic techniques and rarely induce full recovery.

Pharmacological interventions using hypnotics provide a rapid and short-term relief of the complaints. Because of their effects and side effects, they may be indicated for short-term usage and are not seen as causal therapy. In patients with chronic insomnia, who did not benefited from cogntive-behavioral therapy, might be treated with second-line hypnotics like sedating antidepressants that can be useful because of they show a low risk of addiction and habituation in the long term.

In many cases, *psychotherapeutic* and in particular *cogntive-behavioral interventions* are considered as causal therapy addressing the underlying etiology. Successful behavioral therapies do not require long-term application of hypnotics. The aim is the permanent reduction of the psychovegetative arousal in the sleep situation that may be seen as a precondition for good sleep. Recent studies indicated that cognitive behavioral therapy for insomnia (CBT-I) has similar short-term effects compared to hypnotics. In the long term, however, CBT-I is superior to sleep medication. A few studies have addressed the question to what extent the synergistic effects of CBT-I and pharmacotherapy with hypnotics of the BZD or BZRA type can occur. These reports conclude that there might be a small additional effect, but again, in the long term, CBT-I alone is the superior option. Also, studies with psychiatric and somatic patients with comorbid insomnia indicated, that CBT-I not only alleviates the insomnia complaints but also had positive effects regarding the underlying disorder. First nonrandomized trials and field studies further suggest that CBT-I may also be helpful for shift workers suffering from insomnia.

Over the years, different types of CBT-I were developed and applied by groups with different professional backgrounds in individual or group therapy formats. Furthermore, programs have been developed that provide self-help techniques in the form of manuals or internet-based programs. The first findings showed the effectiveness of these interventions even if they might be less effective than face-to-face formats.

3.7.1 Psychoeducation

Insomnia patients often show behavior patterns that are incompatible with sleep and can enhance the sleep problems. These may be unsuccessful self-treatment attempts to decrease psycho-vegetative arousal levels, or may be conceptualized as part of an underlying mental disorder.

3.7.1.1 Information About Sleep

To reduce inadequate expectations regarding sleep and to correct sleep myths, patient receive basic information about healthy sleep, its phenomenology, age-related changes, and its function. Information on sleep-promoting and sleep-incompatible behaviors enables the patient to become an expert in his own right and can reduce feelings of helplessness regarding the sleep disorder. In addition, knowledge about disturbed sleep and treatment options can decrease insomnia-related distress.

3.7.1.2 Inadequate Behaviors Related to Insomnia

To understand the rules and recommendations of sleep hygiene, the following paragraphs describe some characteristic inadequate behaviors of insomnia patients and their negative effect on sleep.

Insomnia patients tend to *spend more time in bed* to compensate for the lost sleep in order to increase the probability of getting at least some sleep. From an educational point of view, a conditioning of being awake and rumination within the bed occurs, which perpetuate the insomnia via an increasing psycho-vegetative arousal.

Irregular bedtimes, especially going to bed very late, and long sleep episodes in the morning hours and during daytime/evening (falling asleep in front of the TV), are quite typical. From a chronobiological point of view, not adhering to the circadian rhythm contributes to the sleep–wake rhythm problems. Sleep phases in the morning and during the day reduce the sleep pressure and have a negative effect on sleep latency the following night.

Everyday objects in the sleep environment may remind one of daytime stressors and trigger cognitive, emotional arousal and rumination.

Nighttime activities, for example, ironing, cleaning cupboards or the oven, home office work, watching TV, and surfing the internet according to the motto "If I cannot sleep, I will do something useful, distracting, and tiring" activate the sympathetic nervous system and are not compatible with psycho-vegetative relaxation as a precondition for sleep. A sleep–wake rhythm including including nighttime activities, similar to that of shift workers, can augment and maintain the sleep disorder.

Sports and other *physical activities* are typically practiced in the evening hours by insomnia patients with the objective of getting tired. Actually, such behavior activates the sympathetic nervous system, even though the cognitive-emotional stress level is not affected. An appropriate time interval between physical activity and bedtime should be observed. Physical activity at night is typically not beneficial for insomnia problems.

Regular and sometimes high-quantity *alcohol consumption* in the evening is frequently reported by insomnia patients, sometimes as an attempt to self-treat the sleep. Patients experience the alcohol-induced psycho-vegetative relaxation and sedation that facilitate sleep. However, the risk of addiction and increasing the quantity of alcohol because of tolerance is likely. Normal quantities of alcohol may suppress slow wave sleep and REM sleep and can trigger nightmares, sweating, headaches, trembling, arousals, and long wake periods in the second half of the night via withdrawal effects and dehydrating properties of alcohol.

Monitoring repeatedly time of night, possibly an expression of an increased need for control, is a phenomenon frequently observed in individuals with insomnia. Thinking about elapsed time from sleep onset and remaining time available for sleep promotes worries regarding sleep, and the efforts to fall asleep enhance insomnia by increasing distress associated with sleep.

Often, insomnia patients show increased motivation and perfectionism in professional as well as private contexts. Job-related activities and social requirements late in the evening, and actually working at night, are quite frequently observed. The use of smartphones and tablets (new media) during bedtime facilitates professional or private activities that might be stress-increasing. The blue light emitted by those devices reduces melatonin secretion and probably has often a minor effect on insomnia. Moreover, relaxation phases before going to bed to activate the parasympathetic system that is necessary for sleep are not integrated.

3

3.7.1.3 Good Sleep Hygiene

Sleep hygienic interventions aim at reducing sleep-incompatible behaviors and establishing sleep-promoting behaviors. These techniques are a fundamental ingredient of insomnia therapy; however, solely applying sleep hygiene is often not sufficiently effective in reducing insomnia complaints.

Although many patients know in general about appropriate behavior regarding sleep hygiene, they do not always implement these strategies in their daily life.

Sleep Hygiene Tips

- Reduction of bedtimes to the necessary amount: 6 to a maximum of 7 h are sufficient.
- Observe regular sleep–wake schedules, including weekends.
- Sleeping during daytime should be limited to nap of a maximum of 20 min.
- Create a comfortable atmosphere in the bedroom: remove objects that remind you of the daily routines and provide a comfortable room temperature.
- No late and heavy meals.
- Avoid alcohol consumption in the evening; if possible, reduce tobacco consumption in the evening.
- No caffeinated beverages after 1 PM.
- No intensive activities or sports close to bedtime.
- No sleeping in front of the TV.
- No stimulating activities during wake periods at night, for example, working.
- No TV in the bedroom.

The therapist has to motivate the patient and at the same time control whether good sleep hygiene is practiced. It is essential that the patient is encouraged to shift from passive-receptive attitude to an *active attitude*. The aim is to educate the patient, so he or she becomes an expert about his or her disorder. Active cooperation and the "role of an expert in his own interest" help to reduce the feeling of helplessness regarding the insomnia disorder and promote a more relaxed attitude towards sleep.

It is important to notice that the observation of sleep hygienic tips is not limited to insomnia disorders. In most sleep disorders, e.g., restless leg syndrome, sleep hygiene is basic because patients with sleep disorders irrespective of their etiology tend to show sleep-incompatible behaviors. Inappropriate sleep hygiene may be responsible for the persistence or insufficient remission of any sleep disorder.

A *sleep diary* may be kept to support and evaluate the behavioral changes during therapy.

Bedroom and bed should be used exclusively for relaxation, sleeping, and sexual activities. Daytime sleep episodes longer than a brief nap of about 15–20 min can reduce the need to sleep in the evening and should be avoided.

Following the individually required *quantity of sleep* and the optimal *sleep schedule* is sleep promoting. This sentence might sound trivial or even paradoxical, but it makes sense in the context of some typical and frequent behaviors reported by insomnia patients. These patients go to bed early, to increase their chance to get more sleep. They remain in bed too long on work-free days to compensate the sleep deficit accumulated throughout the week. This self-imposed sleep pattern promotes insomnia complaints. Excessively long periods of staying in bed should be avoided. Regular bedtimes should be kept, also on weekends. For insomnia patients, bedtimes should be about 6 h, with a maximum of 7 h.

A *relaxing atmosphere at the end of the day*, without working, and a ritualized sequence of sleep-promoting behaviors, e.g., completing tasks, changing clothes, and body hygiene as rituals before bed time support emotional equilibrium. The increased level of arousal during the day can be reduced. The activities of the next day should be planned, preferably outside the bedroom, before going to bed. Furthermore, the current day with all its events should be reflected on and set aside.

Behavioral Tips for Healthy Sleep

- Create a relaxing atmosphere in the evening hours.
- Before going to bed, reflect on the experiences of the day outside the bedroom and write down the activities planned for the next day.
- Practice rituals of going to bed: write a diary, listen to relaxing music, read relaxing books, do relaxing exercises.

- Position alarm clocks and other clocks outside of view; do not look at your clock or mobile phone at night.
- Maintain a comfortable atmosphere in bed. Be relaxed if you are not fall asleep at once, and observe all thoughts in a relaxed manner, also thoughts about wanting to sleep.
- Let mental and emotional distraction of everyday tasks and events "pass by", engage in enjoyable thoughts supporting a pleasant and relaxed state.

The sleep environment should be organized in that way that the sleeper feels comfortable, and at ease. Objects reminding of work and job, such as a desk in the bedroom, should be avoided if possible.

The *room temperature* must not be at a certain value, the room temperature should be subjectively comfortable. Temperatures subjectively perceived as too low or too high may cause chilling or sweating, which increase stress and thus foster sleep problems. The same rationale is valid for colors in the bedroom: the individual well-being is of importance. Thus, those colors that support subjective wellness and relaxation are recommended.

It is important to sleep on an *comfortable mattress* that does not lead to physical miscomfort or even pain. There is no perfect mattress for everyone. Moreover, individual preferences, somatic conditions and diseases of the musculoskeletal apparatus should be taken into consideration. People who are prone to sweat at night might prefer pocket spring mattresses because of the better aeration. People who are prone to chills would choose cold-foam mattresses.

Attention has to be paid to sufficient *sound proofing*. The subjective levels of perceiving something as unpleasant noise is individually different. People suffering from insomnia, however, are prone to very light sleep and are often sensitive to every noise in their bedrooms, which increase their requirements for sound proofing. Interestingly, some insomnia patients sleep very well in front of the TV despite the background noise and flickering light, and often in an uncomfortable position, which emphasizes the psychological factors relevant in the etiology this type of insomnia.

Furthermore, the *options of darkening* the bedroom should met the individual's needs. Objective criteria regarding the level of darkening that promote good sleep are frequently discussed in the literature; however, they actually do not exist. During sleep, the eyes are closed, the eye balls are directed upward so that the eyes do not perceive much light which might inhibit the production of sleep-promoting melatonin. Suboptimal lighting conditions are often perceived as not comfortable and thus increase stress, exacerbating the sleep problems. The insomnia patient might attributes the sleep problems to the inappropriate light conditions, even though the physiological effect on sleep is often negligible.

In bedrooms, clocks should not be positioned in a way that it is visible from the sleeping position because insomnia patients tend to monitor their sleep extensively and, thus, increase the exaggerated and often paradoxical efforts to fall asleep. The same applies for clocks that procduce auditory signals, e.g., every hour.

3.7.2 Cognitive-behavioral Therapy of Insomnia

In 1809, Jean Paul described 14 procedures to facilitate sleep in his booklet entitled "Dr. Katzenbergers Badereise" (Dr. Katzenberger's Trip to the Medicinal Springs). These procedures can be summarized as follows:

> … they finally are all the art of creating boredom for oneself; this is an art that logically thinking minds see as irrational art, not to think (author's translation).

In addition to the tips for healthy sleep (sleep hygiene), nonpharmacological insomnia therapy includes basic elements of different psychotherapy schools. Elements of cognitive-behavioral therapy are often applied in this context. The target of psychotherapeutic efforts is the increased psychophysiological arousal in insomnia patients that manifests on cognitive, emotional, and vegetative levels. The objective of each psychotherapeutic intervention is to establish a balanced, relaxed state in the sleep situation on all three levels.

On the *cognitive level*, the increased arousal often manifests in the tendency to ruminate about everyday events. Those events may be events perceived as stressful, for example, major life events such as divorce, loss or change of job, moving to another place, loss of a close person, worries about family problems, or interpersonal problems. But also trivial matters of everyday life may maintain an increased psychophysiological arousal level, for example, thinking about the daily tasks or events at home or at work in the near future or recent past.

A focus on sleep with heightened self-monitoring of one's inability to sleep is a second factor that increases psychophysiological stress levels. Characteristic behaviors are frequently checking the time at night (looking at the clock) and thinking about the negative consequences of sleeplessness. Worries about the severity of sleepiness and the increased inner tension during the day are also typical.

On the *emotional level*, rumination and focusing on insomnia problems causes enhanced mood inbalance. Negative emotions such as anxiety, sadness, rage, anger, and inner restlessness are typical. However, positive emotions may also cause an emotional inbalance. Joy, feeling proud, or being in love can also interfere with sleep via an increased psychophysiological arousal.

The intense efforts of patients to fall asleep are based on the frustration and worries about one's own inability to sleep. These anticipatory worries regarding sleep occur not only at bedtime but already show up in the evening hours or even during the day.

On a *vegetative level*, increased arousal for example, motor agitation, tachycardia, and sweating, may be observed. The affected individuals interpret these effects as a direct consequence of the increased cognitive and emotional arousal; however, they are often the only symptoms reported if the patient has low introspection or suffers from a mental disorder.

The vicious circle of insomnia is considered as the etiological and maintaining mechanism of insomnia, i.e., there is a self-reinforcing circle of sleep-incompatible factors (◘ Fig. 3.2).

In cases of short-term insomnia and chronic insomnia, this vicious circle is characteristic and is considered as the significant etiological factor of chronic insomnia. In insomnia therapy, the focus is on identifying and changing the vicious cycle together with the patient. Breaking this self-promoting circle of sleep-incompatible factors might be considered key for successful therapy.

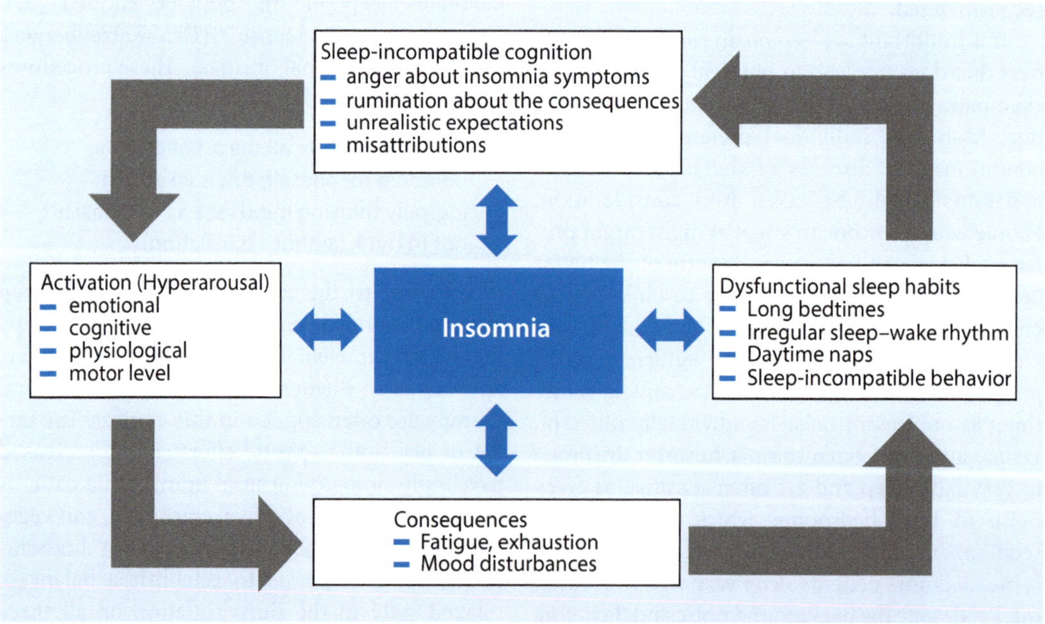

◘ **Fig. 3.2** Vicious circle of insomnia (modified according to Riemann and Backhaus, Schlafstörungen bewältigen, Beltz PVU 1996; courtesy of Beltz-Verlag)

One prerequisite for a successful psychotherapeutic intervention is the insomnia patient's understanding of these associations. This awareness has to be addressed with the patient as a first therapeutic step.

Practical Tip

All psychotherapeutic interventions aim at establishing a relaxed state in the cognitive, emotional, and vegetative domains that is compatible with sleep.

It's important to notice that the ability to sleep itself is not the focus of the psychotherapeutic interventions. An intensive focus of the therapist on sleep might enhance the patient's focusing on his/her sleep and, thus, have a negative effect on sleep.

3.7.2.1 Bedtime Rituals

The *bedtime rituals* aim at establishing a transition period between daily routines and bedtime. The objective is a reduction of the psychophysiological arousal level, promoting a relaxed attitude, and the sensation of letting go from daytime requirements. Generally, all behaviors that are associated with the feeling of comfort support the patient's relaxation, e.g., a hot bath in the evening, bed socks (studies confirm a significant effect on sleep latency), warm beverages (herbal tea, milk), relaxing music, dim light (candles), or reading a relaxing book. In addition, techniques to decrease possible distress related to day-to-day life are beneficial, e.g., reducing rumination about stressing events and the requirements of the (upcoming) day before going to bed. The idea is to solve problems already during the daytime and/or to give these issues enough time before going to bed, so that such issues are no longer distressing during the sleep onset process. Writing memos, keeping a diary, or talking with one's partner may be supportive.

Case Report

After the first day of her attendance of a CTB-I workshop, the participant (insomnia patient) experienced a very good night's sleep. She reported the following bedtime ritual:

- "About 2 hours before going to bed, I took a long hot bath. For this purpose, I decorated the bathroom. I listened to relaxing music, put candles everywhere in the bathroom, put my favorite bath essence into the water, and spread rose petals in the whole bathroom, even into the water. After spending about 45 minutes in the water, I dried myself off thoroughly and rubbed ointments and creams on my body. Then I went into my bedroom.
- Before going through the doorway into the bedroom, I stopped, shook my body, and imagined that I let go all the worries of the day outside the bedroom. When I felt that I had let go all the worries, I stepped through the doorway.
- I had already previously chosen my favorite linen. I had also used candles (safe tea lights that go out unsupervised), and relaxing music, spread rose petals everywhere, and used my favorite perfume on the linen. I felt so comfortable, relaxed, and safe; and I had just forgotten that I had to fall asleep … and suddenly my alarm clock rang this morning."

Relaxation procedures reduce the increased psychophysiological arousal level built up during the day. Relaxation methods like autogenic training, progressive muscle relaxation according to Jacobson, or yoga, can be discussed with the patient. Furthermore, mental relaxation techniques are helpful, for example, soothing images, visualizing relaxing journeys, and mindfulness. It is often quite difficult for insomnia patients to learn those techniques because their difficulties with relaxing are among the main etiological factors in insomnia. It is beneficial to apply specially adapted techniques, practice periods during the day and patience, by both patient and therapist, should be emphasized until the first positive results are achieved.

Relaxing images or visualizations of journeys based on the motto "Be your own TV program" (sleep-disturbed individuals often sleep well in front of the TV because the distraction increases mental relaxation) may support sleep because these techniques distract from negative thoughts and put the focus on pleasant feelings. The relaxing effect on cognitive, emotional, and vegetative domains is the crucial parameter. In addition, sheep counting or something similar (e.g., counting down from 10,000 by subtracting 13 each time until 0 is nearly reached) may be recommended.

Case Report

To visualize a relaxing image, the following measures may be helpful.

> Imagine a situation that is very pleasant for you where you feel entirely comfortable. This situation may be something you have experienced in the past, for example, a vacation, or an imaginary situation. After you have chosen such a situation, please try to imagine it as specific and detailed as possible. This is supported by focusing on different senses:
> - What can you see, hear, feel, smell, and taste?
> - Imagine the season and the time of the day of your situation.
> - How is the weather? Feel how pleasant this imagined scenario is.

The visualized picture may look like this:

> It is a beautiful late summer afternoon at the seaside. The sun is shining, it is comfortably warm but not too hot, the sky is blue. I am sitting in a beach chair looking out on the sea, I am leaning back, my legs and feet are stretched out, and it is very comfortable. The sand on the beach is fine and white, beach grass is on the dunes. I am watching the waves, how they break on the shore. At a distance, several seagulls are flying around a boat. I am hearing kids' voices from far away and sometimes a seagull screech, otherwise I am only hearing the sound of the waves. The sun is warming my skin and every now and again the wind blows gently over my face. I am breathing deeply and I am smelling the salty air. I am enjoying the silence and I am feeling cozy and relaxed.

3.7.2.2 Cognitive Techniques

Cognitive Restructuring

Cognitive restructuring aims at changing dysfunctional thoughts related to sleep. Often, insomnia patients attribute unrealistic expectations and effects to their poor sleep that clearly increase distress, e.g., they have to sleep to avoid negative consequences (Table 3.3). The information about sleep that is necessary for cognitive restructuring has already been outlined in the section about psychoeducation and healthy sleep (see ▸ Sect. 3.7.1).

Rumination Chair

For many bedtime rituals, a rumination chair may be helpful for the patient. It should be placed in a quiet corner of the apartment outside the bedroom that is suitable for self-reflection. The atmosphere should be comfortable. Dim light, a warm blanket, and some soft music may be supportive,

Table 3.3 Dysfunctional thoughts of insomnia patients that might have negative effects on sleep

Dysfunctional thoughts	Functional alternatives
Every human individual needs 8 h of sleep.	The spectrum of individual sleep duration is very broad. In addition, intraindividual differences are observed—even good sleepers sometimes have nights with less amounts of sleep.
If I do not sleep long enough or deep enough, I am inefficient during the daytime.	My efficiency does not only depend on sleep but also on other factors. It has happened quite often that I was able to perform well even after a bad night's sleep.
I have problems to fall asleep. Others do not have problems with sleep; it drives me crazy!	To be angry about not being able to fall asleep is not helpful. Being angry the whole night is even more disstressing than a night of poor sleep.
I have been lying in bed for 1 h and I am still awake. This will be a horrible night.	I will stay in bed calmly, relax, and enjoy the night. Sleep will come sooner or later.
These sleep problems drive me crazy; I do not know what to do.	There are good and bad nights. I will wait, relax, and visualize relaxing images. Even a bad night is not the end of the world.

but TV should not be watched. Within the framework of stimulus control (see ▶ Sect. 3.7.2.4), it is important to choose a place outside the bed where rumination is allowed.

Stopping Thoughts

The thought-stopping technique may help avoid negative thoughts during relaxation exercises, imagination practice, and stimulus control.

The patient is instructed to analyze the significance of the negative thoughts.

- If they are important, it may be helpful to write them down on a piece of paper placed on the night table. If the patients feel the need to handle the thoughts/problems immediately, he or she is encouraged to do so outside the bed and the bedroom. For this purpose, he might use a rumination chair in a quiet corner of his or her home.
- If the thoughts/problems are not that important, imaginations or other relaxation techniques can be practiced, and the thoughts typically dissipate.

3.7.2.3 Sleep Restriction

Sleep restriction is a key element of insomnia therapy because insomnia patients are prone to spend too much time in bed often accompanied by long rumination periods.

The objective is to reduce the time in bed to a figure that a sleep deficit is built up over several days. The increased sleep pressure fosters sleep with in the restricted time in bed. The improved ability to sleep may help to reduce the feelings of helplessness during time in bed and improve the ability to relax.

On the basis of a 2-week sleep diary, the effective sleep duration is assessed. The effective sleep duration, often underestimated by the patient, is chosen as time in bed (however, the minimum is 4.5 h). The *sleep efficiency* is calculated as follows:

$$\text{Sleep efficiency} = \frac{\begin{array}{c}100 \times \text{subjectively estimated sleep duration}\\ \underline{\text{(subtracting all periods with wakefulness)}}\end{array}}{\text{Bedtime}}$$

- If the patient achieves a sleep efficiency of more than 90%, the patient is allowed to extend his or her time in bed by 20 min (typically on a weekly basis).
- If efficiency amounts to 85–90%, the time in bed is kept as is.
- Sleep efficiencies below 85% are indicative that time in bed should be reduced by 15 min.

Sleep restriction is performed over 6 to 8 weeks. The objective is a bedtime of 5 to 6 h with a sleep efficiency of more than 90%.

Practical Tip

In an outpatient setting, times in bed of 4.5 h may result in increased daytime tiredness and the tendency to fall asleep in situations such as at work or when driving a car. The patient should be informed about this risk. If needed, a short-term sick leave may be indicated to reduce the risk of endangerment of the patient and others because of the sleep restriction.

3.7.2.4 Stimulus Control

Stimulus control aims at breaking up the conditioning between bedroom and poor sleep.

Healthy individuals have conditioning between sleep environment and initiating psycho-vegetative relaxation. In insomnia patients, however, a negative conditioning for sleep associated with the stimulus of the bedroom or the bed and increased psycho-vegetative arousal in this situation is found.

Case Report

Many insomnia patients report that they feel tired and relaxed before going to their bed room. However, they report that as soon as they are in bed, all tiredness and relaxation disappear - this is the effect of the negative conditioning. "Doctor, it seems as if a switch is flipped. As soon as I am lying in bed, I am wide awake."

Within the framework of stimulus control, the patient is instructed not to ruminate while lying in bed but to creating a relaxed atmosphere. He is encouraged to apply bedtime rituals, visualizations, or other relaxation exercises and thought-stopping techniques. If the patient does not succeed in creating this relaxed atmosphere, he or she should leave the bed and the bedroom. Outside the bedroom, he or she is allowed to deal with his or her negative thoughts and emotions, for example, in a rumination chair (see ▸ Sect. 3.7.2.2). The atmosphere outside the bedroom should be comfortable, no bright lights, no job-related activities, and in particular no TV watching. If the patient feels more relaxed, he or she is allowed to return to bed. In bed, again creating a relaxed atmosphere is the focus. If this does not work, the patient should get up again. If the patient is in a relaxed psychovegetative state, there is no need to leave the bed, even though some other authors give different recommendations.

3.7.2.5 Group Therapy and Insomnia Workshops

The different elements of psychotherapy for insomnia may be provided as individual therapies but are also highly effective in a group therapy format. Psychoeducative and internet-based programs will gain importance - as the number of patients with insomnia is huge; first trials indicated their effectiveness. In addition, programs offered by healthcare professionals will be more and more important. If those programs do not improve sleep in a sufficient way psychotherapists specialized in sleep medicine should be consulted.

The agenda of a 2-day group workshop based on behavioral therapy for insomnia is described here as an example (◘ Table 3.4). It is offered regularly at the Interdisciplinary Sleep Center of the Pfalzklinikum in Klingenmünster, Germany, for patients coming from all over Germany. Prior to the workshop, patients undergo an intensive diagnostic procedure to ensure that the participation in the behavioral therapeutic group program is indicated.

These 2-day CBT-I workshops show a high effectiveness in the long-term. Being interviewed 1 to 4 years after the workshop, the participants report:

- An increased sleep duration of about 6 h on average
- A mean reduction in sleep latency from 66 to 27 min
- Reduction of time of being a wake after sleep onset from 83 min to 29 min on average

The participants further report:

- The restorative effect of sleep is increased
- Daytime well-being is improved
- Consumption of hypnotics could be significantly reduced

3.7.3 Pharmacotherapy of Insomnia

Pharmacotherapy for insomnia can be an important treatment strategy. However, prior to treatment intensive diagnostics regarding the behavioral, medical, psychiatric, and drug-related factors responsible for the sleep disorder have to be carried out. Pharmacotherapy should be applied in combination with psychoeducation and CBT-I. The prescription of drugs based solely on the patient's complaints about sleep disorders without evaluation by sleep specialists should be avoided. In most cases, pharmacotherapy with hypnotics is symptomatic and should only be applied for a limited time, typically 4 weeks. Only for CBT-I nonresponders and insufficient improvement regarding sleep despite the treatment of an underlying somatic and/or mental disorder should long-term pharmacotherapy be considered. In those cases, side effects and in particular the potential of addiction and habituation of different hypnotic substances must be carefully evaluated.

The hypnotic substances vary with regard to their pharmacodynamics, the effects, and side effects. In prescribing hypnotics, the following *six basic principles* might be helpful.

Six Basic Principles for Prescribing Hypnotics

- Clear indication
- Smallest possible dose
- Shortest possible treatment duration
- No abrupt discontinuation of the drug
- Evaluate possible contraindications
- Combine with nonpharmaceutical methods

Table 3.4 Agenda of a 2-day workshop for patients at the Interdisciplinary Sleep Center of the Pfalzklinikum Klingenmünster, Germany

Topic	Function
Basics of healthy sleep	Information regarding the sleep basics
	Learning to be an expert on one's own sleep
	Information on sleep hygiene
	Reduction of inappropriate expectations toward sleep
	Decatastrophizing the sleep disorder
Most frequent sleep disorders	Information on sleep disorders
	Learning to be an expert on one's own disorder
	Individually tailored information on sleep hygiene
	Realistic assessment of one's own symptoms
Insomnia: Etiology	Recognizing that
	– Focusing on the insomnia complaints
	– Increased psychophysiological arousal and
	– Rumination are the main etiological factors of the disorder
	Awareness that medical factors are often secondary
Self-help methods	Presentation, information, and training of cognitive-behavioral interventions
Drug-related therapy for insomnia	Information about the use and the risk of hypnotics
	How to use hypnotics in a sensible way
	Increase motivation to reduce hypnotics
	Realistic expectations about the therapeutic effects of hypnotics
Stress management	Recognizing that an increased psychophysiological arousal in the evening and at night is also present during daytime
	Training in stress reduction techniques
Relaxation exercises	Instruction and training in relaxation techniques like progressive muscle relaxation, autogenic training, visualization of relaxing images, imagined journeys
Group discussions	Establishing and developing etiological models of the sleep disorder adapted for the individual
	Establishing and developing individual self-help strategies
One-on-one sessions	Recapitulate the course contents and, if needed, tailor the strategies to the specific need of each individual patient

The selection of a hypnotic compound is made after diagnostics addressing somatic and psychiatric factors. The dose should not be higher than recommended; lower doses should be applied if possible. The duration of the treatment should be limited to a maximum of 4 weeks. If the drug is applied intermittently, e.g., in intervals of a maximum of two to three times per week, the treatment can be extended because of the reduced risk of habituation and addiction.

If discontinuation of the drug leads to aggravation of the sleep problems, a second treatment phase may be started. If the insomnia complaints persist, a sleep specialist should be consulted. If hypotics are applied for a longer time, they should not be discontinued abruptly but slowly reduced, especially for benzodiazepines (BZD) and the Z substances like zopiclone, like zolpidem, and zaleplon (benzodiazepine receptor agonists, BZRAs). The duration of the reduction phase depends on the duration of the treatment and, if performed in an outpatient setting, may require several months. For eszopiclone, clinical studies did not show any tolerance or withdrawal effects even after 6 months of treatment: that is the reason why eszopiclone may be prescribed for more than 6 months, in contrast to other BZRAs. In the USA, eszopiclone has been granted FDA approval for long-term application.

First trials showed that chronic application of hypnotics could increase mortality and dementia risk. These findings, however, need to be confirmed by future studies.

Contraindications like the respiration-depressing effects of BZD, which may increase respiratory events during sleep in patients with sleep-related breathing disorders (SRBDs), should be taken into account (◘ Table 3.5).

It has to be taken into account that hypnotics are not a causal therapy. Thus, it is recommended to combine pharmacotherapy with nonpharmaceutical interventions (▶ Sect. 3.7.1).

Basics of Treatment with Hypnotics

- Comprehensive diagnostics with regard to somatic, psychological, and psychiatric factors.
- Establishing a treatment concept combining psychoeducative and cognitive-behavioral interventions, and pharmacotherapy.
- Carefully check the indication. The physician determines the dose, time of intake, and treatment duration.
- Exclude patients from pharmacotherapy who are at risk becoming addicted.
- Exclude patients with contraindications for the respective drug, e.g., specific somatic diseases.
- Evaluate possible interactions with other medications.
- It should be discussed with the patient whether an intermittent drug intake schedule in order to reduce the risk of habituation and addiction is feasible.
- Maximum treatment duration of 4 weeks; consultation after 2 weeks.
- If the sleep disorder persists after a treatment period of 4 weeks, a second treatment period of 4 weeks might be indicated.
- After a total of 8 weeks of pharmacotherapy without sufficient response, a sleep specialist should be consulted.
- Hypnotics after longer intake must not discontinued abruptly. Depending on the treatment duration, step-by-step reduction of the dose is highly recommended.

The ideal hypnotic is characterized by:

- Rapid effect onset
- Large therapeutic spectrum
- Confirmed sleep induction
- Maintenance of the physiological sleep pattern
- Low toxicity
- No side effects, no interactions with other medications, and no hangover in the morning
- No habituation and addiction risk
- No tolerance and withdrawal effects
- Age-independent dosages

The various hypnotics meet these requirements of an ideal hypnotic drug more or less (◘ Table 3.5).

3.7.3.1 Benzodiazepine Receptor Agonists (BZRAs)

The BZRAs (◘ Table 3.6) include the so-called Z substances like *zolpidem*, *zopiclone*, and *zaleplon*. A substantial number of clinical trials over at least 4 weeks confirmed the positive effect of BZRA on

Table 3.5 Pros and cons of different substances applied as hypnotics

Substance	Pros	Cons
Benzodiazepine receptor agonists (BZRA): zolpidem, zopiclone, zaleplon	Good hypnotic effect Short duration of the effect Minor hangover in the morning Sleep-specific effect Rare problems with adaptation and rebound Low toxicity Solid scientific data	Similar side effects as benzodiazepines Some reports about addiction
Eszopiclone	Similar to BZRA	Even after 6 months of treatment, no tolerance development or withdrawal effects
Benzodiazepines (BZD)	Good hypnotic effect Positive clinical experience for years regarding effects and side effects Large therapeutic spectrum Substances with various half-lives are available	Possible addiction Rebound phenomena Anterograde amnesia Muscle relaxation Respiratory suppression Anxiolytic effects Paradoxical effects, slow wave sleep suppression, REM sleep suppression in the first part of the night Scientific evidence somewhat outdated
Antidepressants	Almost no addiction risk Rare withdrawal problems Minor or no slow wave sleep suppression Antidepressive effect, supportive empirical evidence	Relatively high toxicity Anticholinergic and cardiac side effects Cannot be applied in a similar way at different ages Often REM sleep suppression Long duration till the drug works Hangover effects (in particular at the beginning of the treatment) Limited clinical data regarding the effectiveness in insomnia
Antipsychotics/neuroleptics	Neglectable risk of addiction Low cardiotoxicity Antipsychotic effect Reduces arousal	Anticholinergic, extrapyramidal, hematologic, antihypertensive side effects Late dyskinesia Sometimes long delays of the effect Insufficient clinical data regarding the effectiveness in insomnia
Antihistamines	Rather low toxicity	Low hypnotic potential Rapid tolerance development Anticholinergic side effects Questionable addiction potential Studies on the effectiveness for insomnia are missing or insufficient
Alcohol derivatives	Rapid effect onset	Mild hypnotic effect Narrow therapeutic spectrum Tolerance effects Addiction risk Insufficient clinical data regarding effectiveness
Phytotherapeutics	No addiction risk Low toxicity	Mild hypnotic effects Insufficient data situation for insomnia
Melatonin retard	Effect on sleep–wake rhythm Low toxicity Sufficient clinical data	Only approved for patients aged 55 and older

Modified according to Hajak and Riemann [7]

Table 3.6 BZRA for the treatment of insomnia

Substance	Evening dose (mg)[a]	Half-life (hours)	Indication
Zolpidem	10	1.7–2.4	Difficulties in initiating and maintaining sleep
Zopiclone	3.75–7.5	3.5–6.5	Difficulties in initiating and maintaining sleep; waking up early in the morning
Zaleplon	5–10	0.9–1.1	Difficulties in initiating sleep
Eszopiclone	1–3	5–8	Difficulties in initiating and maintaining sleep; waking up early in the morning

[a]Typical dose for patients with primary insomnia

3

sleep. Only eszopiclone has achieved FDA approval for long-term treatment.

- Zopiclone: half-life of 3.5–6.5 h, indicated for difficulties in initiating and maintaining sleep with early awakening
- Eszopiclon: half-life of 5–8 h; indicated for difficulties in initiating and maintaining sleep with waking up early in the morning
- Zolpidem: half-life of 1.7–2.4 h, suitable for difficulties in initiating and maintaining sleep
- Zaleplon: very short half-life of 0.9–1.1 h, particularly suitable for difficulties of initiating sleep. Because waking activities are not affected 4 h after intake, it may also be indicated for problems with maintaining sleep, taking the drug during the night if needed. In 2017 and 2018, it was no longer sold on the German market.

Meta-analyses could not confirm a superiority of the three Z substances compared to the classic BZDs with respect to sleep parameters. However, the profile of side effects is much more favorable. Hangover effects the next morning are rarer, the daytime status is improved, and rebound insomnia after abrupt withdrawal is less frequent.

The addiction risk of the three Z substances, especially in cases of intermittent application schedules, is considered as minor compared to BZD. On the other hand, rare clinical case reports describe the development of addiction during BZRA treatment. A long-term study with zolpidem confirmed high effectiveness without tolerance development, if intermittent applicated (intake for maximum of 5 days per week) over a period of 3 months. Further trials indicate that the intermittent application of the Z substances prevents addiction. A study in patients older than 60 years indicated that the increasing number of side effects outweighs the clinical benefit of BZRA in this age group.

Zopiclone is sold on the European and Asian market, but not in the USA. Eszopiclone is prescribed in the USA, the first Z substance that was FDA approved for long-term application. Studies for treatment periods of 6 months did not show any withdrawal or tolerance effects.

3.7.3.2 Benzodiazepines (BZDs)

BZDs have been on the market since the 1960s. BZDs enhance the inhibiting effect of GABA neurons. About one third of all synapses in the central nervous system are GABAergic. The $GABA_A$ receptor does not only bind to BZD, but also alcohol, barbiturates, and other substances. A small reduction of the GABA inhibition, for example, by toxins, can increase anxiety, excitation, spasms, hypertension, convulsions, and finally even cause death.

BZDs promote the effect of GABA in the sense of leftward shift of the S-shaped GABA dose–response curve. BZD receptors are directly coupled to the $GABA_A$ receptor that may hyperpolarize the postsynaptic membrane potential over the chloride-ion channel. The $GABA_A$-BZD–chloride-ion-channel complex consists of five subunits.

The broad therapeutic spectrum of BZDs and BZRAs (► Sect. 3.7.3.1) is based on their exclusively physiological enhancement of GABA inhibition.

Practical Tip

Four main effects of BZDs:
- Anxiolytic
- Sedation/hypnotic
- Anticonvulsion
- Muscle relaxation

According to the type of BZD, these four main effects are relevant to different extents. In contrast to BZDs, the Z-class substances (BZRA) and eszopiclone have an almost exclusively sedating/hypnotic effect. This selective hypnotic property, the improved profile of side effects, and the probably lower risk of addiction are the reasons why BZRAs replaced BZDs in their application as hypnotics.

Some BZD derivatives were frequently used in the illegal drug scene. This was due not only to availability and low price but also to receptor affinity and rapid effect. Flunitrazepam, diazepam, and lorazepam are the favored drugs in this scene; however, there are also reports that all other BZDs, even ones such as triazolam with short half-lives are consumed.

Current studies estimate that between 1.1 and 1.9 million people are addicted to BZD and BZRA in Germany; predominantly older patients with more women than men. A loss of efficiency may increase significantly the doses used by the patient and result in addiction.

When the medication is abruptly discontinued, the inhibition in the central nervous system due to the medication is suddenly gone, so increased excitatory phenomena may occur, e.g., massive sleep problems, physical withdrawal effects such as trembling, sweating, and vegetative arousal. If high doses have been consumed, deliria, withdrawal psychoses or seizures can occur. Thus, attempts to quit are often frustrating.

Practical Tip

Abrupt discontinuation of BZD medication is contraindicated.

Because of the very low toxicity of BZDs, a slow reduction of the dose over weeks or even months is the correct choice that many patients experience as helpful and even sleep promoting. The original dose can be reduced, for example, by 10% every other week. Switching to liquid diazepam may be helpful because it may be easier to dose if intake is very reduced. However, the long half-life of diazepam has to be taken into account. If the BZD medication is slowly reduced, the cells can express $GABA_A$-BZD receptors until the original concentration is reached. To minimize psychovegetative withdrawal effects, the withdrawal may be supported by giving a sedating antidepressant in a low dose, for example, doxepin.

If anxiolytic effects in cases of psychiatric insomnia are part of the treatment regime, BZDs with short and medium half-lives may be applied. In most patients, no significant hangover effect in the morning occurs. BZDs with longer half-lives should only be applied when anxiolysis during the day is warranted.

One of the most common side effects of BZDs, anterograde amnesia, may be experienced as distressing (◘ Table 3.7).

BZD derivatives have a another common side effect that can be easily diagnosed with EEG. They reduce slow wave sleep stage N3, the frequency of delta waves is not affected in a marked way but the

◘ **Table 3.7** Short- and medium-acting Benzodiazepine hypnotics

Substance	Half-life (in hours, including metabolites)	Evening dose (mg)
Triazolam	1.5–5	0.125–0.25
Lormetazepam	8–15	1–2
Brotizolam	4–7	0.125–0.25
Temazepam	5–14	10–40
Nitrazepam	15–30	5–10
Lorazepam	13–14	0.5–2
Oxazepam	5–15	10–30
Flunitrazepam	10–30	0.5–2

amplitude is reduced; the delta waves no longer reach the criterion of 75 μV that is necessary for classification according to the AASM criteria.

A long-term intake of BZDs also increases beta frequencies during sleep, signifying an increased EEG activity. The spindle density in the beta band correlated significantly with the plasma concentration of the BZD. The suppression of REM sleep during BZD intake is the reason why after abrupt withdrawal rebound insomnia with REM rebound and fractionated sleep occur.

3.7.3.3 Treatment Strategies Regarding BZDs and BZRAs

The treatment strategies for BZDs and BZRAs described in the following paragraphs aim at minimizing the addiction risk by intermittent application, this is not necessary for eszopiclone as it is approved for long-term treatment. Furthermore, long-term treatments with hypnotics for chronic and severe cases are outlined, also combined with second-line hypnotics.

Standard Interval Therapy

The duration of intake is limited to a maximum of 4 weeks. The hypnotic drug is stepwise reduced over several days, and after a drug-free period of at least 4 weeks, an additional treatment period of a maximum of 4 weeks may follow.

Controlled Interval Therapy

Within this regimen, the physician agrees on specific days of the week together with the patient on which hypnotics are taken. A maximum of 3 nights per week, in exceptional cases 4 nights, are recommended.

Quota-Interval Therapy

The physician determines how many nights per week the patient may use a hypnotic, e.g., three times per week. The specific days are selected by the patient.

Low-Dose Long-Term Therapy

The indication for a long-term BZRA therapy can be given in patients with chronic, severe insomnia and significant impairment of the daytime functioning if, after consulting a sleep specialist, no causal therapy, e.g., CBT-I seems to be feasible and/or beneficial and second-line hypnotics are not effective.

For this group of patients, it should be required that a CBT-I treatment has failed at least twice, and no tolerance and dose increases using BZD or BZRA are reported in the medical history. The Z-class hypnotics including zopiclone, zolpidem, and zaleplon are preferred compared to BZD hypnotics.

Low-Dose Combination Therapy

Low-dose combination therapy is reserved for severe and chronic cases that require daily hypnotic intake and where hypnotics as a single treatment strategy are not sufficiently reducing sleep problems.

Low doses of sedating antidepressants or low-potency neuroleptics have proved to be clinically effective. In cases of tri- and tetracyclic drugs, usually the initial dose is 10–25 mg. In individual cases, the dose may be increased to 100 mg. Hangover effects on the next morning, however, should be avoided. If hangover occurs, it is not always necessary to reduce the dose, it might suffice to take the drug earlier. Usually, the medication is applied 2 h before going to bed so that arousal and worries that might interfere with sleep can be reduced. About 30 min before going to bed, a hypnotic, if possible half of the dose, is applied additionally to initiate sleep. Using a interval therapy approach for the additional hypnotic intake, risk for tolerance and addiction can be minimized.

3.7.3.4 Melatonin and Melatonin Receptor Agonists

Melatonin is an endogenous hormone produced by the pineal gland. The release occurs during the dark period between sunset and sunrise. Low doses of melatonin during the day can increase sleepiness that can be objectified by measuring the sleep latency via polysomnography, whereas only large doses given at night induce the same effect. Orally applicated melatonin seems to have a small sleep-promoting effect. Meta-analyses suggest that melatonin is effective in the treatment of jetlag and sleep–wake rhythm disorders such as the delayed sleep-phase syndrome (▶ Chap. 6).

In the USA, melatonin is freely available as an OTC product. In Europe and Germany, it is only available via prescription. Melatonin reaches its maximum concentration after 0.5 h and has a half-life of about 1 h, i.e., the duration of the effect is quite short. Hence, melatonin might be appropriate for less severe problems of initiating sleep.

Currently, the clinical data supporting the efficacy of melatonin in the treatment of short-term insomnia or chronic insomnia are not convincing. Several studies indicated a small positive effect on sleep latency; however, effect sizes have been very small. Since 2008, a retard melatonin compound (Circadin) is approved in Germany for insomnia treatment of patients older than 55 years. It should be applied over a period of 3 weeks.

In the USA, ramelteon is on the market: it is a MT_1 and MT_2 melatonin receptor agonist that reaches its maximum concentration 0.75–1 h after intake with a half-life of 1–2.5 h. Similar to melatonin, based on its pharmacokinetics, ramelteon seems appropriate for problems with initiating sleep. The therapeutic dose of 8 mg about 30 min before going to bed has been recommended.

Tasimelteon, another melatonin receptor agonist, was approved for the European Union for the treatment of blind patients with a non-24-h sleep–wake rhythm disorder. This disorder is chronic; because of not perceiving light, the biological clock cannot be synchronized with the 24-h day–night cycle in blind individuals and typically shows a longer cycle.

The effectiveness of tasimelteon was shown in two clinical trials with 104 participants (blind participants with non-24-h sleep–wake rhythm disorder). In both trials, tasimelteon prolonged night sleep and reduced daytime sleep compared to placebo. The side effects that were most frequently reported in the clinical trials were headaches, increased liver enzymes (alanine aminotransferase), nightmares or strange dreams, disturbed sleep, infection of the upper airways or the urinary tract, and sleepiness.

Tasimelteon may impair activities that require high concentratoin and, therefore, should be taken always at the same time in the evening before going to bed. Tasimelteon has obtained the status of an orphan drug (i.e., medication for rare diseases).

3.7.3.5 Hypocretin/Orexin Antagonists

Orexin A and B, also known as hypocretin A and B, are peptides that are released in the lateral hypothalamus and are important in maintenance of wakefulness. The loss of orexin-producing neurons occurs often narcolepsy; a sleep disorder with increased sleepiness during the day (see ▶ Chap. 5.1). Because orexin is crucial in the control of wakefulness, a blockade of orexin receptors promotes sleep.

Suvorexant, an orexin receptor antagonist, was FDA approved in the USA for treating insomnia. Suvorexant is effective in doses of 10 and 20 mg as antagonist of the orexin receptors in the hypothalamus and thus increases sleepiness. Suvorexant provides a completely new mode of action for pharmaceutical insomnia treatment. Several clinical trials, suvorexant reduced sleep latency and and the time awake after sleep onset compared to placebo. Significant negative effects after discontinuation of the drug were not observed. Suvorexant was not compared to other hypnotics in empirical studies. It is not yet available on the European market.

3.7.3.6 Second-line Hypnotics

Second-line hypnotics include *sedating antidepressants* and *low-potency neuroleptics* that can be applied in chronic insomnia. Another application are insomnia disorders co-morbid with addiction in the medical history. Within combination therapeutic regimes, second-line hypnotics are used in severe cases of refractory insomnia disorders. If the insomnia disorder is co-morbid to a mental disorder, second-line hypnotics are applied to improve the mental disorder that might be partly responsible for the insomnia symptoms.

There is a trend in many countries to treat short-term insomnia and chronic insomnia with sedating antidepressants. In the past 15 years, the percentage of hypnotics (including BZD and BZRA) decreased by more than 50% because of the use of second-line hypnotics. This might be explained by the well-known addiction risk in long-term application of hypnotics. Many second-line hypnotics are effective in insomnia disorders; however, they are not always approved for this indication.

The sedating effect of most second-line hypnotics is based on the high affinity to the central histamine H_1 receptor and also the effect on the serotonergic and norepinephrine system. At the same time, they have an anxiolytic and soothing effect and thus can promote sleep.

Antidepressants

The current clinical data on the effectiveness of antidepressants (Table 3.8) in insomnia are not very extensive. Studies show a sleep-inducing and sleep-maintaining effect of trimipramine, doxepin, amitriptyline, piperazine, mirtazapine, opipramol, and trazodone if applicated for 4 weeks. The sleep-promoting effect is achieved with a much lower dose than it is needed for the treatment of depressive disorders, which has also a positive impact on the rate of side effects , i.e., side effects are quite rare. The characteristic side effects consist of hangover in the morning, low blood pressure, libido problems, xerostomia, weight gain, constipation, urinary retention, glaucoma, and cardiac arhythmias. In the USA, trazodone is one of the most frequently prescribed second-line hypnotic because hangover in the morning emerge are rare as the half-life of trazedone is short. Meta-analyses documented that the positive effects of sedating antidepressants are less pronounced than those of BZDs and BZRAs. Amitriptyline, doxepin, and trimipramine reach their maximum serum concentration after 1.5–6 h following oral intake and have a half-life of 10–50 h.

Table 3.8 Sedating antidepressants as second-line hypnotics

Substance	Half-life (h)	Evening dose (mg)[a]
Trimipramine	15–40	5–100
Doxepin	10–30	3–100
Amitriptyline	16–40	25–100
Mirtazapine	20–40	3.75–15
Trazodone	4–8	25–100
Opipramol	6–11	25–150
Agomelatine	1–2	25–50

Cave: Antidepressants are not approved for the treatment of insomnia disorders in many countries
[a]Usual evening dose in mg

In addition, studies also indicate important substance-specific side effects that have to be taken into consideration. The clinically relevant anticholinergic side effects, e.g., xerostomia, constipation, and accommodation anomalies must be considered. Due to relatively long half-lives plasma concentrations can add up and result in delirium or cognitive problems the anticholinergic effect, especially in older patients.

Regarding doxepin, recent studies showed a positive effect on sleep using very small doses of 3 mg in older and 6 mg in middle-aged patients over a period of at least 4 weeks. Because of the low dose, the aforementioned side effects occur less frequently.

Agomelatine is the first melatonergic antidepressant: it works as an MT_1/MT_2 agonist and $5\text{-}HT_{2C}$ antagonist. Besides its antidepressant effect, several trials indicated a positive effect on sleep and circadian rhythm. It is important to know that agomelatine should be taken while "sitting on the edge of the bed" without any physical activity or exposure to light before going to sleep. Because of its different mode of action, the side effects typical of other antidepressants such as xerostomia, weight gain, reduced libido, and hangover in the morning have not yet been described.

Practical Tip

During initial application of sedating antidepressants, a sedating effect can be observing during the daytime for up to 2 weeks. To improve the patient's compliance, stepwise dose increases of the antidepressant are recommended.

Neuroleptics

Sedating, low-potency neuroleptics can also be applied for the treatment of insomnia disorders: they play a major role in the treatment of insomnia disorders in older persons that

Table 3.9 Low-potency neuroleptics as second-line hypnotics

Substance	Half-life (h)	Evening dose (mg)[a]
Melperone	4–6	25–100
Pipamperone	3	20–120
Perazine	35	10–100
Levomepromazine	16–78	5–50
Quetiapine	12	25–75
Olanzapine	20–54	2.5–20
Promethazine	10–12	10–100
Prothipendyl	2.5	40–120

Note: In different countries, the different compounds have different approval for the treatment of insomnia
[a]Usual evening dose

are characterized by excitation in the evening or at night. Overall, lower doses are required than for the treatment of psychotic disorders (Table 3.9). Neuroleptics such as promethazine have a positive impact on sleep because of their antihistaminergic effect. In many other neuroleptics such as quetiapine and olanzapine antagonistic effects on dopaminergic, serotonergic, muscarinic-cholinergic, and adrenergic receptors are also involved. Risk of developing extrapyramidal side effects is minor as most of the compounds showing low potency. However, treatment options have to be evaluated for each individual because of the nonzero risk of extrapyramidal symptoms.

The most frequently observed side effects of low-potency neuroleptics are low blood pressure, hangover, xerostomia, constipation, urinary retention, increased appetite, and weight gain.

Overall, the scientific data base is not very solid, despite clinically experience showed positive effects in insomnia. Similar observations were reported for atypical antipsychotics such as olanzapine and quetiapine that have been studied as a treatment option in insomnia disorders.

Table 3.10 Antihistamines as secondary hypnotics

Substance	Half-life (h)	Evening dose (mg)[a]
Diphenhydramine	4–6	50–100
Doxylamine	7–9	25–50

[a]Usual evening dose

Antihistamines

The antihistamines doxylamine and diphenhydramine are over-the-counter drugs. Comparable to antihistamines that are only available by prescription, their sedating effect is based on the antagonism at the central histamine H_1 receptors.

Solid scientific evidence of their effectiveness in cases of insomnia is lacking: no meta-analyses are available and no randomized placebo-controlled trials. The hypnotic effect might be minor; the velocity of 2–3 h for reaching peak concentration is clearly slower than that of BZRAs. An early intake in regard to the usual bed time is required. The half-lives correspond to those of some BZDs (Table 3.10). Habituation with loss of effectiveness after several days or weeks is frequently observed. Polysomnographic studies have not been carried out. In older patients, anticholinergic side effects may cause impaired cognitive functioning. As these drugs are freely available, special attention must be paid to interactions with hypnotics, antidepressants, neuroleptics, antiepileptics, opioids, and anticholinergics.

Alcohol Derivatives

The alcohol derivative named chloral hydrate synthesized by Justus von Liebig in 1832 was first systematically investigated as a hypnotic in 1869. Its sleep-promoting effect in dosages of 250–1000 mg with a half-life of 7–9 h was demonstrated. Because of its limited therapeutic spectrum (toxic in higher dosages) and high addiction risk, chloral hydrate is no longer recommended.

Like chloral hydrate, clomethiazole (distraneurin) belongs to the sedatives of the alcohol derivatives. It is applied in the treatment of deliri-

3

ous syndromes. Because of its sedating properties and its half-life of 3–5 h, it can also be applied as a hypnotic, especially in geriatric patients. For patients with day–night reversals, it is the medication of choice. With small doses of 50–250 mg, nighttime sleep can be induced. The addiction risk of clomethiazole, however, is quite high.

Phytotherapeutics

Many herbal products are used for alleviating insomnia symptoms.

The effectiveness of herbal products, mostly combinations of valerian, hop, melissa, St. John's wort, and others, has not sufficiently demonstrated. The few effectiveness studies that are available showed severe methodical limitations. Four meta-analyses indicated a small superiority of valerian compared to placebo. In severe insomnia with increased arousal levels in the evening, the calming and sedating effect of phytotherapeutics might not be strong enough. Except for valerian, polysomnographic studies do not show any relevant effect of phytotherapeutics on sleep parameters. Several studies, however, indicated subjective sleep improvements. For valerian, a review of 19 controlled trials showed that, the results of these studies are contradictory, so that no recommendation may be given.

Practical Tip

Despite the lack of clinical evidence of their effectiveness on measurable sleep parameters, phytotherapeutics may be perceived as subjectively helpful and sleep promoting by patients. However, sleep centers that usually treat severe insomnia disorders should be very careful in recommending phytotherapeutics.

3.8 Questions

1. Which types of insomnia can be classified?
2. Please describe the most important psychodynamic characteristics of the subtype of "psychophysiological insomnia" of chronic insomnia.
3. What are the basic principles that have to be taken into consideration before initiating drug treatment?
4. Which sleep medication types are available for the treatment of primary insomnia? Please state the pros and cons of each type.
5. Please describe the elements of cognitive-behavioral insomnia therapy.

Further Reading

1. American Academy of Sleep Medicine. International classification of sleep disorders, vol 3. Aufl.: Diagnostic and coding manual. Westchester: American Academy of Sleep Medicine; 2014.
2. American Academy of Sleep Medicine. The AASM-manual for the scoring of sleep and associated events: rules, terminology and technical specifications. Version 2.3. Darien: American Academy of Sleep Medicine; 2016.
3. Anothaisintawee T, Reutrakul S, Van Cauter E, Thakkinstian A. Sleep disturbances compared to traditional risk factors for diabetes development: systematic review and meta-analysis. Sleep Med Rev. 2015;30:11–24.
4. Baglioni C, Battagliese G, Feige B, Spiegelhalder K, Nissen C, Voderholzer U, Lombardo C, Riemann D. Insomnia as a predictor of depression: a meta-analytic evaluation of longitudinal epidemiological studies. J Affect Disord. 2011;135:10–9.
5. Benca RM, Obermeyer WH, Thisted RA, Gillin JC. Sleep and psychiatric disorders. A meta-analysis. Arch Gen Psychiatry. 1992;49(8):651–70. https://doi.org/10.1001/archpsyc.1992.01820080059010.
6. Chen X, Beydoun MA, Wang Y. Is sleep duration associated with childhood obesity? A systematic review and meta-analysis. Obesity. 2008;16:265–74.
7. Hajak G, Riemann D. Diagnose und Therapie von Schlafstörungen. Neurologe Psychiater. 2008;9:21–31.
8. Hoffmann F, Scharffetter W, Glaeske G. Verbrauch von Zolpidem und Zopiclon auf Privatrezepten zwischen 1993 und 2007. Nervenarzt. 2009;80:578–83.
9. Hoffmann F. Benefits and risks of benzodiazepines and Z-drugs: comparison of perceptions of GPs and community pharmacists in Germany. Ger Med Sci. 2013;11:1–7.
10. Hohagen F, Rink K, Käppler C, Schramm E, Riemann D, Weyerer S, Berger M. Prevalence and treatment of insomnia in general practice. A longitudinal study. Eur Arch Psychiatry Clin Neurosci. 1993;242(6):329–36.
11. Kryger M, Roth T, Dement WC. Principles and practice of sleep medicine. Philadelphia: Elsevier; 2017.
12. Mayer, et al. S3-Leitlinie Nicht-erholsamer Schlaf/Schlafstörungen. Somnologie. 2009;13(suppl. 1):1–160.

13. Morin CM, Bélanger L, LeBlanc M, Ivers H, Savard J, Espie CA, Mérette C, Baillargeon L, Grégoire J-P. The natural history of insomnia. Arch Intern Med. 2009;169:447–53.
14. Ohayon MM. Epidemiology of insomnia: what we know and what we still need to learn. Sleep Med Rev. 2002;6(2):97–111.
15. Peter H, Penzel T, Peter J-H. Enzyklopädie der Schlafmedizin. Heidelberg: Springer; 2007.
16. Riemann D, Baum E, Cohrs S, Crönlein T, Hajak G, Hertenstein E, Klose J, Langhorst MG, Nissen C, Pollmächer T, Rabstein S, Schlarb A, Sitter H, Weeß H-G, Wetter T, Spiegelhalder K. S3-Leitlinie Nicht erholsamer Schlaf/Schlafstörungen Kapitel "Insomnie bei Erwachsenen" (AWMFRegisternummer 063-003). Update 2016. Somnologie. 2017; https://doi.org/10.1007/s11818-016-0097-x.
17. Sexton CE, Storsve AB, Walhovd KB, et al. Poor sleep quality is associated with increased cortical atrophy in community-dwelling adults. Neurology. 2014;83:967–73.
18. Schlack R, Hapke U, Maske U, et al. Häufigkeit und Verteilung von Schlafproblemen und Insomnie in der deutschen Erwachsenenbevölkerung. Bundesgesundheitsbl. 2013;56:740. https://doi.org/10.1007/s00103-013-1689-2.
19. Weeß H-G. Die schlaflose Gesellschaft. Stuttgart: Schattauer-Verlag; 2016.
20. Weeß H-G, editor. Update Schlafmedizin. Bremen: UniMed Verlag; 2015.
21. Yaffe K, Falvey CM, Hoang T. Connections between sleep and cognition in older adults. Lancet Neurol. 2014;13:1017–28.

Sleep-Related Breathing Disorders

B. A. Stuck and J. T. Maurer

B. A. Stuck et al., *Practice of Sleep Medicine*, https://doi.org/10.1007/978-3-030-17412-5_4

Sleep-related breathing disorders (SRBD) can be classified into breathing disorders with and without obstruction of the upper airway; furthermore, the third edition of the ICSD again lists snoring within the SRBD. Even if there is important overlapping regarding diagnosis and treatment the diseases are very different with regard to their etiology and pathogenesis. In particular, obstructive sleep-related breathing disorders are a widespread phenomenon. Not only the disease itself but also the public perception of obstructive sleep apnea has increased in the past decades. Snoring of adults is of even higher prevalence and nearly ubiquitous in the media.

4.1 Breathing Disorders without Obstruction

Sleep-related breathing disorders without obstruction of the upper airway are subdivided into central sleep apnea syndromes, sleep-related hypoventilation syndromes, and sleep-related hypoxemia.

Central sleep apnea syndromes are characterized by an increased or reduced respiratory drive by which the control loop of breathing induces an alternation between hyperventilation and apnea. The best known type is Cheyne-Stokes respiration. The complaints regarding the central sleep apnea syndrome are rather minor and unspecific. A negative impact of the central sleep apnea syndromes on the mortality of the patients is most probable; however, it is not yet confirmed for all of them.

Sleep-related hypoventilation syndromes are characterized by sleep-related insensitivity toward CO_2, a primary weakness of the respiratory muscles, or by chronic overload of the respiratory pump leading to hypercapnia with or without hypoxemia during sleep. Relevant triggers are severe restrictive and obstructive pulmonary ventilation disorders of various geneses as well as obesity. Primary types are very rare. Because of the underlying disease, the prognosis is mostly poor, and additionally it is influenced in a negative way by the breathing disorder.

Sleep-related hypoxemia is different from the last-mentioned disease by the presence of hypoxemia without simultaneous hypoventilation. It is typically caused by pulmonary or neurological deficits. Frequently, it is accompanied by respiratory partial insufficiency and pulmonary hypertension that determine the prognosis.

4.1.1 Definitions

Sleep-related breathing disorders without obstruction of the upper airway include diseases that are based on different disorders of ventilatory control and mechanics.

These disorders are characterized by intermittent decrease of the respiratory effort of variable duration with a nonobstructed upper airway. In this aspect, they are relevantly different from obstructive sleep apnea (see ▶ Sect. 4.2) that, however, may be found simultaneously as additional breathing disorder.

In the ICSD-3, sleep-related breathing disorders without obstruction are thus classified:

- Central sleep apnea syndromes
- Sleep-related hypoventilation syndromes
- Sleep-related hypoxemia

In all groups, primary (sometimes congenital) as well as secondary types can also be differentiated.

Periodic breathing is defined as the regular sequence of respiration and breathing interruption with constant duration of the cycle over a period of several minutes. However, this term is not exactly defined under all aspects, and different authors use it in different contexts. According to the ICSD-3, this term is exclusively used for breathing in high altitudes.

Classification of Sleep-Related Breathing Disorders without Obstruction of the Upper Airway Adapted from the American Academy of Sleep Medicine (AASM)

1. Central sleep apnea syndromes
   (a) Primary types
   - Primary central sleep apnea
   - Primary central sleep apnea of infancy (see ▶ Chap. 11)
   - Primary central sleep apnea of prematurity (see ▶ Chap. 11)

(b) Secondary types
- Central sleep apnea with Cheyne-Stokes respiration
- Central sleep apnea without Cheyne-Stokes respiration
- Periodic breathing at high altitudes
- Central sleep apnea caused by medication or other substances
- Treatment-emergent central sleep apnea

2. Sleep-related hypoventilation syndromes
   (a) Primary types
   - Congenital central alveolar hypoventilation syndrome (see ▶ Chap. 11)
   - Idiopathic central alveolar hypoventilation

   (b) Secondary types
   - Caused by organic disease
   - Caused by medication or substances
   - Obesity hypoventilation syndrome
   - Late-onset central alveolar hypoventilation (see ▶ Chap. 11)
3. Sleep-related hypoxemia

Regarding pediatric breathing disorders, see ▶ Chap. 11. For exact definition of single respiratory events, see ▶ Chap. 2.

4.1.1.1 Central Sleep Apnea Syndromes

Central sleep apnea syndromes are characterized by intermittently reduced or reflectively increased respiratory drive that leads to continuous alternation of hyperventilation and hypoventilation up to central apnea. The number of central respiratory events has to outweigh the obstructive events.

To diagnose the *primary type* of adult central sleep apnea, five or more central apneas or hypopneas per hour of sleep and the exclusion of the secondary type are required, plus one of the clinical symptoms (daytime sleepiness, insomnia, awakenings with dyspnea).

Because of its pathognomonic breathing pattern, the *Cheyne-Stokes respiration* has a special position within the *secondary types*. At least five central apneas or hypopneas per hour of sleep are required that occur during the characteristic crescendo–decrescendo pattern of the airflow curve and are associated with arousals and sleep fragmentation. For exact definition of the breathing pattern, see ▶ Chap. 2. Insomnia as well as hypersomnia complaints or awakenings with dyspnea may be reported.

An association with a severe disease is required; most frequently, these are manifest heart failure, atrial fibrillation, stroke, or, more rarely, renal failure. The length of the cycle from one ventilation maximum to the next is typically longer than 45 s, which may be used in unclear cases as a differentiation from other central breathing disorders.

Periodic breathing at high altitudes regularly occurs at 4000 m above sea level and can sometimes be already observed at 2500 m above sea level. It mostly occurs in the first night after the climb and is observed nearly exclusively during non-rapid eye movement (non-REM) sleep. The typical respiration pattern is characterized by periodically recurring apneas, mostly without crescendo–decrescendo pattern, in intervals of 12–34 s.

A *secondary central sleep apnea without Cheyne-Stokes respiration* generally occurs as a sequela of brainstem damage (e.g., Arnold-Chiari malformation, stroke).

The diagnosis of *central sleep apnea caused by medication or other substances* requires at least five central apneas or hypopneas without crescendo–decrescendo respiration pattern. Furthermore, long-acting opioids (legal substances such as methadone, retarded morphine, or illegal opiates) have to be consumed over a longer period. Other breathing disorders such as hypoventilation or Biot's respiration do not preclude the diagnosis.

The term *treatment-emergent sleep apnea* defines an originally predominant obstructive sleep apnea in which central apneas occur or aggravate after elimination of the obstructive respiratory events [e.g., from continuous positive airway pressure (CPAP) therapy]. In most cases, it regresses within the first months of therapy. The presence of another type of central sleep apnea excludes the diagnosis.

4.1.1.2 Sleep-Related Hypoventilation and Hypoxemia Syndrome

These sleep-related breathing disorders are defined by reduced ventilation over longer periods during sleep, leading to hypercapnia without or with hypoxemia (definition of hypoventilation, see Sect. 2.7.8). Hypoventilation and its blood gas alterations are first seen or aggravated in REM sleep.

If no underlying disease can be found to explain the episodes of hypoventilation, it is termed *sleep-related idiopathic central alveolar hypoventilation.*

Sleep-related hypoventilation caused by organic disease is found in cases of disturbed pulmonary gas exchange based on an interstitial parenchyma or vascular lesion as well as chronic obstructive pulmonary disease or in cases of neurogenic degeneration or dystrophy of the respiratory muscles (e.g., Duchenne muscle dystrophy) or an insufficient compliance of the thoracic wall (e.g., kyphoscoliosis). In former times, the term of overlap syndrome was used when obstructive sleep apnea occurred simultaneously with sleep-related hypoventilation in the context of chronic obstructive pulmonary disease (COPD). This unspecific and confusing term should no longer be used. Instead, the statement of both single diagnoses is preferred.

If substances, for example, muscle relaxants or long-acting sedatives, attenuate the respiratory center, *sleep-related hypoventilation from medication or other substances* may result.

For the first time, the separate diagnosis of *obesity hypoventilation syndrome* is listed; hereby the hypoventilation is induced by obesity [body mass index (BMI) >30 kg/m^2]. It is the only sleep-related hypoventilation syndrome of which the diagnosis requires hypercapnia during daytime ($PaCO_2$ >45 mmHg) beside hypoventilation during sleep.

In the ICSD-3, sleep-related hypoxemia without simultaneous hypercapnia was differentiated from hypoventilation syndromes. A frequent cause for this constellation is an alveolar diffusion disorder with compensatory hyperventilation. To determine the diagnosis, the oxygen saturation has to be reduced to 88% or less for more than 5 min. It is controversially discussed if it was adequate to create a separate subcategory of the sleep-related breathing disorders.

In the context of sleep-related hypoventilation and hypoxemia syndromes, also the term *chronic respiratory insufficiency* has to be defined.

- The early form is characterized by hypercapnia and hypoxemia that are only found during REM sleep and/or physical strain.
- The manifest chronic respiratory insufficiency, however, is characterized by pathological blood gases already at rest during daytime and during the entire sleep time, independent from the sleep stages.

Practical Tip

The presence of sleep-related breathing disorder does not exclude the synchronous existence of another disorder, which naturally makes diagnosis very difficult. In particular, the differentiation of mild obstructive sleep apnea from snoring may be difficult when at the same time central sleep apnea or sleep-related hypoventilation or hypoxemia syndrome is observed that by definition causes desaturation.

4.1.2 Etiology and Pathophysiology

4.1.2.1 Regulation of Breathing

The functions of breathing during sleep are basically the same as during wakefulness:

- Uptake of oxygen
- Elimination of carbon dioxide
- Stabilization of the acid–base balance

The pulmonary parenchyma, the airways, and the muscular respiratory pump command a large reserve capacity to fulfill these tasks under different conditions (e.g., rest, physical strain, high altitude, diseases).

The regulation of breathing occurs unconsciously, but it can also be cortically overlaid. The respiratory neurons in the brainstem generate the respiratory pattern and determine the necessary respiratory minute volume. Furthermore, they are responsible for the time-coordinated activation of respiratory and the auxiliary respiratory muscles as well as the airway muscles. These neurons reach the relevant afferent nerve pathways from peripheral (primarily oxygen dependent) and central (primarily CO_2 dependent) chemoreceptors, stretch receptors (in particular, thoracic wall), mechanoreceptors (in particular, respiratory muscles), thermoreceptors, and higher central nervous system centers.

The complex regulatory cycle of breathing is basically identical during sleep and wakefulness (see ◘ Fig. 4.1). Thus, it is clear that respiration may be disturbed by many extrinsic and intrinsic factors by which the breathing pattern and/or the blood gases are modified pathologically.

Ventilation mostly depends linearly on the partial pressure of CO_2. An increasing arterial

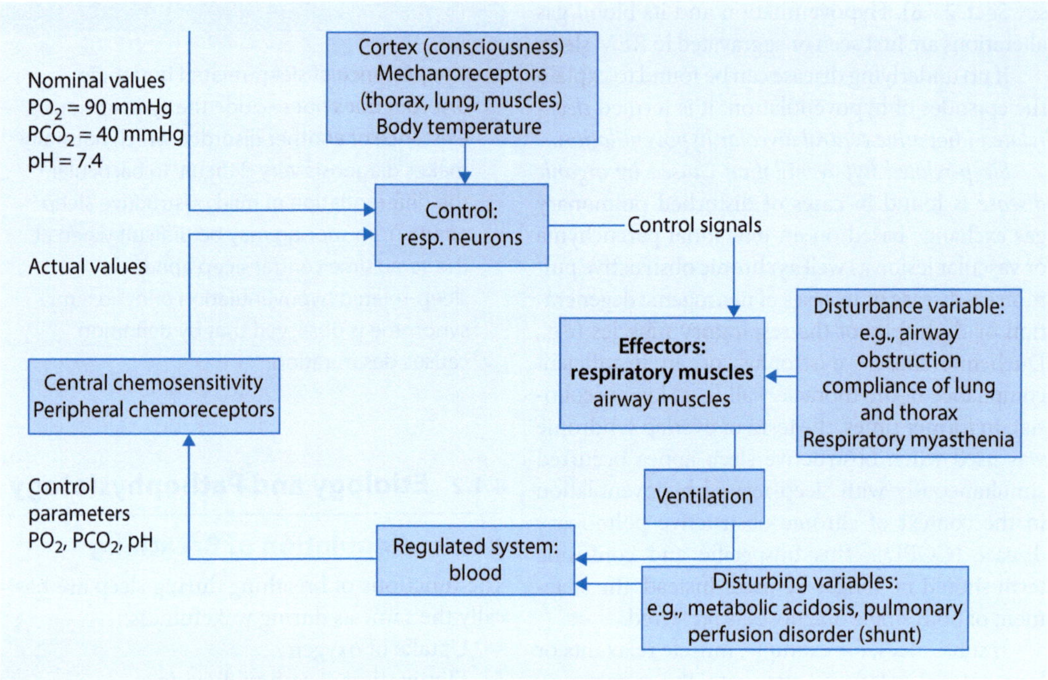

Fig. 4.1 Regulatory cycle of breathing

partial pressure of CO_2 increases the respiratory drive and as a consequence the ventilation. If the pCO_2 drops below a certain value, central apnea is induced. This hypocapnic apnea threshold is individually different. Apnea, however, is mostly avoided in the wakeful state by additional alertness stimuli.

The arterial partial pressure of CO_2 is kept constant at a value of almost exactly 40 mmHg by means of the CO_2 dependent respiratory response. The respiratory response to CO_2 is the stronger the lower the arterial pH value or the partial pressure of O_2 is at the same time. Thus, an identical increase of the arterial partial pressure of CO_2 with lower pH and/or partial pressure of O_2 leads to higher increase of ventilation. In wakefulness, respiration is further modulated by different factors (alertness stimuli) that are subject to consciousness (e.g., speaking) or that take place unconsciously (e.g., emotions). Regarding further details, the authors refer to general textbooks of physiology.

Even if the chemosensory regulation of breathing during sleep is not basically different compared to the awake condition, physiological changes of the control parameters contribute to unstable breathing during sleep. Discontinuation of the alertness stimuli finally, even in healthy individuals, causes numerous alterations of breathing to be observed (see Table 4.1).

The reduced breathing and respiratory minute volume are of particular importance, resulting in an increased end-tidal (at the end of expiration) partial pressure of CO_2 by about 2–3 mmHg, sometimes even 8 mmHg, in non-REM sleep. The hypocapnic apnea threshold is about 2–6 mmHg below the eucapnic pCO_2 during sleep and thus nearly corresponds to the arterial partial pressure of CO_2 in wakefulness. This shift of the nominal values during sleep onset causes irregularities of the respiratory drive with the consequence of physiological central hypopneas and apneas.

The graphs of the CO_2 breathing response during sleep run flat compared to wakefulness. The identical increase of the partial pressure of CO_2 leads to the lowest ventilatory response during REM sleep, increased response during deep sleep, and highest response during light sleep. Besides the CO_2 breathing response, the apnea threshold and the end-tidal partial pressure of CO_2 also depend on the sleep stage.

Table 4.1 Physiological changes of breathing during the transition to non-REM sleep or REM sleep

Parameter	Alteration	Alteration
	Awake → non-REM	Non-REM → REM
Respiratory minute volume	↓	↓→
Breathing volume	↓	↓
Breathing rate	↑↓	→
Inspiration time	↑↓→	↑↓→
Expiration time	↑↓→	↑↓→
Pulmonary compliance	↓	→
Functional residual capacity	↓	→
End-tidal CO_2	↑	↓→
Muscular inspiration force	↑	→
Diaphragmatic pressure	↑	↓
Intercostal activity	↑	↓
Diaphragmatic activity	↑→	↑
Coordination (extrathoracic, intrathoracic, abdominal)	↓	↓
Airflow	↓	
Airway resistance	↑↑↑	→
Genioglossus EMG	↑	↓→

↓ = Decrease, ↑ = Increase, → = no change

Beside the control parameters, the basic activity of the breathing muscles also changes. During non-REM sleep, the activity of the diaphragm and the intercostal muscles increases. During REM sleep, respiration is almost entirely performed by the diaphragm, which favors hypoventilation. Further, the increase of the airflow resistance during sleep of more than 200% is of high relevance for the development of obstructive sleep apnea as well as hypoventilation syndrome.

The change of body position from the sitting to the lying position also influences breathing. In a lying position, the contribution of the diaphragm to breathing significantly increases in relationship to the thoracic and auxiliary respiratory muscles.

The manifold physiological changes of breathing during sleep indicate that in the case of occurrence of predisposing diseases, many breathing disorders first develop during sleep, or are unmasked or aggravated. For central apneas, this is especially true during non-REM sleep, whereas REM sleep is especially susceptible for hypoventilation.

4.1.2.2 Central Sleep Apnea Syndrome

During sleep, the arterial partial pressure of CO_2 is the dominating breathing stimulus. The physiological increase of the nominal value for the partial pressure of CO_2 and the hypocapnic apnea threshold, as well as the reduced respiratory response during sleep, require an adaptation of the control cycle of breathing during sleep onset.

The hypocapnic apnea threshold and the increase of the CO_2 respiratory response itself, as well as the differences between wake and sleep stage, differ between individuals. Patients with a CO_2 apnea threshold that is near the CO_2 nominal value rather tend to drop below this limit value due to small changes in ventilation. During sleep onset, the increase of the nominal value of the partial pressure of CO_2 from 40 to about 45 mmHg causes a relative hypocapnia that leads to a reduction of ventilation and thus an increase of the partial pressure of CO_2. Patients with a CO_2-driven ventilatory overshoot drop very easily below the CO_2 apnea threshold, and central apnea develops. The partial pressure of CO_2 again increases during the apnea until the apnea threshold is exceeded by 1–4 mmHg CO_2. Arousal is typically associated with the onset of breathing. Hereby, the nominal value of the partial pressure of CO_2 is switched shortly to the value of the wake state (40 mmHg). The response to the associated relative hypercapnia causes another increase of ventilation. The normalization of the blood gases of the still-awake patient allows the person to fall asleep again. The de novo shift of the nominal values for hypocapnic apnea threshold and partial pressure of CO_2 in combination with the significant decrease of the partial pressure of CO_2 already induced by the arousal triggers the next respiratory irregularity.

If the patients overcome light sleep, the incidence of central breathing disorders decreases. In deep sleep, the relevantly increased arousal threshold is made responsible; in REM sleep it is the reduced CO_2 respiratory response. However, it is not yet clear whether leaving light sleep is necessary for the development of more stable breathing or, vice versa, if the development of regular breathing allows the transition to deep sleep. A large variety of organic diseases may trigger and maintain the described mechanisms; in many cases, however, the exact pathogenetic correlations are still unknown.

In the context of *Cheyne-Stokes respiration*, the prolonged circulation time with manifest heart failure is another destabilizing factor. Therefore, the detection of the altered blood gas values by central CO_2 receptors is delayed. It has become obvious that the output of the left heart is inversely proportional to the cycle length from one ventilation maximum to the next. The pulmonary edema that is frequently observed in left-sided heart failure stimulates vagal afferent nerve pathways and further increases the chemosensitivity. Regarding the current concept of the complex interactions, see ◘ Fig. 4.2.

Respiration at high altitudes shows a different pathophysiology. When a person climbs to an altitude of 2500 m above sea level, the inspiratory oxygen partial pressure decreases to such an extent that hypoxemia can only be avoided when the respiratory minute volume is increased. With increasing altitude and decreasing oxygen partial pressure in the environmental air, the increased ventilation leads to respiratory alkalosis. Despite the increased respiratory minute volume, the arterial oxygen saturation decreases to about 80% at an altitude of 4000 m above sea level.

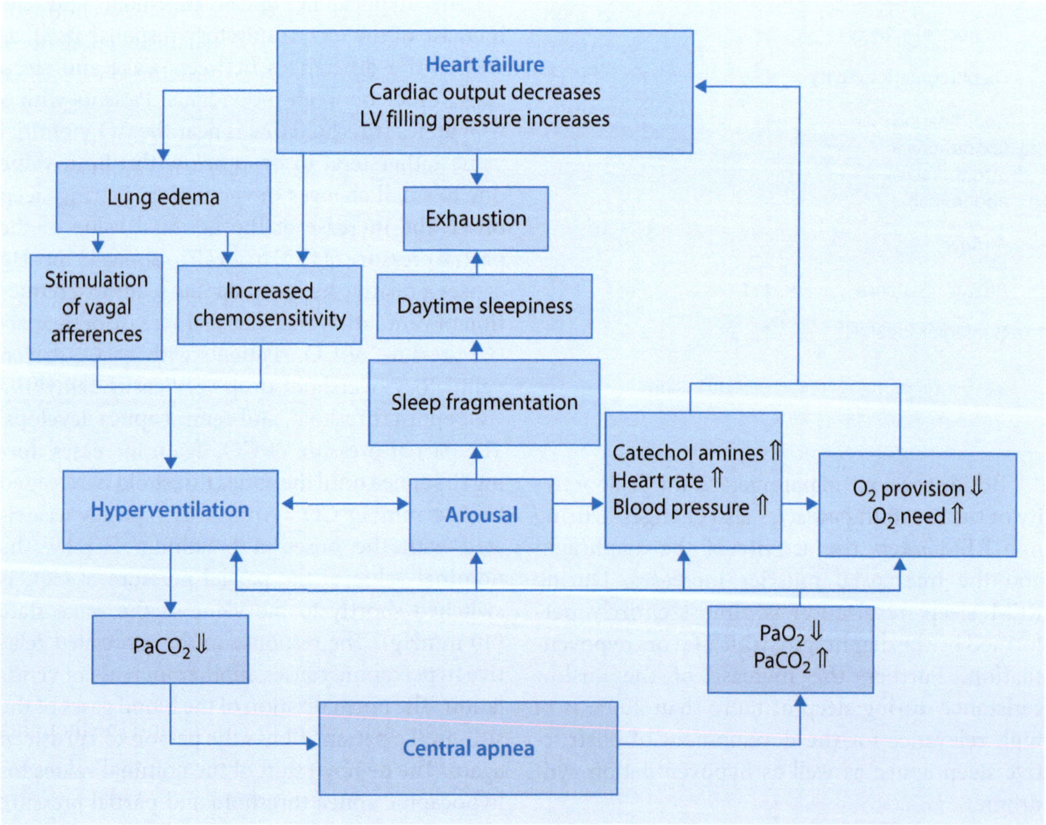

◘ **Fig. 4.2** Influences of left-sided heart failure on breathing and sleep

During sleep, breathing is destabilized by the hypoxic respiratory stimulation and the consecutive hypocapnic inhibition, which is seen in the periodic respiration pattern. As the cardiac function is generally not impaired, cycles are significantly shorter, with 12–34 s, compared to Cheyne-Stokes respiration. Respiratory alkalosis is metabolically compensated within a few days so that the respiratory drive is no longer inhibited.

Over longer periods, polyglobulia is induced by hypoxia, which may reduce or even eliminate periodic breathing at altitudes up to 4500 m above sea level. If an altitude-related pulmonary edema occurs in the context of further climbing, the probability to develop periodic breathing increases further.

Practical Tip

Unstable breathing with central apnea develops or is maintained based on an increased CO_2 chemosensitivity, an accumulation of arousal reactions, and reflex apneas upon different stimuli.

The numerous factors that in single cases may contribute to the development of central apneas during sleep are summarized in the following overview.

Etiology of Central Apneas During Sleep

- Direct functional change of the chemoreceptors
- Degenerative diseases of the central nervous system (CNS), for example, Shy-Drager syndrome
- Diabetic polyneuropathy
- Brainstem lesions
  - Tumors near the brainstem
  - Brainstem infarction
  - Brainstem bleeding
  - Encephalitis
- Increased intracranial pressure
  - Traumatic brain injury
  - Brain tumors
  - Encephalitis
- Chronic consumption of long-acting opioids during at least 3 months
- Idiopathic hypersensitivity of the chemoreceptors
- Arousal induced
  - Movement disorders, for example, periodic limb movement
  - Spontaneous vigilance fluctuations when falling asleep
  - Insomnias of different origins
  - Respiratory arousals with obstructive sleep apnea
- Triggering factors of reflex central apneas
  - Impairment of nasal mechanoreceptors in the context of nasal obstruction or oral breathing
  - Laryngeal stimulation, for example, by gastrolaryngeal reflux
  - Pharyngeal stimulation by negative pharyngeal intraluminal pressure in supine position or during sleep onset
  - Hypoxia-related hyperventilation at high altitudes
  - Pulmonary congestion and vagal stimulation

4.1.2.3 Hypoventilation or Hypoxemia Syndromes

Regular breathing can only be assured when the inhaled air reaches a healthy pulmonary parenchyma, in a normally shaped bony thorax, with adequate CNS breathing stimulation and neuromuscular signal transfer to the functioning respiratory muscles. If one of these components is disturbed and if this disorder cannot be compensated by the organism, finally a reduced uptake of oxygen is always observed as well as reduced elimination of carbon dioxide, leading to a shift of the pH value into the acid range.

In cases of *congenital hypoventilation syndrome* (see ▶ Chap. 11) as well as *idiopathic central alveolar hypoventilation*, a reduced sensitivity to CO_2 is observed, leading to the tolerance of reduced respiration with hypercapnia (respiratory insufficiency) without increasing ventilation. A lesion of the medullar chemoreceptors is assumed as the origin in the idiopathic form without being confirmed. Increased intracerebral pressure or CNS depressant drugs may also lead to functional impairment of the chemoreceptors and thus to hypoventilation. In these cases, the key pathophysiological mechanism consists of a missing central respiratory drive despite a primarily well working respiratory pump.

Respiratory insufficiency may occur as the result of primary weakness as well as exhaustion of the respiratory muscles because of increased strain of the respiratory pump even if the central respiratory drive is adequately present.

4

Origins for *primary respiratory pump weakness* may be such as these:

- Muscular diseases, for example, muscle dystrophy and myopathy
- Neurological diseases, for example, amyotrophic lateral sclerosis and multiple sclerosis
- Neuromuscular disease such as myasthenia gravis

Most common factors leading to *exhaustion of the respiratory pump* are as follows:

- Pulmonary restrictions and obstructions of any type
- Pulmonary perfusion disorders
- Obesity
- Thoracic deformities

Based on the preexisting lesion, absence of the respiratory stimuli of wakefulness during sleep and physiologically coupled reduction of the ventilation are responsible for hypoventilation during sleep. The occurrence of hypoventilation and hypercapnia during sleep is accepted to avoid complete failure of the previously damaged and already maximally stressed respiratory muscles.

The following overview summarizes the particular pathophysiological aspects of hypoventilation in the context of *pulmonary obstruction*, which is the most frequent origin of hypoventilation or hypoxemic syndromes.

Pathophysiological Factors of Sleep-Related Hypoventilation and Hypoxemia with Pulmonary Obstruction (Modified According to Peter et al. 2007)

- Reduced capacity of the respiratory pump
  - Emphysema with dynamic pulmonary hyperinflation
  - Flattening of the diaphragm
  - Impairment of the respiratory muscle capacity caused by hypoxia, hypercapnia, or acidosis
- High stress of the respiratory pump
  - Increased airway resistance
  - Hypersecretion
  - Increased respiratory drive caused by reduced gas-exchange surface
  - Prolonged expiration at the expense of the inspiration time
  - Difficult expiration caused by increased intrinsic positive end expiratory pressure (PEEP) in supine position
- Disturbed physical restoration because of the sleep disorder
  - Repeated arousals
  - Sleep fragmentation

Hypoventilation and hypercapnia occur first and most severely in REM sleep when the diaphragm alone is responsible for all the work of breathing. In cases of impaired diaphragmatic function, for example, a diaphragm in low position because of pulmonary emphysema or unilateral paresis of the diaphragm, the hypoventilation in REM sleep is particularly severe. Later, it extends to the remaining sleep time and finally even the awake stage.

It is assumed that chronic hypercapnia with respiratory acidosis that is metabolically compensated leads to further reduction of the central CO_2 sensitivity and thus further perpetuates hypercapnia.

For all types of hypoventilation, the following statement applies: The severity of the arterial hypercapnia corresponds to the extent of respiratory insufficiency. Hypoventilation is always associated with hypoxemia, and its severity depends on the diffusion properties of the lung. The consequences of progressive blood gas changes are these:

- Pulmonary arterial hypertension, up to pulmonary heart disease
- Polyglobulia
- Cardiac arrhythmia
- Neurocognitive disorders

In that way, it could be confirmed in COPD patients that chronic hypoxemia during sleep contributes significantly to the development of pulmonary arterial hypertension and leads to increased mortality, so that it should be imperatively treated.

Practical Tip

Hypoventilation develops either on the floor of an impaired central CO_2 sensitivity (being able to breathe but not willing to do so) or an impaired respiratory pump (willing to breathe but not being able to do so).

4.1.3 Epidemiology

The incidence of *central sleep apnea syndromes* in the general population is not exactly known. In sleep centers, predominating central sleep apnea dominatin is diagnosed in up to 10% of the patients. However, it must be taken into account that nowadays mostly snoring patients (i.e., patients who suffer rather from obstructive breathing disorders) undergo sleep medical examination. First assessments in high-risk groups reveal central sleep apnea syndromes in 10% of the patients with chronic renal insufficiency and in 24% under chronic opioid therapy. No genetic disposition or high familial incidence is known for central sleep apnea.

Also, data on the incidence of *Cheyne-Stokes respiration* in high-risk cohorts are available. Epidemiological studies state a prevalence of 25 to 40% for patients with heart failure and about 10% for patients with stroke. Cheyne-Stokes respiration is observed more frequently in males than in females and is found nearly exclusively in patients older than 60 years.

Sleep-related *idiopathic central alveolar hypoventilation* is very rare.

No precise data on incidence are available for the more frequently occurring *secondary hypoventilation syndromes*. With a certain severity, they are always present in the context of the underlying diseases. In cases of idiopathic pulmonary hypertension, for example, sleep-related hypoventilation could be found in 75% of cases without consideration of the severity; with a BMI of 50 kg/m^2, an obesity hypoventilation syndrome is found in 50% of the cases.

4.1.4 Clinical Presentation

4.1.4.1 Central Sleep Apnea Syndromes

Central sleep apnea syndromes demonstrate a variable and unspecific clinical presentation that is not surprising in the light of the heterogeneity of the disease group and the variety of predisposing diseases. The predisposing constellations include cardiac and renal failure, cerebral circulatory disturbances, long-term intake of opioids, or residence at high altitudes.

Some patients react on repetitive arousals either with conscious awakening in the sense of disorders of initiating and/or maintaining sleep (insomnia) or with an unconscious sleep fragmentation that manifests only in the form of increased daytime sleepiness (hypersomnia) or tiredness.

Typically, but not obligatorily, affected individuals with insomnia presentation wake up because of dyspnea that generally ceases rapidly after awakening with deep breathing. Often, the bed partner does not even notice the irregular breathing pattern.

In the context of hyperventilation, however, the increased airflow velocity leads to *snoring* because of the turbulences and vibrations of the pharyngeal walls although no breathing noise is heard during regular breathing. It is very likely that the high prevalence of snoring in the adult population often coexists with confirmed central sleep apnea syndrome. Therefore, the symptom of irregular snoring does not at all exclude a central sleep apnea syndrome.

Practical Tip

The symptom of snoring excludes neither the presence of a central sleep apnea syndrome nor the successful elimination of the noise by therapy.

In most cases, disorders in concentration and reduced performance during the daytime are the main complaints. These daytime symptoms, however, are often attributed to the preexisting comorbidities alone without taking into consideration a possible central sleep apnea syndrome.

Because *Cheyne-Stokes respiration* occurs almost exclusively with the presence of a manifest left-sided heart failure or a cerebral insult, the symptoms of the underlying disease are in the focus. In this context, the authors refer to the according manuals of internal medicine and neurology. Rarely is daytime tiredness or even sleepiness the only complaint.

Periodic breathing at high altitudes is the blandest of the four types of altitude sickness occurring with the least altitude difference. It may only manifest with insomnia complaints, increased exhaustibility, headaches, and loss of appetite. Acute altitude sickness with vomiting and impaired diuresis, altitude-related pulmonary edema, and altitude-related cerebral edema, the other three types of this disease, represent life-threatening conditions. Interestingly, neither physical fitness nor smoking nor an individual's age influences the development of altitude sickness.

There are almost no differences regarding the *prognosis and comorbidities* of the central sleep apnea syndromes. Only the cohort of patients suffering from heart failure were examined in this regard. It is considered as evident that Cheyne-Stokes respiration during the daytime is associated with a higher mortality. Some prospective cohort studies have even found increased mortality in patients with heart failure when Cheyne-Stokes respiration occurred exclusively at night. More than 30 central events per hour of sleep are considered as relevant. Because the study results are contradictory, it is not clear if the successful elimination of Cheyne-Stokes respiration reduces mortality.

Practical Tip

The symptoms of central sleep apnea syndrome are typically unspecific; the level of suffering of the patients is mostly low. The significance of central sleep apnea syndromes for general morbidity and mortality is not yet clarified.

4.1.4.2 Hypoventilation or Hypoxemia Syndromes

This group of diseases is always associated with *chronic respiratory insufficiency*.

In the early phase, affected patients notice mostly only a less distinct dyspnea during stress. Symptoms caused by blood gas alterations in REM sleep are the focus.

- Disorders of initiating and maintaining sleep
- Morning headaches
- Daytime sleepiness
- Concentration disorders
- Impaired performance during daytime

Because these symptoms are nonspecific and develop only slowly, patients often do not attribute them to sleep-related breathing disorders. In particular, obese patients explain their complaints by their high body weight.

With the development of manifest chronic respiratory insufficiency, rapid physical exhaustibility during daytime comes to the foreground. The patients are clearly impaired regarding their mobility. Dyspnea in cases of physical strain or even at rest is not obligatory; however, it is often observed. In the further course, secondary polyglobulia, cardiac arrhythmia, and the development of pulmonary heart disease with signs of right-sided heart failure are commonly found. In cases of neuromuscular diseases, furthermore, orthopnea, attenuated coughing, and decreasing phonation time are typical.

The highest number of patients develops hypoventilation on the basis of COPD due to smoking in most cases, pulmonary emphysema is found at the same time. A slight increase in breathing effort, for example, in the context of minor infection of the upper airways, may lead to acute failure of the respiratory pump with severe respiratory acidosis requiring intensive medical treatment. Unfortunately, the condition of many patients only becomes apparent after such a dramatic exacerbation. As smoking is only rarely stopped, the damage to the respiratory pump progresses in most cases. Therefore, the prognosis has to be considered as very poor.

This poor prognosis is true to the same extent for all hypoventilation syndromes, unless the basic disease is reversible. In this context, the *obesity hypoventilation syndrome* has to be mentioned if relevant reduction of body weight is successful. However, it cannot be predicted at which weight an obesity hypoventilation syndrome may occur or can be eliminated by weight reduction.

At very different times of the disease and age, *neuromuscular diseases* lead to respiratory insufficiency. Ventilation therapy may be necessary with birth (spinal muscular atrophy type I), during adolescence (Duchenne muscular dystrophy), in adulthood (myotonic dystrophy), or in older years (spinal muscular atrophy type IV). Initially, amyotrophic lateral sclerosis frequently manifests by acute respiratory insufficiency. Certain diseases from this group, however, are only rarely associated with respiratory insufficiency (e.g., post-polio syndrome, mitochondrial myopathies, central core disease). The weakness of the respiratory muscles, however, impairs not only the respiratory pump but also the power of coughing and thus also bronchial clearance, which significantly influences the prognosis. Therefore, an exact diagnosis of the underlying disease is required to reasonably plan sleep medical and pneumological control intervals.

4.2 Obstructive Sleep-Related Breathing Disorders

Obstructive sleep-related breathing disorders are widely distributed. According to the new classification of the ICSD-3, they are synonymous with obstructive sleep apnea. Based on the increase of the most important risk factor, that is, obesity, further increase may be expected.

Patients suffering from obstructive sleep apnea have a higher cardiovascular risk and are often significantly impaired in their quality of life.

According to the current knowledge, snoring alone, however, is not associated with relevant health-related impairment. The frequently high level of suffering of snoring individuals and the broad distribution emphasize its importance. In the following, obstructive sleep-related breathing disorders of adults are the focus. As pediatric obstructive sleep apnea is still classified as SRBD in the ICSD-3, this disease is discussed in ▶ Chap. 11 (sleep disorders of infancy) (see ▶ Sect. 11.2).

4.2.1 Definitions

In the past, the term obstructive sleep-related breathing disorders summarized obstructive sleep apnea with its different degrees of severity as well as an early type called upper airway resistance syndrome (UARS).

UARS describes a disease that is associated with a pathologically increased resistance of the upper airway leading to respiratory arousal with impairment of the quality of sleep, without being accompanied, however, with noticeable impairment of the airflow curves in the sense of apnea or hypopnea in polysomnography. The broad introduction of dynamic pressure measurement for airflow registration and the increasing understanding of flow limitations, however, have led to a new definition of respiratory events. In this context, the significance of respiratory arousals (RERAs) (▶ Fig. 2.20), which are now also included in the calculation of respiratory events is mentioned. To recognize the respiratory origin of arousals, measurement of the esophageal pressure may be helpful; however, frequently secondary signs of airway obstruction also are found such as flow limitation or increasing snoring that is determined by arousal. Further explanations of the current definition of respiratory events are found in ▶ Chap. 2.

Even if the term of UARS is still broadly distributed, this disease concept has not been pursued in recent years. In the ICSD-2, this syndrome was no longer mentioned and is included in obstructive sleep apnea. The elimination of UARS is consequent because its differentiation from obstructive sleep apnea was finally chosen arbitrarily and there were no relevant differences in diagnostics and therapy.

Not all patients suffering from *obstructive sleep apnea* also complain about subjective symptoms, that is, an obstructive sleep apnea syndrome. In this chapter, the term obstructive sleep apnea is used in a standardized way as it is also found in the current ICSD-3.

Diagnostic Criteria of Obstructive Sleep Apnea According to the American Academy of Sleep Medicine (AASM)

The diagnosis of obstructive sleep apnea can be made when either the conditions A and B or, alternatively, condition C is fulfilled.

A. At least one of the following aspects is found:
   - The patient reports sleepiness, nonrestorative sleep, tiredness, or difficulties of initiating and maintaining sleep.
   - The patient wakes up with breathing interruptions, gasping for breath, or attacks of suffocation.
   - The bed partner or any other observer reports snoring, breathing interruptions, or both during the patient's sleep.
   - The patient is diagnosed with hypertonia, mood swings, cognitive disorder, coronary heart disease,

stroke, heart failure, atrial fibrillation, or type 2 diabetes.

B. Polysomnographic or out-of-center sleep testing (OCST) shows the following conspicuities:
   - Five or more mainly obstructive respiratory events, for example, obstructive or mixed apnea, hypopnea, or RERAs (respiratory effort-related arousal, in the following termed respiratory arousal), per hour of sleep or per hour of monitoring time.

C. Polysomnographic or out-of-center sleep testing shows the following conspicuities:
   - Alternatively, the diagnosis is also confirmed according to the AASM when the following criterion is met:
   - Fifteen or more mainly obstructive respiratory events (e.g., apneas, hypopneas, or RERAs) per hour of sleep or per hour of monitoring time.

Hence, results of out-of-center sleep testing/polysomnography and clinical criteria are important for the diagnosis. Furthermore, not all respiratory events require a clearly definable obstructive genesis that takes into consideration that obstructive sleep apnea is frequently accompanied by central or mixed apneas. The ICSD-3 does not use the term mixed sleep apnea syndrome, which is still applied in many cases.

Compared to the previous version of the ICSD, several innovations are found regarding the diagnostic criteria that are of great significance for the diagnosis of sleep apnea. On one hand, clearly defined comorbidities are found as alternative criteria to clinical symptoms. Thus, in the presence of one of these comorbidities, the diagnosis of obstructive sleep apnea may also be made when more than five respiratory events occur per hour of sleep and the patient, however, does not complain about subjective symptoms. These innovations meet the significance of the mentioned comorbid disorders regarding cardiovascular sequelae of sleep apnea as well as regarding the clinical symptoms and the quality of life of the affected individuals. In addition, this new definition also allows treating (mild) obstructive sleep apnea in those cases in which no symptoms are observed but therapy seems to be indicated because of the (cardiovascular) concomitant disease.

Although polysomnography (PSG) is mentioned as the only objectifying examination procedure in the ICSD-2, the ICSD-3 refers to an alternative "out-of-center sleep testing" (OCST). Accordingly, the limit values for respiratory events refer to the recording time as well as the sleep time. The ICSD-3 recommends using the term respiratory event index (REI) when referring to the OCST and states that OCST is likely to underestimate the severity of the breathing disorders; thus, exclusion of the disease is not possible with OCST alone, especially in the case of clinically suspected obstructive sleep apnea. Respiratory arousal also is not assessed by the OCST. In this way, this new classification significantly upgrades out-of-center sleep testing.

Frequently, the obstructive sleep apnea is classified according to its severity. A binding definition, however, does not exist, and the significance of the subjective symptoms is already reflected in the divided definition of obstructive sleep apnea in the ICSD-3. However, often the following categories are found:

- Mild obstructive sleep apnea with a respiratory disturbance index (RDI) of 5–15
- Moderate obstructive sleep apnea with a RDI of >15–30
- Severe sleep apnea with an index of more than 30

Finally, this classification always remains unsatisfactory so long as it is only oriented to the number of respiratory events and does not take into consideration the complex clinical presentation of the disease.

Practical Tip

The definition of obstructive sleep apnea is oriented by clinical and poly(somno)graphic criteria. The diagnosis, however, can also be made based on the number of respiratory events alone.

4.2.2 Etiology and Pathophysiology

Finally, the origin of obstructive sleep apnea is a functional instability of the upper airway.

During inhalation, the extension of the chest leads to negative pressure in the airways so that the inhaled air may flow into the thorax along this pressure gradient. Although the nose and the lower airways are stabilized by numerous rigid structures (bone, cartilage), the stabilization of the pharyngeal segment of the upper airway mainly depends on muscular structures. In this area, that is, between the choanae and the trachea, a segment is found that is characterized by a comparably high collapsibility. If this pharyngeal muscular segment is no longer able to keep the airway sufficiently open during inhalation, the airway resistance increases with the result of vibrations, snoring, or an increasing obstruction of the airway ranging to obstructive apnea.

In this context, compared to other mammals, humans are particularly at risk. The unparalleled abilities of humans to articulate in multiple ways require a special mobility of the pharyngeal structures. However, this increased mobility and ability of articulation are at the expense of an instability of the upper airway.

Practical Tip

The phenomenon of obstructive sleep apnea results from the special anatomy of the upper airway. The pharyngeal segment of this airway works as a collapsible segment that can only be kept open during inhalation by the activity of the pharyngeal muscles.

This principle also explains why obstructive sleep apnea is generally only found in sleep. With sleep onset, the muscle tone decreases in the area of the dilators of the upper airways with dependence on the sleep stage. This phenomenon itself may exceed the compensatory possibilities of the muscles of the upper airway, especially in REM sleep, and lead to airway obstruction. Furthermore, the supine position during sleep may result in an individually different fluid shift from the inferior parts of the body into the cervical soft tissue that leads to a narrowing of the upper airway and thus to increased collapsibility.

All these factors make clear why obstruction may occur during inhalation, why the upper airway is particularly vulnerable in this context, and why the disorder mainly occurs during sleep. Beyond those general reflections, further triggering factors are of relevance because obstructive sleep apnea does not occur in all individuals but in particularly predisposed subjects and with different levels of severity.

Several triggering factors have been identified in this context whereby anatomical models and functional triggering mechanisms are of high relevance.

4.2.2.1 Anatomical Models

Anatomical models mainly consider the anatomical circumstances and thus the physical laws at the upper airway. Frequently, fluid dynamic reflections are taken as the basis, and the upper airway is considered as the resistor. This model is based on the original condition that a collapsible segment (in humans this is the pharyngeal muscle tube) is located between two rigid tubes (in humans, the nose on one side and the trachea on the other side) and that this collapsible segment is surrounded by a closed space (in humans, the pharyngeal soft tissue).

The condition of this collapsible segment depends on the intraluminal pressure (i.e., from the airway pressure during inhalation) and from tissue pressure. If the negative intraluminal pressure significantly exceeds the environmental pressure, the segment collapses, which clinically corresponds to obstructive apnea. The concept (and thus the measurement) of the critical closing pressure is based on these reflections. The critical closing pressure defines the pressure in the airway at which it closes. In healthy individuals, this pressure is clearly negative, and more negative than the physiological airway pressure occurring during inhalation. Patients suffering from SRBD, however, generally show increasingly less negative or even a positive critical closing pressure with increasing severity of the disease.

Practical Tip

The behavior of the collapsible segment of the upper airway depends on fluid dynamics. To develop the clinical presentation of obstructive sleep apnea, individual triggering factors have to be taken into consideration.

In the context of this anatomical consideration, on one hand the *increasing tissue pressure* is crucial. In the first place, obesity is the most important risk factor for the development of obstructive sleep apnea.

Based on different imaging procedures, numerous studies could confirm that not only is body fat increased in the context of obesity, but especially in the area of the pharynx, fat deposits are found that lead to narrowing the airway in this segment. Other factors that might lead to an increased tissue pressure are, for example, tissue edema, that is often triggered by snoring, or myxedema, which is found in cases of hypothyroidism and that may sometimes be the origin of obstructive sleep apnea in this patient population.

On the other hand, factors are of high relevance that lead to an increased *negative inspiratory pressure*. Those factors include among others anatomical particularities that prone to an obstruction of the upper airway, such as these:

- Nasal obstruction (septal deviation, hyperplastic turbinates)
- Tissue hyperplasia in the oropharynx (tonsillar hyperplasia, uvular hyperplasia, tongue (base) hypertrophy)
- Retrognathia
- Midfacial anomalies (dolichocephalic types)
- Anomaly of the epiglottis

On this basis, the effectiveness of some surgical therapies can be at least partly explained.

These anatomical explanatory models, however, do not fully explain the disease. In particular, in recent times, increasingly functional models have been presented that provide an alternative or complementary explanation for the development of obstructive sleep apnea.

4.2.2.2 Functional Models

In the context of functional consideration of the upper airway, three factors are significant: the capacity of the muscular dilators to respond to pressure alterations in the upper airway, the arousal threshold, and the phenomenon of loop gain.

Generally, the upper airway disposes of the possibility to register intraluminal pressure variations and to counteract an increased airway resistance by means of increasing the muscle tone. However, hereby it could be shown that in particular, the muscular response of the most important dilator of the upper airway, that is, the genioglossus muscle, is individually very different. If the genioglossus muscle does only slightly react on the increased negative intraluminal pressure, the development of obstructions is fostered.

If obstruction of the upper airway occurs, it is generally terminated by arousal; in this context, the increasing airway resistance is mainly responsible for triggering the arousal. Current investigations, however, show that the threshold for triggering an arousal is individually different. If the *arousal threshold* is low, the airway obstruction is terminated early, even before the regulatory mechanisms (e.g., the reflective increase of the muscle tone) may counteract the airway obstruction, which favors the development of respiratory events and contributes to the symptoms of OSA caused by severe sleep fragmentation. The concept of the arousal threshold may provide an explanation why some patients paradoxically experience improvement of the sleep apnea after application of sedatives, at least in the context of clinical studies, because they raise the arousal threshold.

The phenomenon of *loop gain* describes the respiratory response to a respiratory event, such as an apnea. If the respiratory center strongly responds to this event, severe hyperventilation develops during the arousal opening the pharynx. This event may lead to a decrease of CO_2 that reduces the muscular response of the upper airway and favors the development of apneas. Patients with a high loop gain thus show a functional instability of the upper airway.

Practical Tip

The etiology of obstructive sleep apnea is generally multifactorial so that therapeutic approaches also must take into consideration the complexity of this disease.

The mentioned explanatory models and triggering factors are not equally important in all patients. In some patient cohorts anatomical factors are in the focus and thus a pathologically critical closing pressure is in the foreground. In other patient cohorts, however, the mentioned functional aspects are predominant. Finally, it can be assumed that this has also consequences on the effectiveness of different therapeutic procedures and that, for example, surgical procedures are less promising for patients with mainly functional disorders. Thus, in past years, increasing efforts have been undertaken to establish *phenotyping* of the disease, which was intended to optimize the selection of therapeutic procedures.

4.2.3 Epidemiology

The *prevalence* of obstructive sleep apnea depends on age and gender. Furthermore, significant differences exist with regard to genetic and ethnic factors.

The highest prevalence is found in men of middle and older age; however, the data on prevalence clearly vary among studies. Among other reasons, this variation results from the different diagnostic methods and definitions of limit values applied in the investigations. Without any doubt, the prevalence has increased during the past decades, which among other reasons is also caused by increase of the most important risk factor, obesity. Recent population-based studies report prevalences of up to 25% for an apnea-hypopnea index of more than 15. In this context, it must be considered that definitions of the different respiratory events changed over time and the measurement techniques improved; however, the limit values for the diagnosis of obstructive sleep apnea remained the same.

Overall, in the Afro-American population, the prevalence is higher compared to the Caucasian or Asian populations, even independent of the imbalanced distribution of the risk factors (such as obesity).

During the past years, genetic aspects of obstructive sleep apnea were mentioned repeatedly. Finally, a familial association can be observed, with increasing evidence that multifactorial genetic characteristics predispose for this disease. Practical consequences, however, cannot be concluded currently.

4.2.4 Clinical Presentation

The clinical presentation of obstructive sleep apnea is manifold:

- Direct sleep-related symptoms
- Complaints in the context of nonrestorative sleep
- Secondary symptoms caused by secondary diseases

The sleep-related symptoms include numerous phenomena that are often not even noticed by the patient but which are observed and reported by the bed partner:

- Loud and irregular snoring
- Perceptible irregularities of breathing, including apnea
- General restlessness during sleep

Often, the patients wake up abruptly and gasp for breath. Because the arousal or wake phases are of only short duration, the patients do not always remember them, or at least not all the breathing-related wakeup reactions. Nocturnal breathing interruptions and the dramatically appearing gasping for breath especially frighten the bed partner and thus are frequently the reason for medical consultation.

Those nocturnal sleep-related symptoms are often, but not always, accompanied by daytime symptoms, most often by hypersomnia. The severity of the daytime symptoms naturally reveals a correlation with the severity of the sleep-related breathing disorder. Finally, however, patients are also found with only mild sleep apnea who complain about significant impairment of their daytime vigilance and on the other hand patients with severe sleep apnea who mention the relevant symptoms only when being asked or who consider them as "normal." In this context, often a correlation is found with the professional and intellectual requirements of the affected individuals during the daytime.

Practical Tip

Increased daytime sleepiness is the leading symptom of obstructive sleep apnea. It is associated with an increased likeliness to fall asleep during the daytime and has to be differentiated from tiredness or fatigue as it is found, for example, in the context of insomnia or depressive disorders.

The *increased daytime sleepiness* in cases of obstructive sleep apnea is frequently of high social relevance. Patients report that they fall asleep at every available opportunity, for example, in the waiting room of their practitioner and also in the afternoon, after work, during breaks at work in the office, or also on weekends when they are not kept awake by physical activity. Falling asleep in socially undesirable situations is described as being particularly problematic, for example, during meetings or conferences in the presence of one's superior or boss and at the theater or cinema. Often, the severe sleepiness has relevant consequences for social and familial relationships, and the patients become frustrated about their own sleepiness and their impaired physical and mental performance. Obstructive sleep apnea often contributes to stagnation of the professional career. All this, in the complete appearance of the disease, may lead to a relevant change of the personality and to depressive symptoms. The quality of life of the affected individuals is often significantly impaired.

Furthermore, daytime sleepiness can also lead to a significant risk to health or even life of the patients and outside parties. In particular, in road traffic, for example, when driving a car, *micro-sleep attacks* as reported by many patients are a severe problem. Frequently, the patients are able to stop their cars or to take breaks at the roadside just in time, but a relevant number of somewhat severe traffic accidents are assumed to be caused by increased sleepiness. Thus, in some countries, public transportation companies include at least some examinations regarding sleep-related breathing disorders in the context of their occupational medical checkups. Beyond road traffic, workers at potentially dangerous machines who suffer from obstructive sleep apnea also have to be considered as high-risk patients.

Case Report

A 45-year-old bank manager presents for sleep medical consultation. He has been urged by his wife to finally consult a doctor for treatment of his sleep problems.

His wife complains about her husband's loud snoring, which has become intolerable in the past years, being accompanied by significant weight increase (current BMI, 31). Furthermore, he suffers from irregular breathing during sleep associated with long breathing interruptions so that his wife formerly often shook him because she was afraid that he could suffocate. Because of these symptoms, the couple now have separate bedrooms.

The patient further reports that he often suffers from an immense sleepiness during the daytime that forces him to lie down even during the day. He then sleeps longer than he has intended. Recently, he has even fallen asleep during meetings at work. Several times, he has also experienced sudden nodding off while driving in his car, so that frequently he has to stop on his way home in the afternoon to sleep for a while. At work, his boss has already addressed him several times about his decreasing performance, and the boss has even sent him home because he had fallen asleep at his desk. On weekends, he usually sleeps throughout the day so that his social relationships and activities are strongly impaired. Together with a weight increase, severe hypertension became apparent that could not be treated satisfactorily by means of triple antihypertensive medication.

In the further sleep-related examination, obstructive sleep apnea was diagnosed.

The symptoms described by this patient elucidate the classic clinical presentation of obstructive sleep apnea that is typically found in male individuals. However, it must be taken into account that the symptoms differ between the genders and that female patients frequently show less characteristic complaints, in particular, less intensive snoring and less daytime sleepiness. In these cases, often nonspecific symptoms but also insomnia complaints or depressive symptoms are the focus. Patients with cardiovascular diseases who are eminently affected by obstructive sleep apnea often display the according clinical symptoms, which makes it difficult to apply, for example, questionnaires for diagnostic purposes in this patient population.

Besides the individual complaints, *health-related long-term effects* of the disease also must be discussed. Obstructive sleep apnea is associated with a large number of cardiovascular and metabolic diseases or disorders, for example, hypertension, cardiac arrhythmia, arteriosclerosis, coronary heart disease, and accompanying secondary diseases such as heart attack and stroke.

Beyond the mere association, obstructive sleep apnea is meanwhile acknowledged as an independent risk factor for these diseases. In particular, patients suffering from hypertension and obstructive sleep apnea find that it is very difficult to treat hypertension. In this context it is typical that the blood pressure does not decrease at night (so-called nondipping). If the underlying sleep apnea is successfully treated, a reduction in blood pressure or an improved adjustment of hypertension with pharmaceuticals may be observed.

Because of the mutual interaction, sleep-related breathing disorders are often found in cardiologic patients, in particular, in patients suffering from heart failure, who besides typical central breathing disorders with Cheyne-Stokes respiration also frequently suffer from obstructive sleep apnea. If such a breathing disorder is found, it has a significantly negative effect on the morbidity and mortality of this patient population. *Nondipping* or the presence of respective cardiac diseases should by implication also lead to an examination with regard to the presence of sleep-related breathing disorders.

In addition to cardiovascular diseases, increased insulin resistance can also be found in patients suffering from obstructive sleep apnea.

Obstructive sleep apnea is associated with an increased mortality; patients suffering from obstructive sleep apnea that remains untreated have a higher risk to die earlier compared to respective cohorts.

Practical Tip

Beyond the nocturnal breathing disorder and associated daytime symptoms, obstructive sleep apnea is a relevant cardiovascular risk factor associated with increased cardiovascular morbidity and mortality.

4.3 Snoring

In the most recent version of the international classification of sleep disorders (ICSD-3), snoring is again included in the list of sleep-related breathing disorders. Snoring is mentioned in the chapter on "Isolated Symptoms and Normal Variants." The aspects of definitions, etiology and pathophysiology, epidemiology, and clinical presentation are elucidated separately here in the following paragraphs. With regard to the aspects of diagnostics and therapy, however, there is important overlapping with sleep apnea so that the diagnostics and treatment of these two phenomena are discussed together in this manual.

4.3.1 Definitions

A satisfactory definition of *snoring* as an acoustic phenomenon does not exist, because the acoustic phenomenon is always subjective and cannot be clearly defined (the answer on the question what snoring is or which breathing noise can be called snoring will always remain subjective and descriptive). If the patient or bed partner reports an according acoustic annoyance or disturbance during sleep and, if no hints for obstructive sleep apnea are found or the examination for obstructive sleep apnea remains inconsequential, it is most probable to diagnose snoring. Many attempts have been made to establish a terminological differentiation of the acoustic phenomenon of snoring and the epiphenomenon of snoring in the context of obstructive sleep apnea. Hereby, different terminologies such as primary snoring, harmless or benign snoring, non-apneic snoring, or habitual snoring were suggested.

Practical Tip

The definition of snoring per se includes the presence of acoustic phenomena during sleep without the aforementioned criteria for obstructive sleep apnea being fulfilled.

4.3.2 Etiology and Pathophysiology

The origins of snoring are probably less complex than those of obstructive sleep apnea. However,

4

the fact that snoring occurs predominantly in the upper airway and during sleep leads to the assumption that it is also associated with anatomical particularities of the human airway and the decrease of the muscle tone during sleep (see ► Sect. 4.2). Thus, the upper airway with its collapsible segment not only favors obstruction but also allows the development of vibrations and snoring noise. These snoring sounds may generally occur at the soft tissue of the entire upper airway, but the soft tissue of the palate and the base of tongue are most relevant. Compared to obstructive sleep apnea, anatomical factors have a primary role in the context of snoring.

4.3.3 Epidemiology

The *prevalence* of snoring depends on age and gender. The highest prevalence is found in males of middle and older ages. Data on the incidence in this group vary between 20% and 46%. The fact that snoring is neither reliably defined nor do objective characteristics exist may explain the variation in the range of the data. In contrast to the general assumption, the prevalence in women of similar age is also relevant, 8% to 25%, even if it is clearly lower compared to male individuals.

4.3.4 Clinical Presentation

The clinical presentation of snoring results directly: the affected individuals (or the bed partners) report about socially disturbing snoring. Generally, it is a singular phenomenon. If further relevant complaints develop, such as daytime sleepiness or nonrestorative sleep, complementary diagnostics with regard to possible triggering factors or hypersomnia or a general sleep disorder are indicated. Sometimes, snoring may be associated with an extrinsic sleep disorder with daytime sleepiness: this may be the case when the snoring individual is shaken awake by the bed partner or stimulated in another way.

Even if snoring is generally harmless from a medical point of view, many affected people significantly suffer from the social consequences. Not rarely, snoring men present in consultations when they are "chased" from the bedroom. Also, business or holiday trips with snoring colleagues or friends may be stressful for all persons involved. Finally, snoring in men is considered as unattractive, and so young men in particular frequently desire treatment for their complaints.

Practical Tip

From a medical point of view, snoring in adults is harmless. The affected individuals, however, often suffer from the social consequences and feel impaired.

4.4 Diagnostic Procedures

Diagnostic measures to confirm sleep-related breathing disorders are introduced when symptoms such as snoring, breathing interruptions, or awakenings with dyspnea, or when typical high-risk diseases such as obesity, arterial hypertension, or COPD are reported. In daily routine, they are generally based on the guidelines of the respective national healthcare system, but they always consist of the sequence of the following diagnostic elements:

- History taking by means of questionnaires and clinical examination
- Assessment of concomitant diseases such as arterial hypertension, COPD
- Polygraphy or other out-of-center sleep studies
- Polysomnography in lab

Based on new definitions of obstructive sleep apnea with inclusion of respiratory arousals in the respiratory disturbance index (RDI), the severity of breathing disorders can only be assessed correctly by means of PSG. If nonrestorative sleep is the predominant symptom in a snoring individual and if polygraphy does not lead to an appropriate diagnosis, PSG always is required.

The diagnostic guidelines that have been developed by medical societies as well as healthcare institutions differ with regard to the criteria and time when polysomnography should be applied during the diagnostic process.

4.4.1 Examination Procedures and Sleep-Related Medical Diagnostics

Generally, two different diagnostic scenarios can be imagined.

1. In one case, the affected individual seeks medical advice complaining of nonrestorative sleep without further indications of a sleep-related breathing disorder. The possible origins have to be clarified depending on other anamnestic data (e.g., shiftwork; see ▶ Chap. 6), symptoms (e.g., cataplexy; see ▶ Chap. 5), and clinical findings (e.g., hypothyroidism; see ▶ Chap. 10). If this is not possible, PSG is required.
2. In the other case, a disease or symptoms exist that predispose for the development of breathing disorder during sleep, which may occur as a consequence of the disease, or that is simply frequently associated, for example, snoring, obesity, heart failure, or arterial hypertension. The presence of a sleep-related breathing disorder has to be confirmed by out-of-center sleep testing, and diagnostic PSG should complete the examination only in unclear cases. If a disease is found that is typically associated with SRBD without any clinical symptoms, the current guidelines of the man Sleep Society recommend OCST with a reduced number of measurement parameters as adequate examination.

The different diagnostic procedures in the context of sleep disorders are presented in detail in ▶ Chap. 2. In this chapter, those specific diagnostic aspects of sleep-related breathing disorders are discussed that were not presented in ▶ Chap. 2.

The specific diagnostics investigate in particular diseases that lead to secondary alveolar hypoventilation, hypoxemia, or central sleep apnea to achieve an improvement of the breathing disorder by treating the underlying disease. The diagnostics also include the examination of etiopathogenetic factors of obstructive sleep apnea and the resulting therapeutic possibilities, in particular, in cases of incompliance of nasal CPAP therapy.

4.4.1.1 Diagnostics in Cases of Central Sleep Apnea Syndromes

Central sleep apnea syndromes are mostly characterized by *mild sleep-related complaints,* and so they do not become obvious over longer periods of time. They are often discovered incidentally in the context of examining other sleep disorders, for example, obstructive sleep apnea or insomnia. If central apneas are an unexpected incidental finding in sleep-related medical diagnostics, not only should heart or kidney failure and conditions after cerebral insult be excluded, but also other possible triggering factors (see ▶ Sect. 4.1.2) have to be identified and their severity or residual condition defined.

In the context of similar high-risk constellations, *Cheyne-Stokes respiration* has to be differentiated, which is generally not difficult because of the characteristic breathing pattern and the clear definition (see ▶ Sect. 4.1). If, in contrast, a disease is found that is typically associated with central sleep apnea, even mild symptoms should lead to an overnight examination (see scenario 2). This is especially important because not only central apneas but in particular obstructive sleep apnea is found in about 30% of heart failure patients and in about 15% of patients after stroke.

Practical Tip

Generally, a central sleep apnea syndrome is suspected when the patient reports recurrent awakening with dyspnea.

If the *arterial blood gas analysis* shows a low to normal CO_2 partial pressure less than 40 mmHg during daytime, a primary central sleep apnea is diagnosed when the typical central apneas occur in polygraphy or PSG (see ▶ Chaps. 2 and ▶ Sect. 4.1) but no responsible disease can be confirmed.

Central apneas are most frequently found in light sleep, and their incidence decreases via deep sleep to REM sleep.

Single central apneas as sequelae of diseases of the inner organs that do not occur in the context of Cheyne-Stokes respiration patterns may last longest in REM sleep, because in this sleep stage the CO_2 arousal threshold is reduced. In cases of Cheyne-Stokes respiration, the single apneas are not prolonged in REM sleep. In fact, often Cheyne-Stokes respiration is completely suppressed in REM sleep.

Practical Tip

The reduction of apneas in REM sleep makes the difference between central sleep apnea syndromes and hypoventilation or hypoxemia syndromes and obstructive sleep apnea for which an increase of the pathological respiration in REM sleep is typical.

It is not unusual to register a central as well as obstructive breathing disorder in the same night in the same patient by *polygraphy*. If predominantly clearly obstructive breathing disorders are found, obstructive sleep apnea is diagnosed.

If more than 50% of the events are central, *PSG* should be measured in a way that allows a clear assignment of the events. In this context, the following findings especially confirm obstructive events:

- The nasal pressure transducer showing inspiratory flow limitations during hypopneas
- Snoring during hypopnea
- Paradoxical respiratory movements during apnea or hypopnea

If the patient meets the diagnostic criteria for both entities even under observation of these particular measurement parameters, both diagnoses have to be mentioned. In these cases, the obstructive sleep apnea is treated primarily because central events often disappear when the obstructive events no longer unbalance the respiratory regulation.

Sleep-related medical examination is not required in most cases of suspected periodic breathing in high altitudes and central sleep apnea induced by pharmaceuticals or substances because the anamnesis is already substantial and further diagnostics would not have therapeutic consequences.

4.4.1.2 Diagnostics in Cases of Sleep-Related Hypoventilation or Hypoxemia Syndrome

In this group of diseases, the type and the severity of the impairment of the entire gas-exchange system must be assessed.

The patients should be actively questioned regarding *dyspnea* occurring at rest or only during physical activity as well as morning sputum.

In the *clinical examination*, cyanosis, use of the respiratory auxiliary muscles, scoliosis, obesity, and peripheral edema are assessed, and hints of bronchitis, emphysema, or diaphragmatic paresis are investigated by means of percussion and auscultation.

In the *blood count*, the presence of polyglobulia is of high relevance.

In individual cases, *radiology* or if needed also *computed tomography* of the thorax and *bronchoscopy* are helpful for finding the pulmonary diagnosis.

The *ECG* may suggest right heart burden. The right heart stress may be quantified by means of *echocardiography* or *right heart catheter*.

In every case, *pulmonary function testing*, for example, spirometry or body plethysmography, has to be performed to identify the severity of the obstruction or restriction. In the context of a vital capacity of less than 50%, for example, respiratory problems can be expected; if it falls below 30%, respiratory insufficiency is most probable even if hypercapnia is not yet present during daytime. If the forced expiratory volume in 1 s (FEV_1) amounts to less than 70% of the vital capacity, a relevant bronchial obstruction is diagnosed.

It is required as well to conduct a capillary or arterial *blood gas analysis* in the wake stage at rest, which, however, may reveal normal findings in early stages. In cases of early chronic respiratory insufficiency, hypercapnia is revealed at least under physical activity and in REM sleep. In unclear cases, the CO_2 partial pressure during sleep must be monitored continuously in a noninvasive, transcutaneous, or end-tidal manner, or the patient must be awakened so that blood gas analyses may be performed invasively. Pulse oximetry during sleep is only a reliable parameter of respiration during sleep if no diffusion disorder is present, which almost exclusively is the case in neuromuscular diseases without recurrent pneumonia.

Practical Tip

If sleep-related hypoventilation or hypoxemia syndrome is suspected, the following examinations at least must be performed:
- Pulmonary function testing
- Arterial blood gas analysis during daytime
- Polygraphy

The determination of the CO_2 partial pressure during PSG is the decisive examination method in unclear cases.

For further diagnostic procedures, the disciplines of pneumology, endocrinology, hematology, neurology, and orthopedics have to be consulted according to the suspected or known underlying disease.

In cases of hypoventilation syndromes, the chronic respiratory insufficiency is either caused by primary muscle weakness or overload and consecutive fatigue of the respiratory muscles up to exhaustion (see ▸ Sect. 4.2).

Muscular power and strain of the respiratory muscles can be determined noninvasively by the *method of mouth occlusion pressure*. With this method, it is possible to assess more readily if noninvasive home ventilation should be introduced to avoid failure of the respiratory pump. Because most of the respiratory work during sleep is done by the diaphragm, determination of the transdiaphragmatic pressure may be useful in the individual case.

Hypoxemia syndromes can be identified by means of *polygraphy* because of the characteristic tonic decrease of the oxygen saturation over longer periods during nighttime without clear decrease of the airflow (◘ Fig. 4.3). If intermittent hypoxemia is only found in intervals of 60 to 120 min, it is most likely that a REM-associated hypoxemia is found that can be confirmed by PSG. Hypoventilation syndrome, especially when it shows only isolated hypercapnia with normal gas exchange, may be assumed in the standard setting if a decreased oxygen saturation is observed compared to wakefulness in combination with tonic increase of the heart rate at the same time. For exact diagnosis, the CO_2 partial pressure during sleep has to be measured. In this context, the transcutaneous method is preferred to the end-tidal approach as errors may occur unnoticed in the end-tidal measurement because of the open or half-open system.

4.4.1.3 Diagnostics in Cases of Obstructive Sleep Apnea

To assess the classic symptoms during sleep, in particular the *history* compiled by a third party is important because the affected patients are mostly not conscious of either the breathing interruptions or irregular snoring or arousal reactions. It must be actively asked if the breathing disorder increases depending on the patient's position and under the influence of alcohol or benzodiazepine receptor agonists. The incidence and duration of obstructive apneas, however, are regularly underestimated by the bed partners because they only recognize these when they themselves do not sleep. The daytime sleepiness has to be assessed (at least by means of the Epworth Sleepiness Scale, ESS) because severe likelihood of falling asleep during the day may lead to the incapacity to work (see ▸ Chap. 12). Using standardized questionnaires in the corresponding national language, not only the symptoms but also typically associated diseases, mainly arterial hypertension, sequelae of arteriosclerosis, heart failure, diabetes mellitus, and COPD, may be assessed in a detailed and structured way (see ▸ Chap. 2). Single questionnaires that sometimes also include clinical findings (e.g., Berlin Questionnaire) may increase the pretest probability of polygraphy and PSG.

Practical Tip

History taking and clinical and device-based examinations should be performed to confirm the diagnosis as well as concomitant diseases and give therapeutic hints in cases of suspected obstructive sleep apnea.

Clinical and device-based examinations are focused on the identification of concomitant and

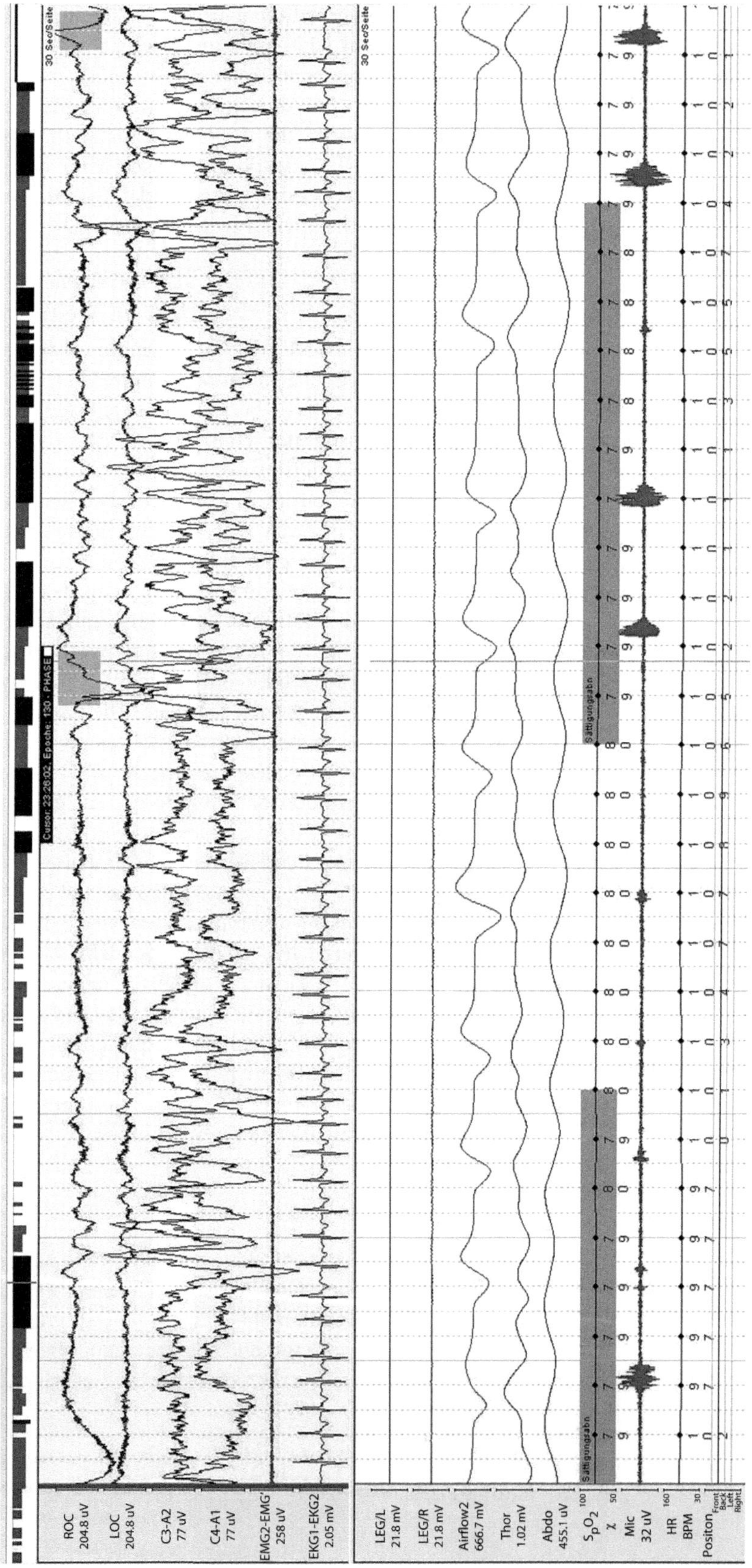

■ **Fig. 4.3** Polysomnographic extract of a hypoventilation phase with hypoxemia secondary diseases of obstructive sleep apnea and the evaluation of the upper airways (see ► Chap. 2). Independently from the discipline involved at the beginning, the diagnostic minimum consists of these:

- Clinical examination
- Calculation of the BMI
- Measurement of the blood pressure according to Riva-Rocci

These examinations are complemented by examinations according to the respective anamnestic profile in an interdisciplinary context.

The *clinical endoscopic examination* of the upper airways is particularly important when ventilation therapy is not tolerated and alternative therapeutic options are discussed (see ► Sects. 4.6.4 and 4.7). Examination of the nose is also significant because each nasal positive pressure ventilation is facilitated when nasal obstruction can be eliminated. Therapeutic consequences are drawn in cases of hypertrophic tonsils (tonsillectomy) and retrognathia of the mandible and/or maxilla (mandibular protrusion splints, maxillo-mandibular advancement).

The *lateral cephalogram of the skull* for two-dimensional measurement of the facial skull, including the oropharyngeal soft parts (cephalometric analysis), is an examination procedure performed before maxillofacial interventions (◘ Fig. 4.4).

To take into account the dynamic processes that take place during the development of apneas and to identify their location as well as their mechanism, *video endoscopy* under sedation, *pharyngoesophageal pressure measurements*, and *snoring sound analyses* are applied. In particular, video endoscopy under sedation (with midazolam or propofol) is increasingly performed worldwide when possible therapeutic alternatives have to be clarified in cases of CPAP noncompliance. The severity (none, partial, or complete) and pattern of obstruction (anteroposterior, lateral, or concentric) are described separately for the levels of the velum, tonsils, base of the tongue, and larynx. In comparison to clinical endoscopic examination alone, the therapeutic concept is changed in many patients by the results of video endoscopy under sedation. However, up to now an improved patient selection with increase of the success rate could be shown only for a few surgical procedures. Pharyngoesophageal pressure measurements and snoring sound analyses still have to be classified as experimental.

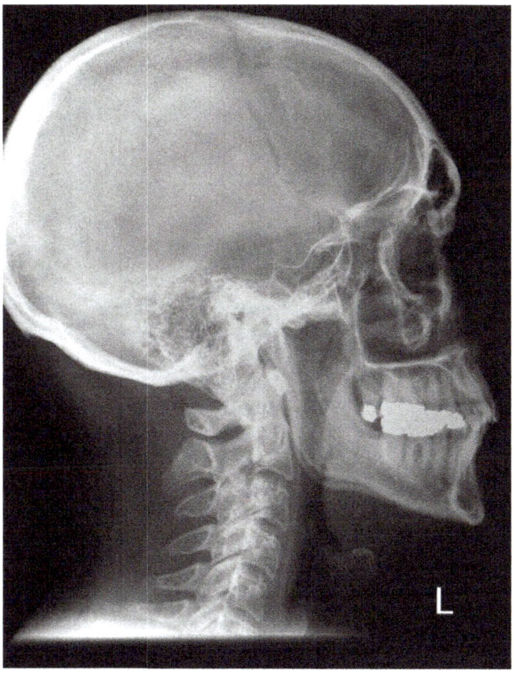

◘ **Fig. 4.4** Cephalometry

In *polygraphy* (see ► Chap. 2), a patient with obstructive sleep apnea typically shows repetitive obstructive apneas and hypopneas in combination with desaturation (partly even below 50%) and increased heart rate (◘ Fig. 4.5).

The last-mentioned symptoms may be missing when beta blockers are taken or a cardiac pacemaker determines the heartbeat. In cases of coexisting heart or lung disease, the desaturation findings are more severe with regard to the duration of the apnea compared to healthy individuals.

The recognition of *respiratory arousals (RERA)* is required for the determination of all respiratory events. Beside the normalization of paradoxical breathing and the abrupt end of increasing snoring (so-called crescendo snoring), increased heart and pulse rates are indirect signs of RERA. RERA may only be clearly identified based on sleep monitoring in the PSG. Thus, it seems obvious that not all patients can be accurately diagnosed by means of polygraphy. In the context of indirect signs for respiratory arousals in the polygraphy and an increased daytime sleepiness, PSG is always indicated.

In cases of obstructive sleep apnea, PSG (see ► Chap. 2) mostly shows a reduction of the deep and dream sleep. The sleep profile is fragmented

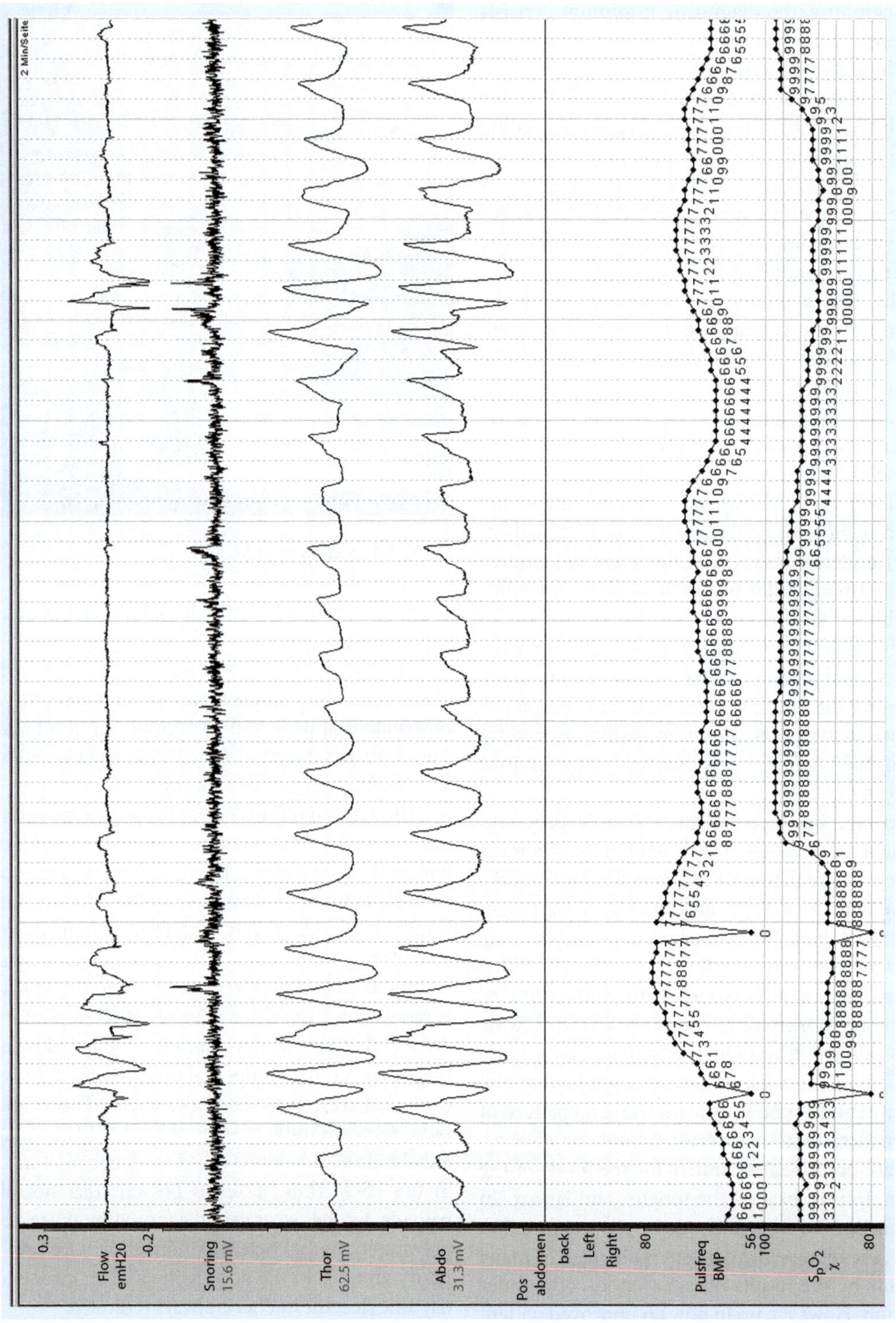

Fig. 4.5 Polygraphy: obstructive sleep apnea, 50 sec duration, delayed drop of oxygen saturation, two arousals with increase of heart rate

by repeated respiratory arousals. In extreme cases, sleep cycles are no longer seen at all.

Obstructive sleep apnea is the most frequently and best examined sleep-related breathing disorder. Snoring is the leading symptom that is the most frequent complaint based on which diagnostic procedures are initiated.

Because snoring is widespread in the adult population and the consciousness of the population and physicians has increased, the need for examinations is so great that it cannot be covered by available physicians experienced in sleep medicine.

Therefore, attempts have been made for many years to develop simple examination devices with only one or at maximum two channels (e.g., nasal cannula and pulse oximetry) and with simple, automatic evaluation algorithms that are not intrusive. Each of these new systems has to be validated in comparison to PSG because the sensors and algorithms cannot be easily transferred. As the relevant breathing patterns are often not directly displayed, they cannot yet replace polygraphy or PSG.

4.4.2 Differential Diagnoses

Obstructive sleep apnea and *Cheyne-Stokes respiration* (common predisposition: left-sided heart failure) as well as obstructive sleep apnea and *obesity hypoventilation syndrome* (common predisposition: obesity) are often observed in the same patient. Because of its enormous incidence, *snoring* is also frequently associated with other sleep disorders. Therefore, a careful visual analysis of polygraphy or PSG has to be performed to identify all sleep-related breathing disorders.

If *snoring sounds* are found in a patient suffering from Cheyne-Stokes respiration, the acoustic signals are classically observed on the maximum of ventilation. An increase of the noise during hypopnea, however, corresponds to its obstructive genesis.

The *course of oxygen saturation* in the context of obstructive sleep apnea and most central sleep apnea syndromes is characterized by a slow decrease and a rapid re-increase after breathing onset. In cases of Cheyne-Stokes respiration, the curve of the oxygen saturation has a sinusoidal shape. Tonic desaturations with exacerbation in REM sleep indicate a hypoventilation or hypoxemia syndrome.

In the context of arousals, frequently *limb movements* are observed that might (mis-)lead to the diagnosis of a periodic limb movement syndrome. Whether the leg movements occur independently from respiratory events can only be detected by a very detailed analysis of the PSG registration. These leg movements are not examined further, because in many cases they disappear or do not cause complaints after successful therapy of the obstructive sleep apnea.

In the course of their lives, patients suffering from *narcolepsy* develop coping strategies to better live with its symptoms. If sleep-related breathing disorders occur additionally, this new sleep disorder finally leads to the necessary diagnostic steps in many cases. Therefore, therapy control in the context of sleep-related breathing disorders has the special purpose to identify other sleep disorders if patients continue to complain about nonrestorative sleep despite the successful treatment of a sleep-related breathing disorder.

Practical Tip

Intensive sleep-related differential diagnostics are of high importance, especially when the patients continue complaining about nonrestorative sleep despite successful treatment of a sleep-related breathing disorder.

Because of the identical complaints of nonrestorative sleep with the coexisting symptom of snoring, it is sometimes very difficult to differentiate all kinds of *hypersomnia* and *insomnia* from obstructive sleep apnea or central sleep apnea.

4.5 Therapeutic Principles

The treatment of sleep-related breathing disorders is often complex and cannot be performed according to rigid standards. Such diseases are caused by many factors and generally require an individual consideration of therapeutic alternatives. The therapeutic options can be classified into conservative, device-related, and surgical procedures. Of course, a combination of approaches is possible and frequently helpful.

In the most favorable case, the physician is able to provide the whole spectrum of possible therapeutic options. If this is not the case, it should be in the patients' interest to consult external specialists or to transfer the patients to the respective institution. As the objective of therapeutic intervention is completely different with regard to snoring and sleep apnea, the therapeutic principles of both phenomena are discussed separately in the following paragraphs.

In this context, it is mentioned again that patients often reveal more than one sleep-related disease. Especially regarding the high prevalence, *sleep-related medical comorbidities* are particularly frequent in cases of sleep-related breathing disorders. These problems include, among others, movement disorders during sleep (periodic limb movements) or also disorders of initiating and maintaining sleep. In particular when the described complaints (e.g., daytime sleepiness in cases of obstructive sleep apnea) do not improve despite adequate therapy, the corresponding differential diagnostic reflections should be made, and further diagnostic procedures should be initiated.

4.5.1 Therapeutic Principles in Cases of Snoring

As it has already been described, snoring cannot be considered as a disease in the narrow sense of the word. A real medical risk is not found, and generally there is *no medical indication* for treatment. This conclusion corresponds, for example, to the procedure of esthetic interventions so that the basic reflections in this context overlap in a series of aspects. The affected individuals are often significantly stressed, and the level of suffering must not be underestimated. However, it must be stated that with this background, the indication of invasive measures must be made very strictly.

Of course, the indication of treatment can only be made in cases of snoring when the affected persons express their wish for therapy. Frequently, for example, patients present who are worried because of their severe snoring and who are afraid of suffering from obstructive sleep apnea. If the sleep-related examination can exclude obstructive sleep apnea, those patients are sufficiently reassured, and there is no need for further diagnostics or therapy. In no case should the patient be urged to undergo therapy for snoring or a necessity for therapy be suggested. Currently, there is no convincing evidence that early therapy for snoring might avoid a possible progression to obstructive sleep apnea.

Practical Tip

The diagnosis of snoring cannot be made with sufficient certainty based only on the clinical presentation. In particular, sleep-related diagnostics are essential before therapeutic interventions.

If a patient presents with the complaint of "snoring," the authors think that a competent *sleep-related examination* should be performed in any case even without the presence of other risk factors or indications of sleep apnea.

An objectifying sleep-related examination in the sense of a home sleep apnea test should be performed in those cases in which another sleep-related breathing disorder (e.g., obstructive sleep apnea) is suspected, where relevant comorbidities are found, or if the patient desires treatment of snoring. If no hints to a breathing disorder are revealed and the structured sleep-related history is inconspicuous, the diagnosis can be made with sufficient certainty.

If after respective diagnostics a snoring patient desires to be treated, it is the task of the sleep specialist to discuss the available therapeutic options with the affected individual. Generally, invasive measures should be considered very critically, and the patient should be informed accordingly. Regarding the selection of a possible surgical procedure, minimally invasive procedures should generally be preferred. Also in the context of conservative procedures (e.g., mandibular advancement devices), long-term risks should be particularly taken into consideration. If the patient decides on a therapeutic intervention, generally all ensuing costs are borne by the patient.

In contrast to obstructive sleep apnea, objectifying sleep-related diagnostics are not required after therapy because the final result is irrelevant. If the patient or the partner is satisfied with the result, the therapeutic objective has been achieved.

In recent years, numerous attempts have been made to objectify snoring or its acoustic components. For clinical application, however, the satisfaction of the patient or bed partner is decisive.

Nonetheless, the patient should be informed that even after successful therapy, snoring may recur in further years, and even the progression to obstructive sleep apnea is possible. Therefore, the respective symptoms or complaints should again lead to presentation and consultation of a sleep specialist.

4.5.2 Therapeutic Principles in Cases of Sleep Apnea

Also, in the context of sleep apnea, therapeutic necessity is not given in every case. In single cases, therapy may be completely avoided, and follow-up examinations are recommended. Sometimes primary weight reduction may be indicated even if no rapid therapeutic success can be expected in this regard.

Practical Tip

Whether a specific therapy is indicated in cases of sleep apnea and its urgency generally depend on three main factors:

- Individual symptoms
- Severity of the breathing disorder
- Individual comorbidities

As already mentioned, there is a correlation between the objectively measured severity of the breathing disorder and the subjective symptoms. In single cases, however, often surprising deviations are found.

According to the individual cognitive demands of the patient, a comparably *low-grade* or *marginal obstructive sleep apnea* may lead to relevant impairment of the daytime performance with increased daytime sleepiness that already in itself represents a need for therapy. Of course, such a constellation should give reason to investigate other origins of a daytime sleepiness.

If a *moderate* or *severe sleep apnea* is found, generally therapeutic necessity is indicated even if no subjective impairment of sleep or daytime performance is observed.

In the context of obstructive sleep apnea, corresponding epidemiological trials show an increase in the cardiovascular risk from a *respiratory disturbance index* of above 5. Regarding the assessment of the therapeutic necessity or urgency, however, a holistic consideration has to be performed. It is not sufficient to base the therapeutic decision exclusively on the number of respiratory events. In an otherwise healthy young man who does not complain about other symptoms, no treatment may be necessary even with an index of more than 15. On the other hand, however, a patient with severe cardiovascular disease should undergo early and appropriate treatment of the breathing disorder.

Practical Tip

A general limit for the respiratory disturbance index for which therapy is basically needed independently from individual factors and concomitant diseases cannot be clearly defined.

This lack is not only true for obstructive sleep apnea but in particular also for hypoventilation syndromes and central sleep apnea because here the correlation between the objective severity of the breathing disorder, the subjective symptoms, cardiovascular morbidity, and especially mortality is even less clear than in cases of obstructive sleep apnea.

Regarding the indication to treat obstructive sleep apnea in elderly patients, a higher reluctance seems to be justifiable in consideration of the high prevalence in this age group. Even if the ICSD-3 does not indicate different definitions or limit values for the different age groups in adults, there seems to be a higher number of respiratory events in particular in patients older than 80 years expressing a physiological decrease of the airway stability. If these patients do not complain about symptoms in the sense of increased daytime sleepiness, a wait-and-see strategy seems to be justified in the individual case, even with an index of more than 15. This mode is especially true with the background that in patients older than 80 years long-term cardiovascular risk is a relative issue and only a limited number of studies on the reduction of the cardiovascular risk in higher ages are available. Of course, however, the complaints in the sense of daytime sleepiness or reduced performance should be an indication for treatment also in the elderly.

In cases of sleep apnea, the aim of treatment is different from that in the case of snoring. Besides the improvement of the subjective complaints, the treatment should also:

- Reduce the number of respiratory events.
- Improve cardiovascular risk.
- Finally, extend patient survival.

Thus, an according *objectifying sleep-related follow-up* always has to be performed in cases of sleep apnea after treatment. The subjective report of the patient alone never suffices. Furthermore, the available therapeutic options may be expected to be effective and to meet all aspects of the disease. However, so far this is not the case for all therapies.

4.6 Ventilation Therapy

Noninvasive ventilation therapy is currently the gold standard for the treatment of sleep-related breathing disorders because it allows eliminating every type of breathing disorder independently from the genesis. It is a symptomatic and not a causal therapy. A ventilator, tube, and mask are permanently needed. The precondition for the effectiveness of this symptomatic therapy is the acceptance and regular use by the patient. Ventilation therapy is best titrated and its efficacy confirmed under polysomnographic control. In some countries (e.g., France), APAP therapy in cases of OSA is only introduced on an outpatient basis and exclusively controlled by polygraphy under certain circumstances.

The development of the first device for nasal ventilation therapy with continuous positive airway pressure (nCPAP) by Colin Sullivan in Australia in 1981 was a milestone in the treatment of sleep-related breathing disorders. Until then, ventilation devices were not suitable for use at home nor were masks available that would have allowed a noninvasive ventilation over several hours.

Although the first device was suitable only for the treatment of obstructive sleep apnea, in recent decades, smaller, more powerful, and more flexible devices have been developed as well as a multitude of accessories that improved the acceptance and significantly extended the possible applications of noninvasive ventilation therapy. Development is still continuing so that new procedures and indications are continuously tested besides the treatment procedures that are meanwhile confirmed on a very high evidence level.

4.6.1 Different Types of Noninvasive Ventilation Therapy

All procedures applied in sleep medicine work with positive pressure that is generated by a fan and transferred via a tube and a mask to the airways. So, it is a positive pressure ventilation in a potentially or planned half-open system. The multitude of the ventilation devices that are nowadays available can barely be imagined. Generally, however, two principles can be differentiated.

- Positive pressure ventilation in spontaneously breathing patients
- Positive pressure ventilation in cases of disturbed respiratory drive of the patient

For both principles, automatic systems are available that by means of special sensors recognize pathological breathing patterns or airway changes of the patient in the limits preset by the physician and that automatically respond to it according to manufacturer-specific algorithms.

For better overview, all relevant ventilation variants available in sleep medicine are summarized in ◘ Table 4.2.

4.6.1.1 Positive Pressure Ventilation in Cases of Spontaneously Breathing Patients

The procedures can only be applied when the patient still has a sufficient respiratory drive.

CPAP

Positive pressure ventilation with continuous positive airway pressure (CPAP) is the simplest, oldest, and most frequently applied technique in the context of sleep-related breathing disorders.

The applied pressure has the same level during inhalation and expiration and can be set in a range between 3 and 20 mbar. With sufficient positive pressure, the upper airways are kept open to that extent that the obstruction is eliminated in

Table 4.2 Scheme of different ventilation variants

Name and abbreviation	Description	Relevant parameters
Continuous positive airway pressure (CPAP)	Identical positive pressure during inhalation and expiration	Airway pressure
Automatic positive airway pressure (APAP, auto-CPAP)	Automatic increase of the pressure if airway obstructions are detected	Upper and lower pressure limit
Positive airway pressure with two pressure levels (bilevel-S)	Different pressure during inhalation and expiration in spontaneous breathing	EPAP, IPAP, trigger, rise time/edge
Positive airway pressure with two pressure levels and back-up respiratory frequency (bilevel-S/T)	Different pressure during inhalation and expiration in spontaneous breathing; pressure-controlled ventilation only if the breathing frequency drops below a minimum value	EPAP, IPAP, trigger, rise time/edge, minimum respiratory frequency, I/E ratio
Positive airway pressure with two pressure levels and fixed respiratory frequency (bilevel-T)	Pressure-controlled ventilation	EPAP, IPAP, rise time/edge, fixed respiratory frequency, I/E ratio
Adaptive servoventilation (autoset-CS, auto-SV)	Pressure-controlled ventilation adapted to Cheyne-Stokes respiration	EPAP, maximum IPAP
Impulse-positive airway pressure (ImPAP)	APAP with pressure impulse as pharyngeal receptor stimulus in cases of central apneas	Pressure limits, duration of apnea

E expiration, *EPAP* expiratory positive airway pressure, *I* inspiration, *IPAP* inspiratory positive airway pressure
Manufacturers often use different terms for the same general ventilation variants and continue developing new modifications. Therefore, this list does not claim to be complete. Missing listing does not mean deficient quality

the sense of pneumatic splinting. The necessary pressure is assessed under polysomnographic control to secure the effectiveness of the treatment in all body positions and sleep stages. With effective CPAP, the patient is able to breathe regularly during sleep. *Obstructive sleep apnea* is reliably eliminated.

The patient can self-determine if the system starts immediately with the effective pressure or with lower pressure (ramp function). If the ramp is activated, the pressure increases to the effective pressure over a period of 5 to 45 min, which may facilitate sleep onset.

Via the open airway, CPAP also increases the positive end-expiratory pressure (PEEP), which leads to a decrease of the preload in cases of patients with heart failure, and over this mechanism, it can reduce the cardiac performance and the pulmonary congestion (see ▶ Sect. 4.1). So, CPAP can eliminate the breathing disorder in one third of the cases of *central sleep apnea syndromes as well.*

APAP

Regarding the application of constant CPAP, it became obvious that the pressure which is necessary to keep the airways open is often higher in the supine position as well as in REM sleep compared to other body positions and sleep stages. Based on these reflections, devices have been developed that continuously measure the *pressure requirement* and *set it automatically*. Therefore, the term auto-CPAP or APAP (automatic positive airway pressure) is used.

The applied systems have to react reliably and sufficiently quickly with pressure increase before obstructive respiratory events occur. On the other hand, they must not react on central events or hypoventilation. This distinction is made possible by measuring the *airflow signal* and the *oscillatory impedance*.

Analysis of the airflow signals is most widely spread. If the pneumatographs integrated in the devices register an inspiratory flow limitation, the pressure is increased stepwise (e.g., 0.2 mbar/s) until the flow curve regains its normal shape. For completion, additionally the airway resistance may be measured by impressing an oscillating pressure wave to the airways via the ventilation tube and the mask and assessing its reflection. The higher the resistance, the stronger the pressure wave that is reflected. If this so-called oscillatory impedance goes beyond the value measured for each individual in tidal breathing, the pressure is increased until the oscillatory impedance reaches again the individual normal values. After a certain time with normal breathing, all APAP devices slowly and stepwise reduce the pressure until the pathological signal is again registered and the pressure has to be raised (◘ Fig. 4.6).

The algorithms applied in single cases for controlling the pressure course sometimes vary significantly according to the manufacturer. The effectiveness of APAP therapy must always be verified for the patient's device. A change of the device type without at least polygraphic verification may thus be responsible for an insufficient therapy outcome.

Both techniques have the effect that the average pressure requirement of the night is about 1–2 mbar lower than with constant CPAP; however, the maximum pressure may be higher. Malfunction is mainly caused by mask leakages and may lead to high-pressure peaks. To avoid this phenomenon, a lower and an upper pressure limit is set for the permanent use based on the pressure course measured during the first night. The pressure limits set in this way allow the best compromise between effectiveness and tolerance.

Bilevel-S

The *inspiratory (IPAP)* as well as the *expiratory (EPAP)* pressure may be set separately to values generally between 3 and 20 mbar (hence the term bilevel). Inspiration is facilitated by the higher and expiration by the lower pressure. The pressure difference may be set at arbitrary intervals. In this way, spontaneous breathing of the patient is actively supported by the device (hence, bilevel-S). To allow this, the necessary pressure or airflow change has to be measured correctly and with the required sensitivity (trigger) by the device. On the other hand, the pressure increase or decrease (edge) has to be sufficiently steep to secure an optimal breathing support without being perceived as too abrupt. The set pressures are then kept at a constant value until the end of the respective breathing phase.

A *modification (auto-bilevel)* measures the EPAP in a variable way such as the APAP device to secure an open pharynx. For this purpose, a fixed inspiratory pressure increase is set so that the IPAP changes parallel to the EPAP and hypoventilation is avoided. The clinical relevance of this modification has remained unknown until now.

C-Flex, EPR, SoftPAP, and A-Flex

C-Flex, EPR (expiratory pressure relief), and SoftPAP are manufacturer-specific variants between CPAP and bilevel-S, in which the pressure at the beginning of expiration is decreased proportionally to the expiratory flow. During expiration, the pressure approaches asymptotically the set CPAP pressure, which is finally reached at the beginning of the next inhalation.

In contrast to the classic bilevel therapy, the expiratory pressure cannot be arbitrarily selected but varies from breath to breath. Generally, three levels may be set that lead to a maximum pressure decrease of about 3–4 mbar. The patient can select the levels.

A further development is the A-Flex mode where not only the expiratory pressure is reduced but also the inspiratory pressure is proportionally increased. Whether this modification is associated with further benefit for the patients has not yet been investigated.

4.6.1.2 Positive Pressure Ventilation in Cases of Disturbed Respiratory Drive

In cases of central sleep apnea syndromes and hypoventilation or hypoxemia syndromes, no sufficient respiratory drive is found, or the respiratory pump itself is damaged.

In these cases, the positive pressure ventilation has to completely perform breathing, either transitorily (e.g., only during nighttime) or intermittently (e.g., only under certain respiratory conditions). In this way inspiratory and expiratory pressures and times as well as respiratory frequencies can be preset by the ventilation device. The controlled positive pressure ventilation is complex and is much more difficult to manage than simple CPAP ventilation.

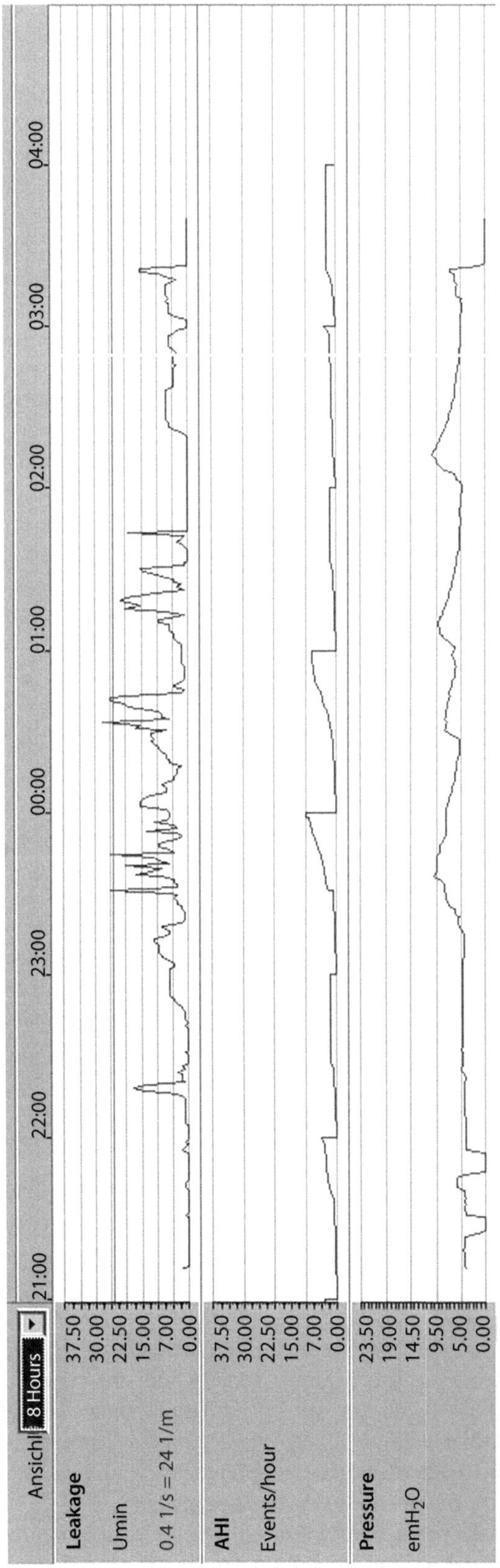

Fig. 4.6 Example of a nocturnal registration of an APAP device

Bilevel-T

Bilevel-T is a timed pressure-controlled ventilation method in which the respiratory frequency and the time relationship from inhalation to expiration are strictly preset by the physician. The patient has to completely adjust the respiratory rhythm to the ventilation system or be ventilated by the system.

Practical Tip

In the context of timed pressure-controlled ventilation (bilevel-T), the patients cannot change the preset parameters by means of their own respiration.

With increasing pressure difference between inhalation and expiration and increasing respiratory frequency, minute ventilation increases. In the context of this ventilation variant, incorrect setting may very rapidly lead to relevant deterioration of the blood gases or even to complete noncompliance and therapy refusal.

Bilevel-S/T

In the context of this variant, the positive pressure ventilation occurs alternating in the *assisted* (spontaneous) or *controlled* (timed) mode. The system initially starts in the spontaneous mode. If a breathing interruption is registered with a minimum duration predetermined by the physician or if the respiratory frequency falls under a certain preset value, the system automatically switches to the controlled mode. As soon as the patient triggers breathing sufficiently, the system switches back to the assisted mode.

4.6.1.3 Positive Pressure Ventilation in Cases of Cheyne-Stokes Respiration

Currently, two different techniques are applied to stabilize Cheyne-Stokes respiration.

In the context of *adaptive servoventilation*, the EPAP and the maximally allowed inspiratory pressure support are predetermined. The inspiratory pressure is close to the EPAP when no breathing disorders occur. If the tidal volume slowly decreases, the IPAP is stepwise increased from breath to breath so that 90% of the previous tidal volume is always achieved. If the patient slips into central apnea, 90% of the tidal volume is still secured by the system; however, this takes place in the controlled mode, and the respiratory frequency is adjusted to the previous respiratory rhythm. With increasing respiration, the IPAP is reversely decreased stepwise.

Because the adaptive servoventilation is set against one's own respiration in cases of Cheyne-Stokes respiration, the actual pulmonary respiration becomes more balanced. Hyperventilation as well as a decrease of the CO_2 below the hypocapnic apnea threshold can thus be avoided.

The *ImPAP mode* (impulse-modulated positive airway pressure) influences the respiration by impressing a short pressure impulse on an APAP pressure after a preset duration of apnea. The pressure impulse stimulates pharyngeal receptors and induces reflectively the patient's own breathing, which terminates the apnea earlier. Arousals should not be triggered in this way. In the course of the application, respiration becomes more regular and the typical crescendo–decrescendo pattern disappears.

Both procedures reliably eliminate Cheyne-Stokes respiration; however, they are still in the stage of evaluation with regard to their therapeutic effects.

Practical Tip

Noninvasive positive pressure ventilation is able to eliminate each type of sleep-related breathing disorder because it acts independently from the genesis of the disorder. Corresponding to the indication, however, different ventilation variants are required.

4.6.1.4 Practical Aspects

The basic precondition for a good acceptance and compliance of the therapy is the *intensive coaching* of the patients, in particular in the initial phase.

In the first place, *information* must be provided about the type and the realization of the ventilation therapy that may be supported by different media. It might be helpful to thoroughly prepare the patients in the context of the diagnostic procedures.

On the day before the first night with ventilation therapy, the patient has to be familiarized with the device and its accessories. When a well-fitting mask is found, it is suitable to let the awake patient breathe with a low pressure (e.g., 4 mbar) as well as a just tolerable pressure in different body positions to allow optimal conditions for the start of ventilation therapy.

This step is particularly important for patients who need bilevel ventilation. The sensation of a too high pressure may be caused by an unnecessarily high EPAP or IPAP, but at the same time, a too sensitive trigger for inhalation, a too insensitive trigger for expiration, a too rapid pressure increase, or a too slow pressure decrease might be responsible for corresponding noncompliance. Too slow respiratory frequency causes dyspnea; too high respiratory frequency leads to hyperventilation with possibly hypocapnia and tetany. If bilevel ventilation in the assisted-controlled or controlled mode is required, the setting of the adaptation phase that the patient perceived as subjectively tolerable is the pressure parameter set at the beginning of the first night.

The training phase with the automatic systems, however, is mainly limited to the adjustment of a well-fitting mask and a short breathing phase in the wake stage.

In the *sleep lab*, the procedure with manually settable devices is started with a low pressure that is well tolerated by the patient. When the patient has fallen asleep, the pressure is increased until respiration is completely normalized. If the patient wakes up because of a pressure that is subjectively perceived as being too high, the titration may have to be restarted with a lower pressure. All body positions and sleep stages should be taken into account.

The therapeutic range of effective settings of just about ineffective to no longer tolerable parameter settings is different in dependence of the present breathing disorder and other individual factors. The effectiveness of the identified pressure may need to be verified during a second night. This procedure is generally sufficient for the treatment of obstructive sleep apnea. In cases of central breathing disorders or hypoventilation or hypoxemia syndromes, often several nights are needed to find the optimal setting of all parameters.

In cases of problems to initiate sleep because of the unfamiliar situation, usually 25–50 mg trimipramine may be helpful or, if a heart disease is found, also hypnotics, for example, zolpidem.

The effectiveness and tolerance of C-Flex, EPR, or SoftPAP do not provide an advantage for this patient population in comparison to constant CPAP; however, those procedures may be suitable in single cases when the pressure is perceived as being too high. If the pressure is perceived as too high only during short wake phases at night, the patient may reduce it to a preset level by activating the ramp function to facilitate falling asleep again. Then the pressure slowly increases again to the effective pressure.

Some manufacturers have developed new devices that are not yet validated and which are of questionable benefit for the patients. These devices try to automatically recognize wake phases via the airflow signal to specifically reduce the pressure to a lower level.

4.6.1.5 Accessories and Masks

Because ventilation therapy can only achieve its full effectiveness when it is applied every night for a sufficiently long period, tolerability of the therapy is a major concern.

Finding the ideal mask for the patients is the most important issue in this context. Silicone-containing masks are generally well tolerated. Most frequently nasal masks are applied that fit airtight around the nose. Alternatively, in particular in cases of claustrophobia or bruises, a nasal pillow mask may be used. Hereby, the air from the fan reaches directly the nasal entrances via soft nasal olives.

In cases of oral leakages, a chinstrap is used that avoids jaw opening, or the interface is immediately switched to an oronasal mask or full-face mask (◘ Fig. 4.7). The last-mentioned ones are also suitable when severe nasal obstruction is found and the patient either permanently or transitorily refuses correction, or correction cannot be performed for medical reasons. Because of the strap fastenings, full-face masks may cause retrusion of the mandible, which sometimes leads to significant narrowing of the pharynx and thus to necessary pressure increase. The resulting leakages then induce further pressure increase that may make the therapy impossible.

It is extremely rare that patients and physicians alternatively decide to apply an oral mask that is fixed via a silicone shield positioned in the oral vestibulum. In sleep medicine, the ventilation mask used in intensive care medicine that

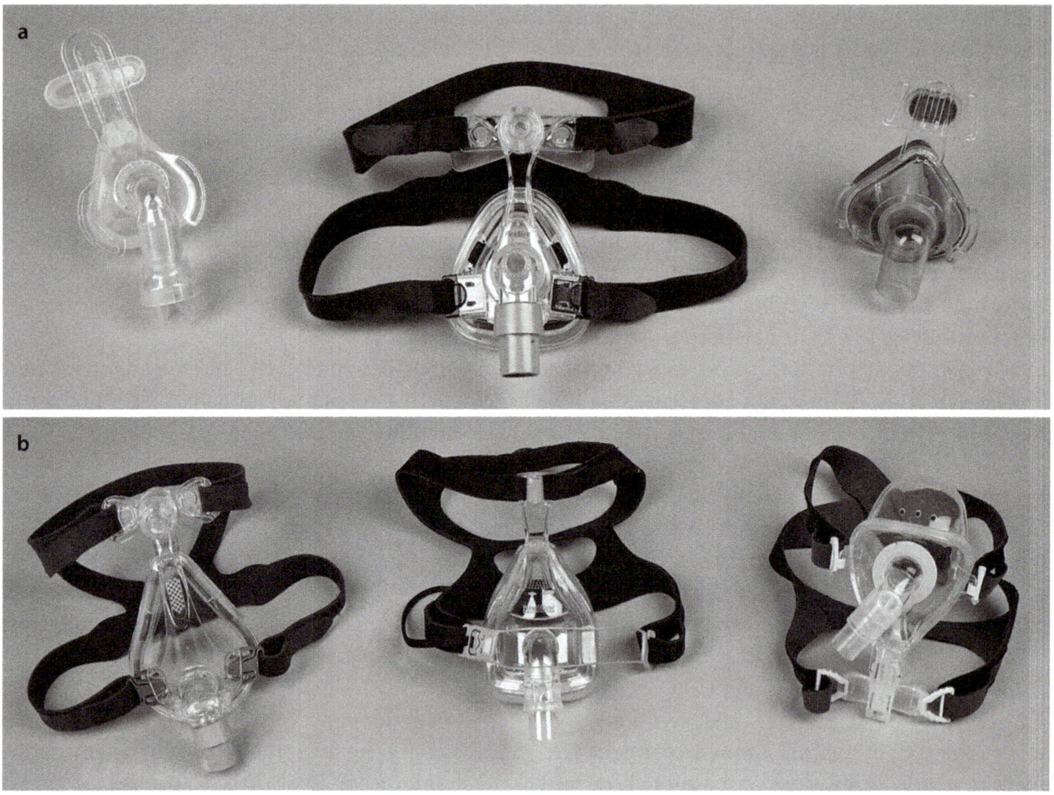

Fig. 4.7 **a** Different nasal masks. **b** Different full-face masks

encloses the entire head and seals cervically is not relevant.

As many masks are currently available, individually manufactured masks based on a facial mold are almost never needed.

Practical Tip

The treatment adherence in cases of noninvasive positive pressure ventilation does not only depend on the subjectively experienced therapeutic benefit but also relevantly on the intensive care of the patient by physicians and device service providers.

To allow sufficient emission of CO_2, a valve is found in or at the mask for the exhaled air. The shape of the valves (slits, wholes, pores) and thus the noise characteristics (loudness and frequency) are different (vented mask).

If patients complain about dry mucosa of the nose and the pharynx, in single cases *nasal ointments* or *nasal oil* products or a *heated humidifier* that is easily coupled to the device may provide relief. If these measures do not suffice, an oral leakage may be responsible that may be eliminated by a chinstrap or an oronasal mask.

In cold environments (open bedroom windows in winter), relevant *condensation water* may develop in the tube and the mask so that real puddles may occur in the sagging tube parts. This occurrence is not only disturbing for the patient as well as the bed partner because of bubbling noises, but in unfavorable cases, aspiration of the condensation water may occur. The ventilation device with humidifier has to be placed lower than the patient's head so that no puddles may develop but the condensation water has to flow back into the humidifier. Furthermore, heated tubes are available reducing condensation. Cold air humidifiers are not recommended because the humidification output is insufficient.

The patient has to be instructed that the mask, valve, tube, and humidifier have to be cleaned every day. For the ventilation device and the headgear as well as the straps, longer intervals are sufficient.

The size and the weight of the CPAP devices no longer play a major role. In the course of the past decades, they became significantly smaller, and nearly all weigh less than 3 kg, sometimes even less than 1 kg. For transportation in airplanes, specific passports for medical devices are available in different languages that classify the devices as medical aids. All devices may be used with a voltage of 220 V as well as 110 V. For use in trucks and caravans, or campers, adapters are available for 24 V and 12 V outlets. In this way, modern CPAP devices can be taken almost anywhere without difficulties.

Bilevel devices for noninvasive home ventilation are usually larger and heavier than CPAP devices, in particular because they contain a battery so that they may work for several hours in cases of power failure.

4.6.1.6 Undesired Side Effects of Positive Pressure Ventilation

In the first night with noninvasive positive pressure ventilation, side effects may already occur. In most cases these are harmless (◘ Table 4.3); however, they may complicate the adjustment of pressure or even make it impossible. Sometimes the mask has to be changed because of *leakages* or

◘ **Table 4.3** Side effects of nasal positive pressure ventilation in long-term use

Side effect	Incidence	Therapeutic options
Xerostomy, dry pharynx	53%	Chinstrap, oronasal mask, heated humidifier
Dry nose	52%	Nasal ointment, heated humidifier
Formation of crusts	38%	Nasal ointment, heated humidifier
Nasal obstruction	36%	Nasal corticoids, nasal surgery
Xerophthalmia	30%	Optimized adjustment of the mask, different mask
Rhinorrhea	28%	Heated humidifier, topical anticholinergics, topical corticoids, turbinate reduction
Epiphora	19%	Optimized adjustment of the mask, different mask
Epistaxis	13%	Nasal ointment, heated humidifier
Sinusitis	8%	Therapy of the sinusitis, disinfection of tube and mask
Hearing impairment, tinnitus	~15%	Otological therapy
Pressure sensation in the ears	~10%	Otological therapy, pressure decrease, APAP, bilevel, C-flex/EPR
Skin irritations, bruises	>50%	Optimized adjustment of the mask, daily alternation of two different masks
Pain	22%	Loosening of the headgear, optimized adjustment of the mask
Aerophagia	11%	Pressure reduction, APAP, bilevel, C-flex/EPR
Leakage	36%	Optimized adjustment of the mask, chinstrap, oronasal mask
Impairment from high noise level	~30%	Longer tube, optimized adjustment of the mask, change of the valve
Too large device	~20%	Smaller device as soon as a follow-up prescription is necessary
Difficult expiration	~10%	Pressure reduction, APAP, bilevel, C-flex/EPR

Source: Modified according to Verse (2000)

claustrophobia despite training during the daytime. In some cases an expiratory pressure reduction is required because the patient perceives the expiration pressure as being too high. The *nasal mucosa* may acutely swell from the airflow, and nasal breathing may be relevantly impaired. A decongestant nasal spray may provide short-term relief.

In very rare cases, *central apneas* and long *hypoventilations* occur under CPAP that can mostly be eliminated by switching to the bilevel-S/T mode. In single cases, however, they have to be interrupted by wakening the patient to avoid CO_2 anesthesia. As it is possible that acute airway obstruction may develop if a floppy epiglottis prolapses into the larynx and left-sided cardiac decompensation (pressure-related) or hypertensive derailment (psychologically caused) occurs, the authors think that the initial pressure titration should be performed under monitored conditions with physicians on duty.

In the long-term course, undesired side effects are often reported, but they can mostly be classified as not being dangerous (◘ Table 4.3, ◘ Fig. 4.8). In most cases, these are *irritations of the skin and the mucosa* of the head and directly mask- or device-related complaints. Such may nearly always be eliminated easily by simple measures. However, if they cannot be removed, consultation of an ENT specialist or dermatologist is recommended.

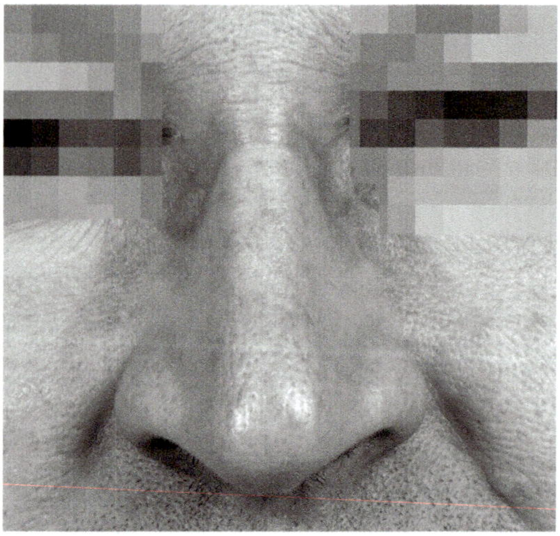

◘ **Fig. 4.8** Patient suffering from bruises at the ridge of the nose caused by nasal mask

Because current devices are very quiet (less than 30 dB, sometimes even less than 24 dB of sound pressure level at 10 mbar), the bed partner is mostly only disturbed by the exhalation valves near the mask. The patient sometimes hears the noise of the fan via the air column in the tube and mask.

The regular follow-up of the patients by competent physicians and healthcare providers is crucial to avoid therapy interruption because of those annoying side effects. If the side effects cannot be eliminated and if relevant insomnia or therapy incompliance is observed for this reason, alternative therapeutic options have to be discussed (see ▶ Sect. 4.7).

4.6.2 Ventilation Therapy in Cases of Central Sleep Apnea Syndromes

In the context of central sleep apnea syndrome, the therapy of the underlying disease is in the main focus.

Therefore, periodic breathing at high altitudes and central sleep apnea with drug or substance abuse are not reasonably treated by means of positive pressure ventilation.

Also, central sleep apnea due to a medical disorder or Cheyne-Stoke respiration may be relevantly reduced if the underlying causes are improved, for example, by optimized medication of heart failure, surgical treatment of nasal obstruction, or neurological rehabilitation after traumatic brain injury.

However, if more than 30 central apneas persist per hour of sleep and if the patient reports further symptoms (see ▶ Sect. 4.1), generally the indication of specific ventilation therapy is given.

The evidence on the prognostic significance of a therapy of central sleep apnea syndromes and in particular Cheyne-Stokes respiration is still unclear. Since a large controlled study reported increased mortality for patients with ejection fraction of less than 45% who were additionally treated with adaptive servoventilation besides optimal cardiac therapy, these patients are now rather treated with other positive pressure techniques, phrenic nerve stimulation, or exclusively with pharmaceuticals.

4.6.2.1 Primary Central Sleep Apnea and Central Sleep Apnea Due to a Medical Disorder

If the following measures do not lead to an elimination of the symptomatic central sleep apnea, different noninvasive positive pressure ventilation techniques are available:

- Improving of the nasal breathing in cases of nasal obstruction
- Avoiding a supine position
- Oxygen administration at night

Apneas may be eliminated by CPAP therapy for as many as 30% of the patients. The necessary pressures generally amount to 5–10 mbar. Different mechanisms are discussed for the stabilizing effect of CPAP therapy on respiration. On one hand, the reflexes triggered by pharyngeal obstructions should be avoided; on the other hand, the oxygen storage should be filled more intensively by increasing the pulmonary volume, which reduces the respiratory drive.

If the CPAP therapy fails, bilevel therapy is applied in the spontaneous or assisted-controlled mode, which seems to lead to the best results. However, unfortunately some patients experience even more respiratory events. Until now, this unpredictable response of the patients with central sleep apnea on the therapeutic interventions has not been understood. Thus, often probatory adjustments of positive pressure ventilation cannot be avoided.

Because the primary central sleep apnea shows *spontaneous remission* in about 20% of the cases, follow-up sleep studies without therapy at certain intervals are always recommended.

4.6.2.2 Cheyne-Stokes Respiration

Cheyne-Stokes respiration is treated according to a *gradual concept*. After each therapeutic step, respiration may normalize. In the majority of the cases, a subjective or objective improvement of the quality of sleep and the daytime sleepiness or fatigue is observed.

The *treatment of the underlying disease* (heart failure, diabetes mellitus, renal failure) is the first priority, followed by *oxygen therapy* (2–4 l/min), which successfully eliminates the breathing disorder in about one third of the patients.

CPAP therapy shows comparable success rates. However, in contrast to obstructive sleep apnea, there is no parameter revealing the necessary pressure for elimination of Cheyne-Stokes respiration, nor are studies available that might have found an optimal pressure for all patients. In practice, pressures between 8 and 10 mbar are most often applied.

Besides the aspect described for primary central sleep apnea, improvement of the hemodynamics of heart failure patients seems to play a major role for the effectiveness of CPAP therapy. The improvement of the cardiac function further supports the performance during daytime. However, patients with heart failure and Cheyne-Stokes respiration belong to a high-risk patient population because of reduction of the preload from the increased intrathoracic pressure, and as a consequence an acute systemic arterial hypotension may develop during the initiation of CPAP therapy. In particular, patients with volume deficiency and atrial fibrillation are at high risk.

If oxygen and CPAP are not sufficiently effective, *bilevel therapy* is mostly applied in the assisted-controlled or completely controlled mode. The setting of the ventilation parameters is initially oriented at the tolerance of the patient and during the nights of adjustment primarily at respiratory parameters. Finally, the selection of the pressure occurs empirically in the same way as for CPAP therapy. Tolerance of the bilevel therapy is generally poorer than that of CPAP therapy.

Up to now it has not been clear if the new automatic procedures of *adaptive servoventilation* and *ImPAP* should be applied exclusively in cases of failed bilevel techniques. At least they not only seem to be better tolerated, but the elimination of the central apneas is most effective. Also further cardiac parameters (ejection fraction, 6-min walking distance, nocturia, quality of life) were most significantly improved by means of adaptive servoventilation. In contrast, patients with severe heart failure (NYHA III–IV) revealed an increased mortality of 34% under adaptive servoventilation in comparison to an untreated control group. Since then, ASV therapy is contraindicated in those patients.

It must be realized that several nights or even weeks may be required until breathing is stabilized after induction of the positive pressure ventilation in cases of Cheyne-Stokes respiration. An almost low-grade improvement during the adjustment phase to a ventilation system does not necessarily mean that elimination of Cheyne-Stokes respiration is not successful. The effectiveness of the treatment must always be verified after the first 3 to 6 months to identify treatment failure early and to introduce alternative procedures.

Practical Tip

In cases of Cheyne-Stokes respiration, therapy of the underlying disease is the first priority. Regarding all applied types of ventilation therapy, no improvement of the mortality rate could be proven for Cheyne-Stokes respiration.

4.6.3 Ventilation Therapy in Cases of Sleep-Related Hypoventilation and Hypoxemia

Such as for central sleep apnea syndromes, the amelioration of the underlying disease is the focus because nearly all hypoventilation syndromes in adults are of secondary origin. Because most of these are progressive diseases, nearly all patients experience hypoventilation in the further course of their disease despite optimal cause-oriented treatment or rehabilitation.

Hypoventilation syndromes are ventilated in an assisted, assisted-controlled, or controlled mode. Negative pressure procedures (iron lung) are almost never used and volume-controlled ventilation is rarely (e.g., in cases of weak coughing) applied. The tendency is to use more and more pressure-controlled techniques.

The daily *duration of ventilation* generally increases during the further progression of the underlying disease. Whereas at the beginning usually ventilation exclusively at night suffices because it leads to a relevant restoration of the respiratory pump and thus to an improvement of the breathing function during daytime, an intermittent or continuous ventilation also during the day cannot be avoided in the later course.

In this context, in many cases invasive ventilation via a *tracheostoma* has to be preferred to noninvasive ventilation because of practical reasons. For example, nutrition under permanent ventilation with a nasal or oronasal mask is almost impossible, and in cases of proneness of aspiration, there is the increased risk of aspiration pneumonia.

The aim of ventilation is not only the elimination of hypercapnia and hypoxemia at night but also an improvement of the quality of sleep as well as the blood gases and performance and quality of life during the daytime.

However, often the symptoms observed during the day cannot be completely and permanently eliminated.

Because ventilation therapy is more difficult to apply in the context of the following indications and becomes frequently necessary in severely ill and care-dependent patients who cannot care for themselves, special attention has to be given to the home environment of the patients and the available care.

4.6.3.1 Sleep-Related Hypoventilation and Hypoxemia Syndromes that Are Not Caused by Bronchial Obstruction

In general, assisted up to controlled noninvasive positive pressure ventilation may be applied in wakefulness as well as during sleep. The indication for ventilation during sleep, however, is made more easily and generously. In cases of a confirmed basic disease, the occurrence of REM-associated hypoventilations and a disturbed quality of sleep with consecutive daytime sleepiness or fatigue without hypercapnia during daytime is considered as sufficient for the introduction of ventilation during sleep by many experts because the relief of the respiratory pump at night often leads to an increased performance during daytime.

If further symptoms are found (see ▶ Sect. 4.1.4), the expected positive effects are initially even more clearly perceived by the patient. Ventilation is mostly perceived immediately as very relaxing. Thus, in general, compliance is very good.

Ventilation is always recommended when CO_2 partial pressure during daytime exceeds 45 mmHg, 50 mmHg during sleep, or oxygen saturation during sleep falls below 88% at least for 5 min or 10% of the monitoring time, and the patient is symptomatic.

Practical Tip

The indication for noninvasive ventilation is based on the symptoms of nonrestorative sleep, clinical signs of right-sided heart failure in combination with nocturnal hypercapnia and hypoxemia, or hypercapnia also during daytime.

In any case, the basic precondition for introduction of noninvasive ventilation therapy is comprehensive written *information* considering the alternative of palliative therapy (oxygen, benzodiazepine, opioids) and the request for treatment of the patient. In the final stage of many neuromuscular or thoracic-restrictive diseases, the patient's desire to terminate an already initiated ventilation therapy also has to be respected.

Bilevel ventilation is trained during the day. With a well-fitting mask, the lowest possible expiration pressure is selected, mostly 4 mbar. The inspiration pressure is initially chosen 5 mbar higher and then set to a pressure difference of 8–10 mbar. The ratio between the duration of inspiration and expiration is set to 1:2. Depending on the ventilation mode, optimally tolerated pressure values, trigger, edges, and/or ventilation frequencies have to be determined very carefully and in close interaction with the patient.

During sleep, based on the optimal setting defined during daytime, the inspiratory pressure is increased to a level at which the oxygen saturation under ambient conditions amounts to more than 90% during REM sleep also. In most cases, pressure differences of 10–15 mbar are sufficient to achieve a decrease of hypercapnia at night and during the day. In single cases, however, differences of more than 20 mbar may be required, particularly in obesity hypoventilation syndrome patients. Here also the expiratory pressure has to be increased to values of more than 10 mbar because often a simultaneous pharyngeal obstruction is observed. By means of the therapy, the CO_2 partial pressure is intended to be reduced to 50 mmHg or less. If hypoxemia persists, additional *oxygen therapy* must be discussed. However, this only seems to be suitable when a pulmonary lesion is diagnosed, and thus it is rarely necessary in cases where obesity hypoventilation is the only disorder.

Assisted ventilation may be sufficient when ventilation therapy is early introduced, so patients benefit more from *bilevel T ventilation* in the further course because the respiratory pump is even more significantly relieved when the pressure change no longer needs to be triggered by the patient. To achieve this effect also in the assisted-controlled mode (bilevel-S/T), the respiratory frequency or the respirator has to be set slightly above the patient's own frequency.

According to the dynamics of the basic disease, a regular *follow-up* of the ventilation therapy is necessary at various intervals. In the context of amyotrophic lateral sclerosis, it is performed, for example, every 3 months, and in cases of stable neuromuscular diseases, scoliosis, or obesity ventilation, it may also be performed once a year.

By noninvasive positive pressure ventilation, the quality of sleep, daytime sleepiness, quality of life, pulmonary function, and blood gases during the daytime, the incidence of respiratory complications, and hospitalization rate as well as the survival of the patients could be significantly improved. Also, secondary pulmonary hypertension as it is frequently found in thoracic-restrictive diseases may be regressive.

Practical Tip

Nowadays, noninvasive ventilation is an essential treatment option for diagnosed respiratory pump weakness.

Controlled studies are still missing, but today they can no longer be justified for ethical reasons.

4.6.3.2 Sleep-Related Hypoventilation and Hypoxemia Caused by Bronchial Obstruction

In Europe, about one third of all patients ventilated at home suffer from chronic obstructive pulmonary disease (COPD), which is frequently associated with emphysema. On average, the patients are of older age, and males are affected more frequently compared to other indications. In stable phases, the patients succeed rather well in maintaining respiration with maximum efforts of the respiratory muscles. Hypoxemia and hypercapnia are accepted.

However, *oxygen administration* via a nasal cannula that is used in many cases for improvement of the hypoxemia and that is rather comfortable for the patient is not sufficient to allow a relevant relief of the respiratory pump. In this way, low-grade additional efforts (e.g., in the context of an infection) lead to decompensation of the respiratory pump. Most frequently, the *noninvasive ventilation* is introduced for therapy of acute respiratory failure occurring in this context, which results in an intensive care hospitalization. For this indication, the benefit of noninvasive ventilation is proven. Under this aspect, a transition to a permanent nocturnal *ventilation at home* is expected to lead to a reduction of COPD exacerbations and as a consequence to reduced hospitalization rates.

If a nocturnal ventilation at home is started in the context of chronic respiratory failure based on stable COPD, the data situation is inconsistent regarding respiratory efforts, pressure of the pulmonary artery, blood gas alterations, structure of sleep, and physical capacity. Only the quality of life seems to improve. In particular, a decrease of the mortality rate in comparison to conservative therapy, however, could not be confirmed.

On one hand, this is not astonishing because ventilation therapy cannot reverse the causative lesion of the pulmonary parenchyma. However, on the other hand, short duration of use, a too low pressure peak, and a too short follow-up are criticized in the studies. At least, however, it seems that better clinical results may be achieved when severe hypercapnia is found preceding therapy and when the pressure difference between inspiration and expiration is set high, that is, to more than 18 mbar.

Furthermore, it has become obvious that the reduction of the CO_2 partial pressure correlates with the daily duration of ventilation. Ventilation in the controlled mode may reduce diaphragmatic activity more significantly compared to the assisted mode, which may be interpreted as a more effective relief of the respiratory pump. Overall, the primary acceptance of ventilation at home amounts to about 80%; the daily duration of use is 6 h on average, which can be evaluated as extremely good.

In this context, a reluctant indication takes account of all this. In Germany, the following criteria are recommended for the introduction of *noninvasive ventilation because of COPD*: clear symptoms of chronic respiratory failure (see ▶ Sect. 4.1.4) and pathological blood gas values with either CO_2 partial pressure over 55 mmHg during daytime or CO_2 partial pressure of 50–54 mmHg during daytime and oxygen saturation below 88% for at least 5 min at night, despite the administration of 2 l/min of oxygen, or CO_2 partial pressure of 50–54 mmHg during daytime and at least two hospitalizations per year because of hypercapnic exacerbations.

In cases of severe symptoms only may those criteria be disregarded.

Ventilation therapy is always initiated in a similar way as for the aforementioned indications in an assisted-controlled or controlled mode. The training and habituation phase during the day are followed by verification at night. Blood-based or not blood-based controls of the CO_2 partial pressure under therapy are required during the day as well as at night. In all cases, a test phase has to be pursued during 1 to 2 months previously to make the decision for permanent ventilation at home to take into consideration the therapeutic success, acceptance, and compliance.

Case Report

A 67-year-old obese nonsmoker (BMI = 39 kg/m^2), female, who receives high-dose opioids because of a stable anterior pelvic ring fracture, is transferred to an intensive care unit with massive dyspnea and respiratory insufficiency. The opioid therapy is substituted by nonrespiratory depressive analgesics, which leads to an improved condition of the patient so that she may be released home with oxygen therapy of 2 l/min. She refuses to undergo further diagnostics.

Some weeks later, she is transferred again requiring intubation and invasive ventilation over 48 h because massive hypercapnia (pCO_2 of 90 mmHg) and hypoxemia (pO_2 of 48 mmHg) are measured, which are expected to be the result of the opioid therapy that the patient had restarted arbitrarily. After weaning off the respirator, the patient is continuously treated with oxygen (2 l/min) via a nasal cannula without receiving further opioids. She still complains of dyspnea at rest, cephalgia in the morning, and severe impairment of her physical performance. Edema of the legs is not observed. She suffers from concomitant diseases such as diabetes mellitus type 2, systemic arterial hypertension, absolute arrhythmia, and a low-grade to moderately reduced left ventricular function.

The blood gas analysis during daytime shows a respiratory global insufficiency (pCO_2 of 46 mmHg, pO_2 of 50 mmHg) with metabolically partly compensated acidosis. The pulmonary function shows a restrictive ventilation disorder (VC of 53%, FEV_1/FVC of 105%). In the cardiorespiratory PSG, severe hypoxemia with an average oxygen saturation of 80% and a minimum of 68% in REM can be measured. The oxygen saturation amounts to less than 90% during 93.6% of the total sleep time. A total of 173 hypopneas are counted; the RDI amounts to 35.

During three fourths of the monitoring time, the patient snores, and tachycardia with an average heart rate of 101 beat per minute is recorded. The sleep profile shows a reduction of the REM percentage to 6%. Deep sleep and light sleep are sufficient. Many sleep stage changes are observed but few arousals (14/h). During deep sleep, the blood gas analysis is repeated; hereby pCO_2 amounts to 60 mmHg and pO_2 to 46 mmHg (▪ Fig. 4.9).

The diagnosis is obesity hypoventilation syndrome with initially additional central sleep apnea caused by opioid overdose.

Over three nights, a bilevel therapy with oronasal mask is introduced in the assisted-controlled mode with an inspiratory pressure of 15 mbar, an expiratory pressure of 5 mbar, and a respiratory frequency of 14/min. Further pressure increase or modification of the respiratory frequency is not accepted by the patient. Based on these parameter settings, the average saturation during sleep in ambient air increases to 87% (▪ Fig. 4.10), and the hypercapnia at night decreases to 50 mmHg. The oxygen saturation, however, is still lower than 90% during 42% of the sleep time. Furthermore, a decrease of the average heart rate to 93 beats per minute is observed. If the patient decides to continue the therapy after the test phase, further pressure optimization and if needed controlled ventilation with adjuvant oxygen administration must be attempted.

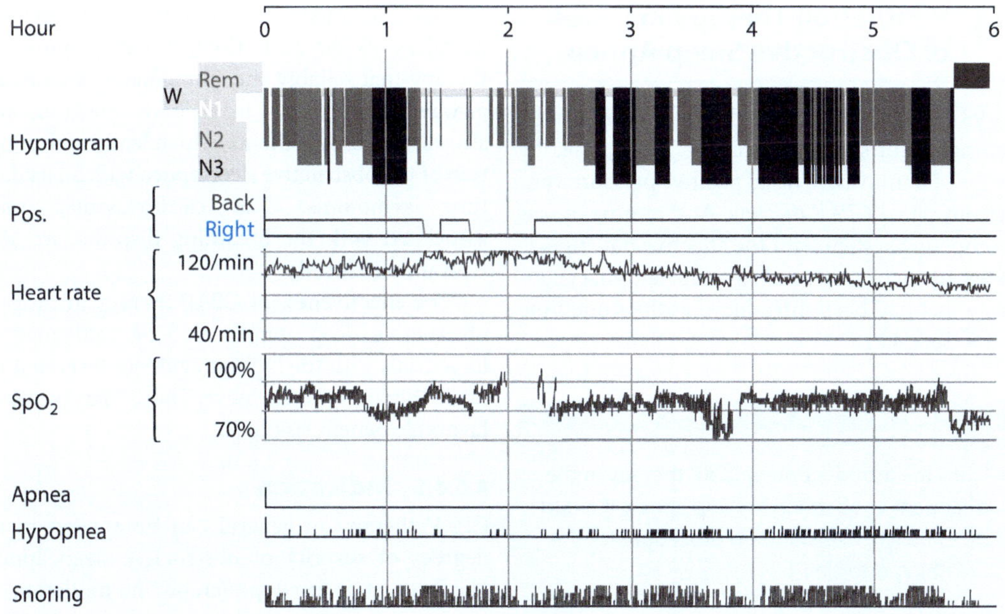

▪ **Fig. 4.9** Nighttime report of the patient with severe obesity hypoventilation

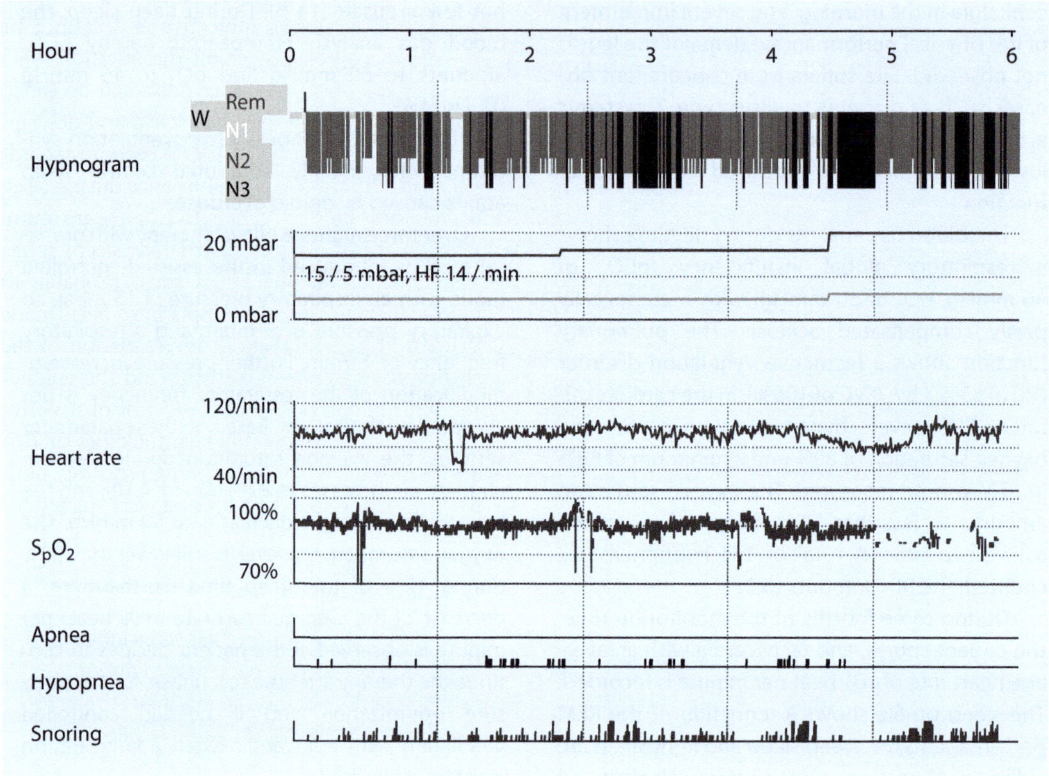

Fig. 4.10 Nighttime report of the patient with severe obesity hypoventilation under therapy

4.6.4 Ventilation Therapy in Cases of Obstructive Sleep Apnea

In 1981, Colin Sullivan was the first to publish the elimination of severe obstructive sleep apnea by means of noninvasive nasal positive pressure ventilation, called *CPAP therapy*. At that time, it was a competing system with the effective but stigmatizing tracheostomy and uvulopalatopharyngoplasty that had been introduced at the same time (see ▶ Sect. 4.7).

Practical Tip

Since the introduction of CPAP therapy in the treatment of obstructive sleep apnea, it could be established as standard procedure for this breathing disorder.

Several reasons may be responsible. CPAP devices and their accessories could be technically improved, which significantly increased the comfort so that undesired side effects are generally harmless. At the same time, it is a symptomatic therapy that reliably and immediately splints the airway pneumatically in all body positions and sleep stages of all patients, which leads to elimination of the obstructive sleep apnea with all its daytime symptoms. The cardiovascular risks associated with the breathing disorder are also relevantly reduced.

The effectiveness of CPAP therapy in cases of obstructive sleep apnea could be confirmed in large trials with the highest evidence level that no other therapy could achieve. Thus, it has the most favorable benefit:risk ratio.

4.6.4.1 Indication

CPAP therapy in general can be applied in all degrees of severity of obstructive sleep apnea. However, it is used preferably in moderate to severe obstructive sleep apnea, whereas alternative therapies also can be used for low-grade types taking into account their morbidity and the patient's individual circumstances.

However, no generally accepted classification of the severity of obstructive sleep apnea could be established so far. Moreover, the severity is defined according to individual criteria based on the following three aspects:

- Severity of the breathing disorder during sleep, that is, RDI (respiratory disturbance index), oxygen saturation, sleep structure
- Daytime symptoms and sociodemographic status, that is, daytime sleepiness, age, job
- Concomitant diseases, such as arterial hypertension and diabetes mellitus, especially if difficult to control

For a young truck driver, for example, with an RDI of only 10 who suffers from relevant daytime sleepiness, CPAP therapy is indicated, whereas for a 70-year-old pensioner with hypertension that is well regulated with medication and otherwise the same constellation, this might not be the treatment of first choice.

With an RDI of 30, the risk is confirmed for the development of cardiovascular secondary diseases, so that under those conditions, CPAP therapy is always indicated.

Practical Tip

Nasal CPAP therapy is the treatment of first choice in moderate to severe obstructive sleep apnea because it reliably eliminates the breathing disorder and does not bear relevant risks for the patient when induced as permanent treatment.

There is no absolute contraindication. But patients with acute heart failure should first be stabilized by means of medication before CPAP therapy is initiated.

4.6.4.2 Practical Aspects

The treatment is started as described in ▶ Sect. 4.6.1. At night, the initial pressure after sleep onset of the patient is only increased if obstructive events occur. It is increased until all obstructive apneas and hypopneas, flow limitations, respiratory arousals, desaturations, and snoring sounds have disappeared. In the ideal case, depending on the tolerance of the therapy, this may take only a few minutes or occur slowly within several hours. In the supine position and in REM sleep, the effective pressure frequently has to be further increased to overcome the increased collapsibility of the pharynx in these phases (◘ Fig. 4.11).

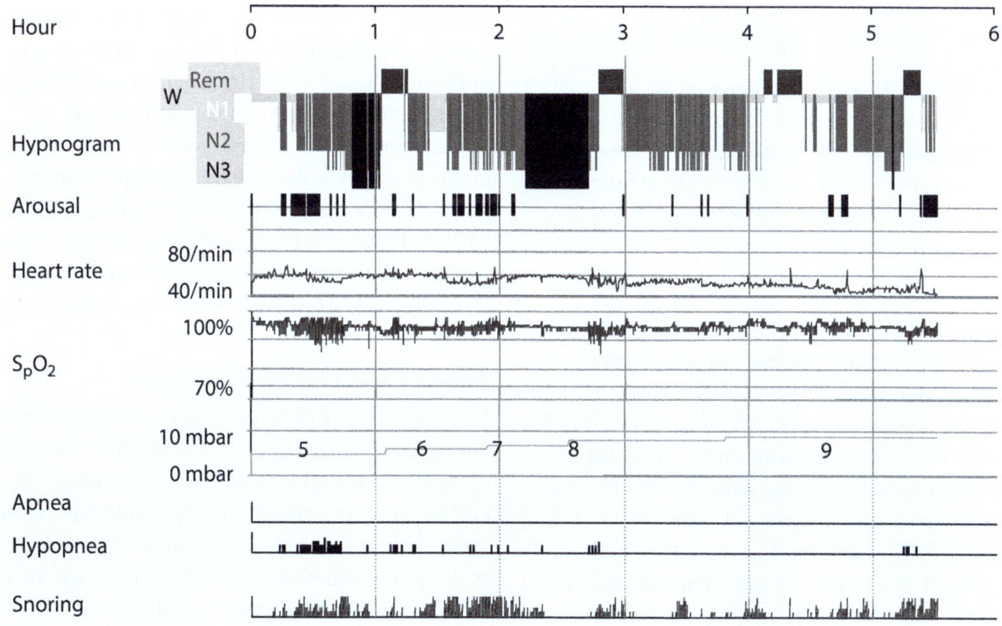

◘ **Fig. 4.11** Nighttime report of a patient with obstructive sleep apnea under CPAP titration

4

If patients with obstructive sleep apnea and a low REM sleep percentage experience a particularly long REM phase under CPAP therapy initiation (REM rebound), this may serve as orientation for good parameter settings.

However, *noise caused by leakage* may be interpreted as snoring sounds by the nursing staff and erroneously induce them to further increase the pressure. If the pressure is increased too much, even more mainly expiratory noise develops, and central apneas and hypopneas are observed. Ideally, the optimal pressure is verified regarding its effectiveness by means of polysomnography during another night.

If the patient does not tolerate the required pressure, further therapeutic options are available including auto-CPAP, C-flex/EPR/SoftPAP, and bilevel-S that may be successfully applied in those situations. Many sleep centers directly initiate auto-CPAP as most APAP-devices available today eliminate respiratory events successfully.

Afterward, the *test phase in the home environment* starts for the patient. Especially at the beginning of the treatment, several changes of the mask, and use of nasal ointment, warm air humidifier, etc., may be necessary to facilitate CPAP therapy that is often perceived as uncomfortable and thus to allow the regular use during the whole sleep time (however, at least for 4–5 h) every night.

Practical Tip

Especially in the initial phase of the treatment, competent and intensive care of the patient by the sleep lab, sleep experts, and manufacturer's staff is essential for the acceptance and thus the effectiveness of ventilation therapy.

In the context of a complication-free course, patients without increased risk profile (e.g., heart failure, excessive daytime sleepiness, occupation) are invited to present after 6 months for *control* with clinical examination and outpatient polygraphy, including the assessment of the subjective sleepiness (Epworth Sleepiness Scale) under CPAP therapy. It is then particularly important to assess the treatment adherence and compliance, which now may be easily read out in nearly all devices with integrated memory chips and thus reasonably complete the patients' subjective reports.

If a risk profile is confirmed, the first CPAP control has to be performed earlier. If a patient has to be declared incapacitated for work because of excessive sleepiness based on obstructive sleep apnea, the control examination should obligatorily include PSG with subsequent vigilance diagnostics (see ► Chaps. 2 and 12).

Further controls are performed by polygraphy or polysomnography every 12 to 18 months in complication-free courses to subjectively and objectively assess the therapeutic success. In cases of pathological polygraphy, PSG in a sleep lab is necessarily indicated where the pressure can be optimized if needed.

If the original symptoms reoccur during therapy, therapy-related reasons (insufficient use, leakage, device failure) have to be differentiated from patient-related reasons (weight increase, progression of obstructive sleep apnea, development of other sleep disorders, or sleep-related breathing disorders). Although therapy-related origins may usually be eliminated on an outpatient basis, the patient-related reasons should suggest PSG because under CPAP therapy they can neither be identified nor be treated by means of polygraphy. In about one third of the patients with effective CPAP therapy and reoccurring daytime sleepiness, however, no reason is found, and symptomatic drug treatment of the complaints is required in the individual case. Sometimes modafinil or Solriamfetol may be applied; in some countries, such as the USA, they are explicitly approved for this indication.

The *long-term compliance* of CPAP therapy could be increased by technical improvements or ventilation devices and masks, amounting to 60% to 80%. If the treatment is interrupted, the breathing disorders redevelop their full severity during the first night, or at the latest, in the second night.

4.6.4.3 Therapeutic Effects

In nearly all patients, ventilation therapy reliably eliminates sleep-related obstructive breathing disorders. An RDI of less than 5 per hour can usually be achieved. Elimination of respiratory arousals leads immediately to an increase of the portion of deep and REM sleep and to a decrease of the percentage of wake phases and light sleep. The macro- and microstructure of sleep normalize.

The improvement of daytime sleepiness and quality of life could be confirmed in randomized trials. However, the premorbid scores are not always achieved. It is assumed that irreversible damage of the central nervous system can be considered responsible for those residual conditions.

The elimination of the obstructive events by means of CPAP also immediately suppresses the associated increases of blood pressure and heart rate that are otherwise induced by the arousal and reflect the activation of the sympathetic nervous system. A significant reduction of the catecholamine level under CPAP could be revealed. The improved oxygenation from CPAP is also responsible for reduction of the catecholamine level, which could also be confirmed during the daytime after longer treatment. In several placebo-controlled trials, a reduction of the systolic, diastolic, and average blood pressure of 5–10 mmHg could be found in patients suffering from hypertension as the result of effective CPAP therapy, which corresponds to the effect of a potent antihypertensive medication.

Several prospective studies could show a relevant increase of the cardiovascular morbidity and mortality (strokes, heart attacks) in cases of severe obstructive sleep apnea. In accordance with the aforementioned results, patients with effective CPAP therapy, however, achieved values that are as low as for patients suffering from snoring. In contrast to this phenomenon, a recent randomized controlled trial with a large patient cohort was not able to confirm these results, which may be explained by the reduced duration of use of only 3.3 h per night.

In patients suffering from heart failure, it is confirmed that CPAP therapy reduces the cardiac preload as well as the afterload. In this way, the cardiac function typically is improved, which could be documented in several noncontrolled trials by an increased ejection fraction of about 10%. However, careful attention must be paid in this patient population because heart failure may decompensate by inducing CPAP therapy.

Recent investigations allow expecting an improvement of insulin sensitivity and thus the diabetic metabolic condition because of CPAP therapy.

Overall, CPAP therapy is best investigated regarding the treatment of obstructive sleep apnea; its positive results could be confirmed in trials with highest evidence level.

Case Report

The 45-year-old bank employee already described in ▶ Sect. 4.2.4 achieves an RDI of 37 in the PSG with an average oxygen saturation of 93% and a minimum of 88%.

On the same day, a nasal mask was adjusted, and ventilation therapy with CPAP was trained. At night, the pressure was manually titrated to 7 mbar, and no further respiratory events were registered. The oxygen saturation at this pressure amounted to more than 92%. However, the patient reported that it was difficult for him to wear the mask because it pinched on the nasal bridge. Frequently, air blew into his eyes. But he was surprised that he felt less tired than previously. The patient was informed that he was still not fit to drive, and the CPAP therapy with a pressure of 7 mbar was recommended for a test period or 4 weeks.

The company responsible for his care delivered the device to his home, instructed him about the use, and adjusted the mask again. After 2 weeks, the mask had to be changed again, and the patient was then able to finally sleep for 5 h without interruption.

During an outpatient presentation after 4 weeks in the sleep medical consultation, the patient stated that he had meanwhile fully accepted the device and wanted to use it further because he felt much better during the daytime. Sometimes he snored, but he complained more about his dry pharynx. Nasal ointment was only partly successful. Consequently, a warm air humidifier was prescribed.

Eight weeks after induction of CPAP therapy, the patient reported that he felt like a new person and did not want to do without the device and the humidifier. Bruises were not observed. His blood pressure had improved; he needed less sleep and was as efficient as he had not been for many years. At work, "things were running smoothly again" and he did not fall asleep. Driving his car was no problem for him. Even the erectile dysfunction observed before induction of the CPAP therapy had disappeared.

In the outpatient polygraphic control examination, only five hypopneas and two central apneas were registered at a constant pressure of 7 mbar. According to the patient, the night had been representative for the past weeks. The ESS was significantly better with 8 points compared to the score before therapy, and the pupillometry in the morning after measurement revealed normal findings. So, his fitness to drive was completely restored.

Further follow-up examinations were set for 12- to 18-month intervals.

4.7 Therapeutic Alternatives

Ventilation therapy for snoring is indicated neither from a medical point of view nor under practical aspects. Numerous conservative and surgical procedures may be taken into consideration. Even in the context of sleep-related breathing disorders going beyond snoring, accompanying or alternative measures may be indicated together with ventilation. Most therapeutic options are applied in the same or modified way for snoring as well as for other sleep-related breathing disorders, in particular for obstructive sleep apnea. Therefore, the therapeutic alternatives and their indication are described together in the following paragraphs.

Generally, it can be stated that therapeutic procedures developed for the purpose of mechanical stabilization or dilation of the airway may only be appropriate for snoring or for sleep-related breathing disorders with mechanical obstruction. The surgical procedures are presented in a separate chapter.

In the following, only procedures that showed a certain effectiveness in clinical trials for at least some indications, or procedures that have been verified reliably in studies, allowing scientifically sound conclusions, are presented.

Especially in the context of snoring and obstructive sleep apnea, a large variety of questionable and frequently even dubious therapeutic procedures are offered and sometimes very aggressively promoted in the lay press. In contrast to pharmaceutical products, these presumptive medical aids often do not need to undergo intensive clinical approval procedures and can be launched into the market mostly without control. Such aids include different types of sprays, drops, or oils, pillows, or also several wakening devices and other sometimes curious constructions. Generally, no clinical trials are available for those products, and the authors' experience has shown that usually even the manufacturers are not really interested in scientific verifications of their products. Nonetheless, a critical discussion of all these products is required because patients often report about having undergone those therapies or seek advice regarding these products.

4.7.1 Conservative Procedures

The following therapeutic alternatives are included in the conservative procedures:

- Weight loss
- Behavioral change
- Medication
- Nocturnal oxygen therapy

4.7.1.1 Weight Loss

Except for central sleep apnea, a high body mass index is associated with all sleep-related breathing disorders and also with snoring. The pathophysiological significance of obesity for obstructive sleep apnea syndrome has already been described in detail; it is fully evident for the obesity hypoventilation syndrome. Correspondingly, clinical trials could document an improvement for nearly all these respiratory phenomena after reduction of body mass index.

Practical Tip

In cases of overweight or obesity, weight reduction should be attempted as an accompanying measure. Except for central sleep apnea syndromes, nearly all other sleep-related breathing disorders experience an improvement after the reduction of body mass index.

Often the patients' history shows that preexisting snoring or a known nocturnal breathing disorder is relevantly aggravated in the context of weight increase. An suitable treatment recommendation in these cases is mostly directly plausible for the patients. Of course, it cannot be guaranteed that the disease completely disappears after successful weight reduction, except for hypoventilation that is only based on obesity. However, in nearly all cases, an improvement may be expected. Sometimes after such an improvement, alternative therapies are available for the breathing disorder that were considered as not being promising because of obesity.

In clinical trials, even relatively small weight reductions often lead to a decrease of the respiratory events. This finding is important because unrealistic requirements for weight reduction down to normal weight are only rarely motivating and effective for very obese patients. Weight reduction is also important because obesity is another independent risk factor that in combination with a sleep-related breathing disorder has a potentiating effect on cardiovascular morbidity and mortality.

Despite the significance of weight reduction in the treatment of sleep-related breathing disorders, the clinical experience is mostly frustrating. As with obesity therapy in general, usually only a few patients succeed in achieving a relevant weight loss or in maintaining their reduced weight over a longer period of time. In cases of high-grade obesity, bariatric surgery (partial gastric resection, gastric banding, etc.) should also be discussed after exploitation of all conservative measures. Our own experiences from cooperation with a specific center for bariatric surgery confirm the positive data reported in the literature regarding the effect of body weight reduction on nocturnal respiratory events. On the other hand, randomized clinical trials are not available, the treatment is not without risk, and even after initial therapy response, reoccurring of the breathing disorder is always possible after a certain time even without weight increase. Despite those limitations, the American Academy of Sleep Medicine emphasizes the significance of surgical weight reduction in its practice parameters.

4.7.1.2 Behavioral Changes

Numerous general behavioral changes are frequently recommended for patients with sleep-related breathing disorders, including avoiding *hypnotics* or *alcohol* in the evening as well as observing a stable sleep–wake rhythm with respective *sleep hygiene*. Avoiding hypnotic intake and alcohol in the evening is generally justified with the explanation that these substances have a muscle-relaxing effect that might aggravate an existing sleep-related breathing disorder, in particular, obstructive sleep apnea.

However, the study situation is contradictory. It is rather improbable that alcohol in the evening really aggravates or unmasks an existing sleep-related breathing disorder to a clinically relevant extent, even if single cases are reported in which obstructive sleep apnea is only manifest even in the sleep lab after respective alcohol provocation. In analogy, the same is true for the intake of sedatives.

Finally, neither alcohol in the evening nor the intake of sedatives is desirable from a sleep medical point of view. Hereby, an impairment of the sleep profile or the impaired daytime vigilance may be expected. Intake of sedatives over a longer period is only indicated in rare cases. On the general sleep medical aspect, the recommendation can only be supported to avoid drinking alcohol in the evening or consuming hypnotics. In analogy, this applies for the observation of a stable sleep–wake rhythm and sufficient sleep hygiene (see ▶ Sect. 3.2.1).

4.7.1.3 Medication

In particular for the treatment of *snoring*, a large variety of partly suspect therapeutics are offered, among them various pharyngeal sprays that promise to improve snoring. None of those pharmaceutical products has demonstrated its effectiveness.

Also in the context of *sleep-related breathing disorders*, several attempts have been made to establish medical therapy. Of course, in cases of different types of secondary alveolar hypoventilation, medical treatment of the underlying disease may lead to an improvement of the sleep-related breathing disorder (e.g., beta-2 sympathomimetics for chronic obstructive pulmonary disease or medication for the treatment of heart failure).

A specific medical treatment of sleep-related breathing disorders, however, is currently not available, although in the context of phenotyping of obstructive sleep apnea medical treatment for distinct phenotypes has recently been tested in clinical trials with positive initial results.

Practical Tip

Effective medical treatment of snoring and obstructive sleep-related breathing disorders is currently not available.

4.7.1.4 Nocturnal Oxygen Therapy

The administration of oxygen at night may be indicated in all sleep-related breathing disorders that are associated with nocturnal desaturation. Although nocturnal respiratory events generally cannot be avoided by the administration of oxygen, its use may be successful to avoid or at least to attenuate the accompanying desaturations.

In cases of obstructive or central sleep apnea, however, an indication is only given in exceptional cases even if the severity of the desaturations can be reduced based by nocturnal oxygen therapy. Here, the available therapeutic alternatives, with nocturnal ventilation therapy in first place, are generally very effective so that a nocturnal oxygen administration is not required or may be taken into account only as adjuvant measure in patients with accompanying pulmonary diseases. Treatment of sleep apnea with oxygen alone is not recommended.

The treatment of hypoventilation syndromes, however, can also be difficult with ventilation therapy, so that in this context, the accompanying administration of nocturnal oxygen may be considered. In the practice, especially patients are concerned who suffer from secondary alveolar hypoventilation in cases of or in combination with chronic pulmonary disease, for example, COPD. In particular, nocturnal oxygen therapy may be discussed if the respiratory arousals are less in the focus of the disease than the associated desaturations.

4.7.2 Device-Based Procedures

Device-based procedures have been developed to counteract an obstruction of the airways in cases of obstructive sleep apnea and to reduce the vibration of the soft tissue in cases of snoring. Currently available devices limited to these indications are:

- Procedures to increase muscle tone
- Technical aids to avoid supine position
- Mandibular advancement devices

4.7.2.1 Increase of Muscle Tone

In past years, various procedures for stimulation and toning the muscles have been tested, all aiming at ameliorating snoring and obstructive breathing disorders. The therapeutic approach was based on considerations regarding the pathophysiology of airway obstruction (see ▶ Sect. 4.2). Finally, it is a question of the dilators of the upper airway that have to counteract the negative inspiratory pressure and keep the airway open. Furthermore, it could be demonstrated that patients with obstructive sleep apnea have an increased muscle tone of the suprahyoidal muscles even during wakefulness, which seems to be necessary to avoid an airway collapse when awake. It was assumed that strengthening or toning of these dilators could be beneficial for the treatment of obstructive breathing disorders.

Numerous publications exist, for example, on *electrical muscle stimulation*. The clinical results, however, have been disappointing in the past. Although some trials showed an improvement of snoring in patients with obstructive sleep apnea, the expectations regarding an effect on respiratory disorders could not be met. Until now, the effectiveness of electrical muscle stimulation could not be proven for obstructive sleep apnea, although new technical development and new device were recently introduced into the market with positive initial results.

A comparable approach was pursued by procedures that promote *training* of the pharyngeal muscles. In this context, some attention was paid to a publication on regularly playing a digeridoo (a tube-shaped wind instrument of the Australian aborigines). For this kind of therapy as well as for special training of the oral and pharyngeal muscles, a limited number of randomized trials is available that confirms the effectiveness in comparison to a control group. Whether the success reported there can be realized in daily practice may be questioned, also considering the time-consuming training phases that are necessary to maintain the effect. Sometimes, other training procedures originating from the field of speech therapy are propagated (e.g., singing exercises and voice training) without that reliable trials would have been published on this topic.

4.7.2.2 Avoiding the Supine Position

Deterioration of obstructive sleep apnea caused by the supine position (so-called positional sleep apnea) is regularly observed, and according to the literature, it occurs in about half of the patients with different severity. Many patients suffering from snoring report, for example, an aggravation of snoring in this position. Generally, mechanical factors are considered responsible for this phenomenon, in first place the gravity-related airway obstruction with the soft tissue (soft palate, tongue) falling into the pharynx but also because of the change in position of the mandible. An improvement of snoring in lateral positions is certainly an experience that most adults have made who had to suffer from a snoring bed partner.

With this background, it seems to be highly interesting to avoid a supine position especially for patients who suffer from obstructive sleep apnea or snoring that is predominantly or exclusively manifest in the supine position. In the context of obstructive sleep apnea, these patients have a respiratory disturbance index during the entire night that requires treatment but present with a tolerable number of respiratory events in the nonsupine position. From a practical point of view, snoring should also disappear in the lateral position because the acceptance by the bed partner would be limited despite a possibly successful reduction of the respiratory events. Avoiding the supine position, however, may also be part of the therapeutic concept when the breathing disorder in the supine position can only be improved but not completely eliminated. In these cases, procedures for avoiding the supine position may be complementarily effective and be of great value in combination with other procedures.

Practical Tip

In cases of snoring that occurs in the supine position, or obstructive sleep apnea that is only observed in the supine position, avoiding this position may be successful as the only or adjuvant measure of treatment.

To avoid the supine position during sleep, numerous anecdotal and also historical reports have been published. Self-constructed aids (e.g., inserting a tennis ball into the back part of the pajamas), however, generally do not provide sufficiently reliable support to avoid the supine position. In addition, turning around one's own axis should still be possible.

Some manufacturers present respective aids, including, for example, vests in which foam half-cylinders are inserted or sewn in. Their effectiveness could be documented in clinical trials with this special patient population (◘ Fig. 4.12). Long-term therapy adherence, however, was disappointing in clinical trials. Furthermore, diseases of the musculoskeletal system or the spine may make their application impossible. Recent publications describe the treatment of position-related sleep apnea with an electronic device that is fixed at the chest wall by means of a belt registering the body position and generating a

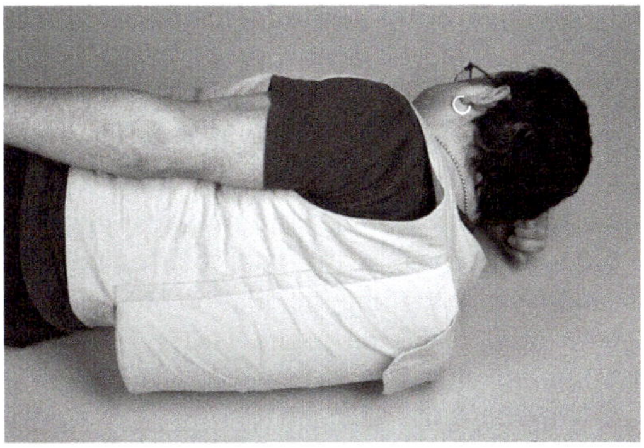

◘ **Fig. 4.12** Example of a vest designed to avoid the supine position

vibration stimulus with increasing intensity when in supine position (labeled as sleep position trainer). From a practical point of view, this technique seems to be an interesting alternative to current aids, and clinical trials confirm the effectiveness and good compliance. Comparable therapeutic approaches are currently offered by different smartphone apps even if in most cases a scientific evaluation is not available.

If a patient is diagnosed with positional obstructive sleep apnea, these measures that are nearly without any side effect, well tolerable, and inexpensive should be discussed and provided. Also, the American Academy of Sleep Medicine recommends the positional therapy as a secondary or accompanying measure in patients with a position-dependent breathing disorder. In particular in cases of obstructive sleep apnea, however, an objectifying control of the therapeutic outcome and a regular verification of the compliance are of relevance.

4.7.2.3 Mandibular Advancement Devices

Mandibular advancement devices (MAD) generally pursue the objective of mechanically dilating and stabilizing the upper airway. They are inserted into the mouth and adhere to the dental arches of the maxilla and the mandible. Both occlusal surfaces are either fixed in one piece (so-called monobloc systems) or flexibly linked via splints, strips, or joints; hereby, the two-splint system seems to be more advantageous. Both occlusal surfaces are positioned in that way that the insertion of the mouthpiece is only possible when the mandible is advanced (i.e., protruded). If the mouthpiece is inserted in this way, an advancement of the mandible results, and thus the airway is mechanically dilated on the level of the soft palate and the base of tongue.

Although the retrolingual dilation due to the fixation of the tongue to the inner surface of the mandible via the genioglossus muscle is immediately understandable, the particular anatomical relationships regarding the dilation of the airway on the level of the soft palate have to be considered in more detail. First, the soft palate with the uvula lies dorsally on the base of tongue so that an advancement of the base of tongue also dilates the space of the palatal soft tissue. Second, the anterior palatal arch is also linked with the base of tongue via the origin of the palatoglossus muscle at the transverse muscle of the tongue, so that a dilation of the airway results in two respects. Furthermore, the functional effects are discussed because an increased pretension of the mentioned muscles also leads to a change of their function.

Practical Aspects

The advancement devices are applied in the treatment of snoring as well as of obstructive sleep apnea. Most promising is their application when the patient has a good *protrusion of the mandible* because these cases are most likely to achieve a therapeutically effective advancement. Even if no recommendation can be given that may be applied to all patients, a maximally possible advancement of less than 1 cm rarely does lead to satisfactory results. In this context, it must be taken into account that the adjustment of advancement devices is not performed with the maximal protrusion because otherwise disorders of the temperomandibular joint may result and the wearing comfort is impaired.

Practical Tip

Treatment with an advancement device is only possible with sufficient mandibular protrusion. In particular, in cases of permanent therapy, cooperation with a dental specialist trained in sleep medicine is recommended.

Besides sufficient mandibular protrusion, dental status should also be satisfactory. Of course, what can be considered as sufficient in the individual case depends on the individual conformation, the compliance of the patient, and the experience of the user. Cooperation with a dental specialist qualified in sleep medicine, however, often allows an appropriate treatment even in cases of difficult findings, and in particular for permanent treatment with MPD it is the precondition for a safe and effective therapy.

Furthermore, it should be mentioned here that besides advancement devices that are custom-made based on dental imprints, *thermoplastic devices* are also available that can be individually adjusted in a relatively simple way and are generally less expensive. For these thermoplastic devices (so-called boil-and-bite devices), good results are documented in clinical treatment; however, they should be applied carefully. Even if great care is taken to adjust the device regarding the protrusion, the individual particularities of the teeth and the periodontal apparatus can only be considered to a limited extent. In addition, the durability of these splints is limited, and an ineffective friction, that is, adhesion of the device at the teeth, may impair the effectiveness. In its current guideline, the American Academy of Sleep Medicine comes to the conclusion that "When oral appliance therapy is prescribed by a sleep physician for an adult patient with obstructive sleep apnea, we suggest that a qualified dentist use a custom, titratable appliance over non-custom oral devices."

However, thermoplastic devices may provide valuable input as test systems. The patient is treated very soon with relatively low financial effort, and the appliance under daily conditions can be tested for a limited period. Furthermore, a first estimation of the effectiveness of advancement devices can be performed before a permanent treatment is induced. The lack of therapeutic success with thermoplastic devices, however, does not necessarily mean that advancement devices are generally not effective in the individual patient.

The spectrum of available systems has been continuously increased, and some significant differences are found between products. In this context, not all such products have been scientifically investigated. Hence, study results on specific device systems cannot be directly transferred to other products or manufacturers.

Patient Selection

Regarding the selection of suitable patients, anatomical conditions have to be taken into consideration. Most suitable are those patients displaying the following characteristics:

- Only slightly overweight (BMI <30 kg/m2)
- Sufficient mandibular protrusion
- Intact dental status
- No other relevant obstruction sites in the clinical examination
- Snoring or mild to moderate (position-related) obstructive sleep apnea (RDI ≤30)

According to the current S3 guideline of the DGSM on sleep-related breathing disorders, mandibular protrusion devices may be applied in cases of mild to moderate obstructive sleep apnea as an alternative to CPAP/APAP treatment. In cases of severe sleep apnea, mandibular advancement devices may be considered when positive pressure therapy is not sufficiently effective or is not tolerated despite the application of all supporting measures.

Case Report

In a sleep medical consultation, a 37-year-old man presents who has a history of being a notorious snorer for many years (on the occasions of private trips with his diving club, his friends refuse to share a room with him). However, the patient is not symptomatic, and he does not complain about daytime sleepiness: sleep is perceived as restorative. A sleep medical examination reveals mild obstructive sleep apnea with an RDI of 17; ventilation therapy is induced. Not least because of the lack of symptoms, the patient subjectively does not benefit from the treatment and uses the ventilation device only very irregularly. He is interested in therapeutic alternatives.

Clinical examination of this slightly overweight patient (BMI, 27) does not show anatomical anomalies. Because of a good mandibular protrusion of 1.5 cm and a healthy dental status, the indication for a treatment with a mandibular advancement devices is made. The patient is presented to a dental specialist qualified in sleep medicine who provides an individually manufactured intraoral device.

After a period of 4 weeks during which the patient had continuously used the device, he reports that the initial difficulties with the device have disappeared and that his girlfriend told him his snoring has significantly improved. The control PSG with the advancement device revealed an RDI of 3.

Acceptance and Side Effects

Not all patients tolerate advancement devices as permanent treatment. Long-term compliance rates between 48% and 90% are reported, whereas assessment of compliance, for example, by means of temperature sensors, has not been implemented in the daily routine. Comparative studies, however, confirm a better compliance of the advancement devices in comparison to CPAP therapy.

Hypersalivation that is disturbing for the patient may occur because of the devices, or the devices may be removed unconsciously during sleep. Furthermore, many patients report disturbing cramps of the masticatory muscles in the morning, so that the mandible or the joint has to be relaxed after taking out the advancement device. Additionally, clinically relevant disorders of the temperomandibular joint may occur, or an already existing disorder may be aggravated. In particular, in cases of longer use, loosening of the periodontium of single teeth may be observed, to which strong acting forces are applied and or occlusion disorders may develop.

The majority of initially occurring complaints disappear in the further course. Data on persisting or clinically relevant side effects vary enormously in the literature (between 0% and 75%). In a long-term trial, a change of the dental position could be documented by means of repeatedly performed imprints in 14% of the patients after 5 years. Therefore, regular follow-up examinations should be performed by qualified dental specialists.

Therapeutic Effects

With specific treatment by means of advancement devices, socially disturbing snoring as well as obstructive sleep apnea may be treated successfully.

Data on the success rates in the context of snoring are naturally subjective, and the data situation is less reliable than for the treatment of sleep apnea. A substantial improvement of snoring, however, can be expected in suitable patient populations. Because snoring is not a disease in the proper sense of the word, possible complications of the treatment should be considered critically.

Regarding the treatment of obstructive sleep apnea, comprehensive and partly even placebo-controlled studies are available documenting the effectiveness on a subjective as well as objective level. Although compliance concerning advancement devices in clinical trials is more favorable in comparison to CPAP therapy, respiratory therapy seems to be superior regarding the absolute reduction of respiratory events.

Practical Tip

According to current guidelines, advancement devices are considered as equivalent therapeutic approaches to ventilation therapy for mild to moderate sleep apnea. Sleep medical follow-up examinations for control of the treatment success are essential.

4.8 Surgical Therapy

Conservative therapeutic measures, in particular ventilation therapy, are still considered as standard and are generally the measure of first choice in the treatment of sleep-related breathing disorders. Nonetheless, patient interest in surgical alternatives is still very high, which may be explained by the limited acceptance and the often insufficient compliance with regard to conservative procedures. Frequently patients ask for effective treatment without the need for a daily or nocturnal intervention (e.g., protrusion devices, ventilation therapy). Surgical procedures may represent an interesting alternative in the context of snoring or obstructive sleep apnea (nonobstructive breathing disorders are generally not suitable for surgical treatment). Their application, however, has to be discussed critically and individually.

4.8.1 Indications and Contraindications

The general aspects indicating the treatment of sleep-related breathing disorders have already been discussed comprehensively (see ▶ Sect. 4.4.2). With regard to surgical therapy, it must be stated that an indication for surgery can only be made if the patient refuses to undergo conservative procedures, or if such measures are not tolerated, or if no satisfactory outcome is achieved. Thus, surgical therapy is usually not the treatment of first choice, and conservative approaches have to be discussed first of all with the patient. This step corresponds to the recommendations of the American Academy of Sleep Medicine that published respective recommendations on the surgical therapy of sleep apnea in its practice parameters on surgical modifications of the upper airway for obstructive sleep apnea. Regarding obstructive sleep apnea, the authors generally offer conservative treatment to the patient, and they mostly succeed in convincing them to at least make an attempt. Frequently, the initial wish for surgical treatment is then dropped.

On the other hand, consequently all therapeutic and thus also surgical alternatives that are available should be clarified and offered when no satisfactory effect or compliance can be achieved with conservative procedures despite all reasonable efforts. For example, not all patients tolerate nocturnal ventilation therapy even if initially expressing a positive attitude regarding this therapeutic approach. In these cases, an interdisciplinary cooperation should allow offering all available therapeutic alternatives. Surgical therapy may frequently lead to substantial improvement in symptoms even if the underlying breathing disorder has not been completely eliminated and surgery has only led to a reduction of the respiratory events. So, if the patients refuse to undergo conservative therapy, surgical therapy is often better even under less favorable circumstances than therapeutic nihilism. With this background, consultation of a sleep specialist with surgical qualification (typically otolaryngologists or maxillofacial surgeons) may often be helpful.

Regarding *contraindications* of surgical therapy, obesity must be mentioned in the first place. Increasing overweight leads to a linear decrease of the success rates of nearly all surgical treatments. Even if no generally applicable limit can be defined, and always the individual findings as a whole have to be considered, it can be stated that surgical therapy is successful with a BMI of >32 kg/m^2 in only rare cases. Finally, the general contraindications for surgical interventions apply, in particular when general anesthesia is required. In this context, the expected therapeutic effects always have to be weighed against the individually existing risk.

Practical Tip

Generally, surgical treatment strategies are only indicated in cases of obstructive sleep-related breathing disorders or snoring. A higher-grade obesity is usually a contraindication for the procedures that are currently available.

The success rates of many surgical alternatives are limited; frequently only a few long-term results are available, and not all procedures have yet been sufficiently evaluated. However, in recent years, the number of high-quality clinical trials on surgical procedures has significantly increased so that now randomized controlled trials are also available for a series of interventions. Meanwhile, the understanding prevails that compliance must not be excluded from the assessment of the effectiveness of therapeutic approaches because it is generally superior for surgical procedures.

4.8.2 Selection of the Surgical Therapy

Selection of the suitable therapeutic approach has substantial relevance. If an intervention has not led to the desired effect, in most cases it is not a technically insufficient performance but more frequently the inappropriate selection of the procedure. If the most suitable therapy is not available, the surgeon must not hesitate to refer the patient to another institution.

In all cases, the selection of the procedure must be based on these concerns:

- The type of the breathing disorder
- The severity of the breathing disorder
- Individual anatomical findings

The significance of the *type of breathing disorders* becomes very clear, for example, in the context of snoring. According to the authors, predominantly minimally invasive procedures should be applied for surgical treatment of snoring that may be performed under local anesthesia and that are associated with a low intra- and postoperative morbidity. Thus, the indication of, for example, laser-assisted uvulopalatoplasty (LAUP) or uvulopalatopharyngoplasty (UPPP) must be made very strictly in cases of snoring and should be reserved for exceptional cases, in particular because generally a less invasive alternative is available for the treatment of snoring.

With increasing *severity of the disease*, the probability of successful surgical treatment of obstructive sleep apnea decreases. Also, in this context no rigid limit value can be defined. In individual cases, for example, severe obstructive sleep apnea due to tonsillar hyperplasia may be successfully treated by means of tonsillectomy in an adult patient, if needed in combination with UPPP.

Finally, clinical assessment of the *individual anatomical findings* is crucial for successful surgical therapy. Hereby, it is important to identify every possible anatomical obstruction:

- Skeletal deformities/retrognathia
- Clinically relevant nasal obstruction
- Hyperplastic tonsils
- Hyperplastic uvula/soft tissue surplus at the soft palate
- Retrolingual obstruction
- Laryngeal obstruction/floppy epiglottis

Only based on these anatomical findings can a reasonable selection of the surgical approach be made.

Additional examinations may improve the selection of the appropriate therapy:

- Different clinical *scoring systems* or Müller's maneuver consist of the attempt to detect the site of obstruction by means of endoscopy or imaging procedures during inspiration against the occluded airway.
- An attempt to identify the location of the airway obstruction via *multichannel pressure probes* that are placed into the esophagus and the pharynx. For this purpose, different rigid and dynamic imaging procedures have also been promoted.
- Finally, endoscopy of the upper airway allows visual assessment of the airway or the airway obstruction during spontaneous or drug-induced sleep (drug-induced *sleep endoscopy*, DISE).

For some interventions, it was possible to show that better patient selection could be achieved by means of these examination procedures. For example, the success rates for tonsillectomy with uvulopalatopharyngoplasty are higher when obstruction on the level of the soft palate or a "high" obstruction could be documented by a clinical score or pressure probe measurements. For breathing-synchronized upper airway stimulation ("hypoglossus stimulation"), obstruction patterns defined in DISE were predictive for the effectiveness of the procedure. Finally, sleep endoscopy is essential for the diagnosis of laryngeal obstruction.

The routinely performed examination of all patients with DISE however is currently not yet evidence based. Regarding a detailed discussion of the topic of assessing the upper airway, the authors refer to the literature listed at the end of this chapter.

4.8.3 Surgery of the Nose

The surgical procedures to treat nasal obstruction are identical to those applied otherwise in the clinical routine. There are no specific surgical procedures or nasal interventions for the treatment of sleep-related breathing disorders. The most common procedures include these:

- Surgical correction of septal deviation (septoplasty)
- Surgical correction of functionally relevant nasal deformities [functional (septo)-rhinoplasty]
- Reduction of hyperplastic inferior turbinates (turbinate reduction or turbinoplasty)

In cases of obstructing inflammatory processes (nasal polyposis), surgical therapy of the paranasal sinuses may also be indicated. However, the different surgical techniques are not discussed in this chapter.

Surgery of nasal obstruction generally improves the subjective nasal breathing and the subjective sleep quality and consecutively also daytime sleepiness. It may furthermore improve a treatment with nasal ventilation (e.g., nCPAP) or even only allow it. Especially in cases of CPAP incompliance with nasal obstruction, consultation of an ENT surgeon is often helpful, and surgical intervention can contribute to increased acceptance of nasal ventilation therapy.

However, surgical treatment of nasal obstruction alone is only rarely effective in the treatment of sleep-related breathing disorders. Although a substantial improvement of snoring is observed in up to 40% of snoring subjects with nasal obstruction, only about 20% of the patients suffering from obstructive sleep apnea experience a relevant improvement (uncontrolled case series). A recently published controlled trial could not confirm a superiority of nasal surgery in comparison to sham surgery.

In summary, it can be concluded that surgical correction of nasal obstruction may improve nasal breathing and subjective sleep quality and may optimize nasal CPAP therapy or even only allow it. In some patients, also snoring or nocturnal sleep apnea may improve in this way. However, therapy is only indicated when nasal obstruction is also subjectively perceived as disturbing. An indication to perform nasal surgery cannot be made based on conspicuous clinical findings or functional measurement alone (e.g., rhinomanometry).

Practical Tip

The indication of surgical correction of a malformation of the shape of the outer or inner nose is generally only given in cases of corresponding CPAP incompliance or subjective nasal obstruction.

4.8.4 Surgery of the Soft Palate

The soft palate is still in the focus of general interest when discussing surgical therapy for sleep-related breathing disorders. There are certainly several reasons for this phenomenon. First, the soft palate is typically the origin of snoring sounds, and obstruction on the level of the soft palate is one of the most frequently observed particularities in patients suffering from sleep-related breathing disorders. Second, the first surgical techniques, in particular uvulopalatopharyngoplasty (UPPP), were initially only extensions of conventional tonsillectomy, so these interventions were rapidly accepted by ENT surgeons.

Compared to first publications, however, surgery of the soft palate was significantly modified. At the beginning radical surgical techniques were applied, but this radicalism was abandoned in favor of increasingly function-preserving and careful techniques. Radical resections at the soft palate, which in the past resulted in severe disorders of these functionally relevant structures on occasion, are obsolete. Careful and function-preserving surgery is now of first priority.

Practical Tip

Radical surgical techniques at the soft palate may be associated with very uncomfortable complications that are difficult to treat and are generally not indicated.

In the following, surgical procedures for the treatment of snoring and obstructive sleep apnea are described separately for didactic reasons. The authors are aware that placebo-controlled trials are available in particular for minimally invasive therapies that document significant reduction of respiratory events in the treatment of mild obstructive sleep apnea. On the other hand, tonsillectomy or UPPP may also be indicated for an individual patient suffering from snoring. Generally, the authors believe that minimally invasive surgical techniques should be applied for the treatment of snoring. Minimally invasive techniques may be indicated in patients with mild obstructive sleep apnea who are otherwise healthy and unimpaired when snoring is in the focus of the complaints. However, these procedures are only rarely suitable as isolated measures in cases of manifest obstructive sleep apnea.

4.8.4.1 Surgical Treatment of the Soft Palate in Cases of Snoring

Regarding surgical treatment of the soft palate in the context of snoring, different minimally invasive procedures must be mentioned. They all aim at mechanically stabilizing the soft palate or removing a mucosal surplus to reduce vibrations of the soft palate and thus also snoring.

Besides numerous modifications and variations, those procedures mainly include electrosurgical procedures (radiofrequency surgery) and soft palate implants. Because of technical disadvantages and a higher postoperative morbidity and complication rate, *laser-assisted surgery* of the soft palate (laser-assisted uvulopalatoplasty, LAUP) is now rarely applied for surgical interventions at the soft palate. It is already contraindicated for mild obstructive sleep apnea because it may lead to reduction of the pharyngeal diameter and aggravation of airway obstruction by scarring.

Radiofrequency Surgery

Radiofrequency surgery is an electrosurgical procedure. According to the configuration of the electrodes and the technical settings, defined (interstitial) thermal lesions may be caused in the tissue or the electrodes may be used for cutting tissue.

To interstitially achieve a thermal treatment of the soft palate, the application needle is inserted under local anesthesia into predefined points of the soft palate and energy is applied submucosally. This procedure results in *scarring of the tissue* with only minimal trauma of the mucosal surface. The subsequent scarring leads to stiffening of the tissue with resulting reduction of the vibration capacity and finally to a reduction of snoring under the clinical aspect.

The effectiveness of this procedure with only minimal intra- and postoperative morbidity could also be confirmed by means of placebo-controlled trials. Even if snoring can only be reduced and not really eliminated in this way, it is nonetheless a safe and effective option.

The effectiveness of this treatment can be increased when an additional *resection of a mucosal surplus* is performed by means of radiofrequency-assisted procedures (radiofrequency-assisted uvulopalatoplasty, RF-UPP). The resection includes exclusively the mucosal surplus, for example, at the posterior palatal arch or at the uvula. Resection and destruction of the palatal muscles must be strictly avoided. Postoperative pain is clearly more severe with the additional resection, but also in this context, postoperative complications are minimal if the intervention is performed appropriately.

The reduction of snoring is even more significant in this context compared to interstitial treatment alone (schematic overview of the surgical procedures, ◘ Fig. 4.13).

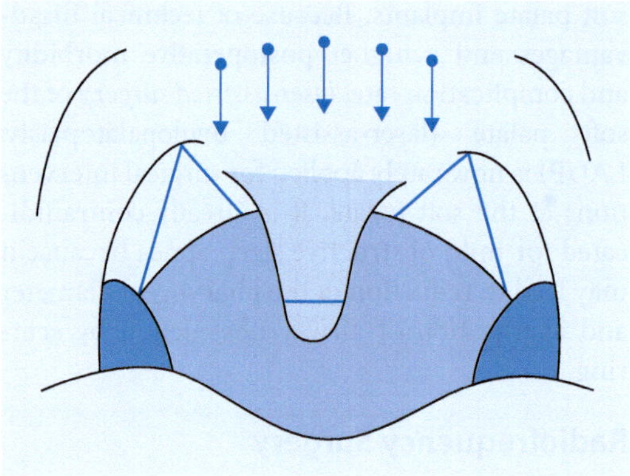

■ Fig. 4.13 Procedure of radiofrequency-assisted uvulopalatoplasty (RF-UPP)

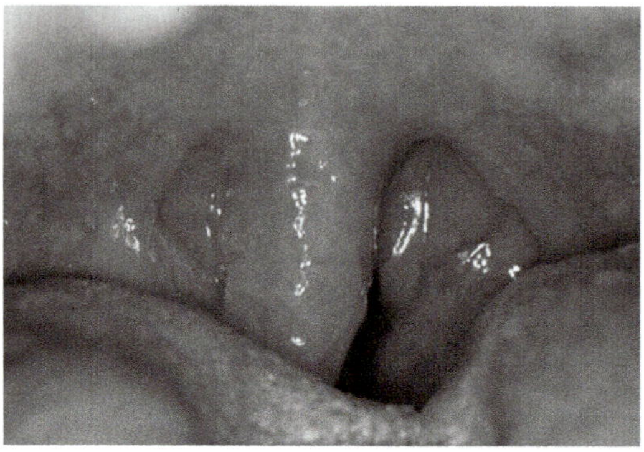

■ Fig. 4.14 Pharyngeal findings with hyperplasia of the tonsils and the soft palate

After both procedures (interstitial as well as combined radiofrequency surgery), a relapse in snoring has been documented in some patients in the context of long-term evaluations. If needed, re-operation may be performed after some years. Which patients benefit permanently from this intervention is still under discussion.

Soft Palate Implants

With the idea to achieve *permanent stabilization of the soft palate* and a permanent improvement of snoring, pin-shaped implants have been developed for the soft palate. These implants, made of Dacron, are inserted under local anesthesia at three different points of the soft palate. Stiffening is achieved on one hand by the mechanical effect of the implants; on the other hand, it is also explained by the scarring that is induced in the process of implant integration.

Also, with those implants, improvement of snoring may be achieved with minimal postoperative morbidity and almost no complications. Some of the patients describe recurrent snoring after initially successful therapy. Tissue surplus cannot be reduced with this technique. In those cases, for example, carefully performed resection of the soft tissue in combination with implantation may be appropriate.

4.8.4.2 Surgical Treatment of the Soft Palate in Obstructive Sleep Apnea

The aforementioned procedures primarily aim at reinforcing the soft palate, whereas procedures for treatment of obstructive sleep apnea are intended to *increase pharyngeal volume*. In nearly all cases when the palatal tonsils are still present, tonsillectomy contributes significantly to the success of treatment, so that respective procedures are regularly combined with tonsillectomy. Sometimes, tonsillectomy as an isolated procedure eliminates the airway obstruction in the context of according tonsillar hyperplasia (■ Fig. 4.14).

The most important procedure of pharyngeal enlargement on the level of the palate is *uvulopalatopharyngoplasty (UPPP)*. UPPP was one of the first procedures in this context, and it is still standard in the surgical therapy of obstructive sleep apnea. After tonsillectomy, the posterior palatal arches are sutured to the anterior ones in such a way that pharyngeal enlargement results. Generally, in addition a too long or hyperplastic uvula is shortened.

Tonsillectomy with UPPP could also prove to be effective for the decrease of respiratory events and for the improvement of daytime symptoms in controlled clinical trials. Furthermore, numerous positive effects, for example, with regard to the cardiovascular function and overall survival, were documented. Even in long-term investigations of as much as 10 years after the intervention, the effects turned out to be stable. With the background of techniques developed for careful muscle and function-preserving surgery, larger patient populations show comparably low complication rates that mainly correspond to the complication rates after tonsillectomy.

In the past, numerous modifications and variants have been described with regard to classic UPPP (lateral pharyngoplasty, palatal advancement, etc.) that are not covered in this chapter. The authors refer to respective review articles.

Case Report

After some months, the 45-year-old bank employee described in the abovementioned example who had been provided a CPAP device no longer would tolerate ventilation therapy although the ventilation therapy had initially developed very positively. Testing other masks and the prescription of a CPAP device with expiratory pressure relief could only moderately improve his complaints (dermal irritation/ulceration, conjunctival irritation, aerophagia). He sensed a continuously increasing aversion against ventilation therapy so that he no longer used the device. According to his report, the daytime sleepiness that had significantly improved initially had again increased.

The clinical examination reveals a relevant hyperplasia of the palatal tonsils with enlargement of the uvula and notable mucosal surplus (◻ Fig. 4.14).

Despite his increased body mass index, the indication for surgical intervention is made, and the surgery date is fixed. The patient is asked to reduce weight up to the date of the intervention.

The patient undergoes tonsillectomy with UPPP under general anesthesia. On the fifth postoperative day, bleeding from the tonsillar bed occurs that can be controlled by conservative measures. The further postoperative course is without complications; after 1 week, the pain has nearly disappeared. Six weeks after surgery, control PSG is performed with a resulting RDI of 17. Now, sleep apnea is observed that is exclusively caused in the supine position during sleep. Therefore, the patient additionally receives a sleep position trainer to avoid the supine position, which finally leads to complete elimination of the apneic phases.

The subjective symptoms are regressive, and snoring no longer occurs, so continuation of the ventilation therapy is no longer indicated.

4.8.5 Surgery of the Retrolingual Space

In particular, in cases of moderate or severe *obstructive sleep apnea*, an obstruction of the airway is found on the level of the base of tongue, either as an isolated finding or more frequently in combination with obstruction at the level of the soft palate. Because this area cannot be directly examined clinically (one important diagnostic criterion is the endoscopy of the upper airway) and resection procedures are associated with high morbidity, surgical therapy of this retrolingual obstruction still causes relevant problems. Therefore, the procedures mentioned are reserved for the treatment of obstructive sleep apnea.

Most various procedures have been developed to reinforce this area and to stabilize it (e.g., radiofrequency surgery of the base of tongue) or also to displace relevant structures in this area, aiming at an enlargement of the airway (e.g., genioglossus advancement, tongue suspension sutures, tongue advancement, or hyoid suspension).

In the context of *radiofrequency surgery*, the attempt is made to achieve scarring and stiffening of the base of the tongue according to the described techniques (see ▶ Sect. 4.8.4) to reduce collapsibility in this area. The procedure, which is the only one that can be described as minimally invasive, may be performed under local anesthesia or sedation; however, its effectiveness with regard to obstructive sleep apnea is limited.

All other procedures generally require general anesthesia.

The procedure of *genioglossus advancement* consists of an excision of the bony a portion of the mandible where the genioglossus muscle is attached. This piece of bone is then pulled in the ventral direction, thinned, and fixed to the outer surface of the lower jaw. In this way, the attachment of the muscle is pulled forward and the airway size is increased.

A similar approach is pursued by different procedures of *tongue advancement*. Hereby, depending on the manufacturers, different materials (e.g., nonresorbable sutures or different loops) are inserted into the tongue and fixed at the inner surface of the mandible. The aim of this procedure is less to pull the tongue forward to a relevant measure but rather to stabilize the tongue and to avoid its falling back during sleep.

Practical Tip

Surgery of retrolingual obstruction is still far from being applied as a standard and routinely performed procedure compared to interventions of the soft palate.

Frequently, the mentioned procedures are applied in combination with procedures of the soft palate (so-called multilevel surgery) to increase their effectiveness.

4.8.6 Hypoglossal Nerve Stimulation

Electric stimulation of the hypoglossal nerve (*hypoglossal nerve stimulation or also airway stimulation or "upper airway stimulation"*) is a new and, in this context, innovative surgical procedure that is not based on resection or displacement but on functional treatment by means of stimulation. This procedure consists of implanting an impulse generator for unilateral stimulation of the hypoglossal nerve during sleep. This step activates the muscles protruding the tongue and thus leads to an increased retrolingual airway size. Via passive activation of the palatoglossal muscle, opening at the level of the velopharynx may be achieved. The stimulation systems that are currently available vary with regard to the type of stimulation that may occur in a ventilation synchronized manner. After implantation of the stimulation system and successful integration, titrations are performed under polysomnographic conditions, and the stimulation parameters are optimized until the breathing disorder ceases. ◘ Figure 4.15 graphically displays the ventilation synchronized upper airway stimulation.

In particular for ventilation synchronized upper airway stimulation, a series of methodically high-quality trials have been published in past years that could document an impressive improvement of subjective and objective parameters. Hereby, the improvement of the respiratory parameters and the daytime symptoms as well as the quality of life were observed to be stable even several years after implantation.

Patients without or with mild obesity suffering from moderate to severe sleep apnea are suitable for this procedure. It was possible to demonstrate for ventilation synchronized stimulation that drug-induced sleep endoscopy provides decisive predictive information. In this examination, a complete concentric collapse on the level of the velopharynx has to be excluded because it is a negative predictor for treatment response. Preoperative screening and the subsequent treatment require an interdisciplinary approach and should be performed in an experienced sleep center with the corresponding infrastructure and expertise.

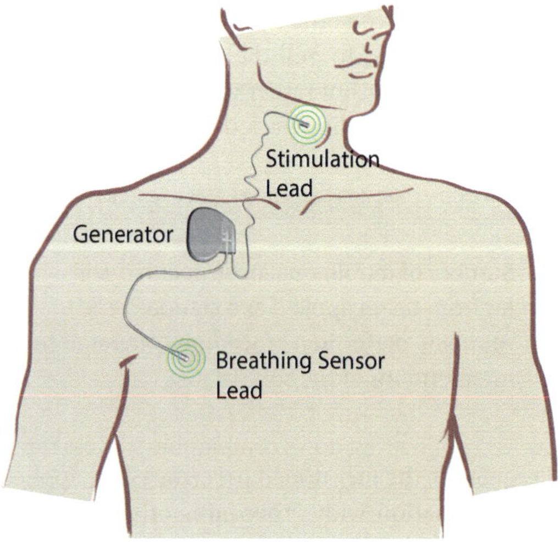

◘ **Fig. 4.15** Principles of upper airway stimulation

4.8.7 Maxillofacial Surgery

The significance of skeletal particularities in patients suffering from sleep-related breathing disorders was emphasized previously (see ▸ Sect. 4.2.2), so it is quite appropriate to return to already established procedures in maxillofacial surgery in cases of patients with skeletal malformations such as dysgnathia. In this context, procedures advancing the mandible (e.g., distraction osteoneogenesis) and also procedures for bimaxillary advancement (maxillomandibular advancement) must be mentioned. Especially for patients with cosmetically unfavorable facial morphology or dysgnathia requiring treatment, these procedures might be beneficial, not only from an aesthetic and functional point of view but also with regard to sleep-related breathing disorders.

Even for patients without visible skeletal malformations, maxillomandibular advancement may significantly increase the airway size. However, acceptance by the patients is limited because of the invasiveness of the intervention. Nonetheless, maxillofacial procedures are the most effective surgical procedures in the treatment of obstructive sleep apnea. Success rates of about 90% are reported, and in a current randomized trial, the effectiveness of bimaxillary advancement also revealed an equivalent outcome compared to CPAP treatment in patients with severe obstructive sleep apnea also. Patients suffering from obstructive sleep apnea who do not accept or tolerate conservative therapy should consider the option of maxillofacial procedures, and they should consult an appropriate specialist.

4.9 Questions

1. Please explain the classification of sleep-related breathing disorders and give an example for each.
2. What are the relevant pathophysiological differences between central sleep apnea syndromes in comparison to sleep-related hypoventilation and hypoxemia?
3. Please list the pathophysiological principles and triggering factors for obstructive sleep apnea.
4. Please describe the diagnostic steps for suspected sleep-related breathing disorder.
5. Which types of ventilation therapy do you know and for which indications are they applied?
6. Which alternatives exist if ventilation therapy has to be terminated because of lack of compliance?

Further Reading

1. American Academy of Sleep Medicine (2014) International classification of sleep disorders, vol 3. American Academy of Sleep Medicine Darien.
2. Aurora RN, Casey KR, Kristo D, Auerbach S, Bista SR, Chowdhuri S, Karippot A, Lamm C, Ramar K, Zak R, Morgenthaler TI, American Academy of Sleep Medicine. Practice parameters for the surgical modifications of the upper airway for obstructive sleep apnea in adults. Sleep. 2010;33:1408–13.
3. Bassetti CL, Milanova M, Gugger M. Sleep-disordered breathing and acute ischemic stroke: diagnosis, risk factors, treatment, evolution, and long-term clinical outcome. Stroke. 2006;37:967–72.
4. Dolan DC, Okonkwo R, Gfullner F, Hansbrough JR, Strobel RJ, Rosenthal L. Longitudinal comparison study of pressure relief (C-Flex) vs. CPAP in OSA patients. Sleep Breath. 2009;13:73–7.
5. Hörmann K, Verse T. Surgery for sleep-disordered breathing. 2nd ed. Heidelberg: Springer; 2010.
6. Mayer G, Arzt M, Braumann B, Ficker JH, Fietze I, Galetke W, Maurer JT, Orth M, Penzel T, Pistner HP, Randerath W, Rösslein M, Sitter J, Stuck BA. S3-Leitlinie Nicht erholsamer Schlaf/Schlafstörungen, Kapitel "Schlafbezogene Atmungsstörungen bei Erwachsenen.". Somnologie. 2017;20(suppl s2):S97–S180.
7. Morgenthaler TI, Kapen S, Lee-Chiong T, Alessi C, Boehlecke B, Brown T, Coleman J, Friedman L, Kapur V, Owens J, Pancer J, Swick T, Standards of Practice Committee, American Academy of Sleep Medicine. Practice parameters for the medical therapy of obstructive sleep apnea. Sleep. 2006;29:1031–5.
8. Owens RL, Edwards BA, Eckert DJ, Jordan AS, Sands SA, Malhotra A, White DP, Loring SH, Butler JP, Wellman A. An integrative model of physiological traits can be used to predict obstructive sleep apnea and response to non positive airway pressure therapy. Sleep. 2015;38:961–70.
9. Peter H, Penzel T, Peter JH. Enzyklopädie der Schlafmedizin. Springer, Heidelberg. 2007.
10. Ramar K, Dort LC, Katz SG, Lettieri CJ, Harrod CG, Thomas SM, Chervin RD. Clinical practice guideline for the treatment of obstructive sleep apnea and snoring with oral appliance therapy: an update for 2015. J Clin Sleep Med. 2015;11:773–827.
11. Schäfer T. Variability of vigilance and ventilation: studies on the control of respiration during sleep. Respir Physiol. 1998;114:37–48.
12. Schulz R, Blau A, Börgel J, Working group Kreislauf und Schlaf of the German Sleep Society (DGSM), et al. Sleep apnea in heart failure. Eur Respir J. 2007;29:1201–5.
13. Sommer JU, Heiser C, Gahleitner C, Herr RM, Hörmann K, Maurer JT, Stuck BA. Tonsillectomy with uvulopalatopharyngoplasty in obstructive sleep apnea – a two center randomized controlled trial. Dtsch Arztebl Int. 2016;113:1–8.
14. Stuck BA, Maurer JT. Airway evaluation in obstructive sleep apnea. Sleep Med Rev. 2008;12:411–36.
15. Stuck BA, Dreher A, Heiser C, Herzog M, Kuehnel T, Maurer JT, Pistner H, Sitter H, Steffen A, Verse T. Diagnosis and treatment of snoring in adults. S2k Guideline of the German Society of Otorhinolaryngology, Head and Neck Surgery. Sleep Breath. 2015;19:135–48.
16. Verse T. Nebenwirkungen der nasalen CPAP-Therapie. HNO. 2000;48:706–715.
17. Yumino D, Bradley TD. Central sleep apnea and Cheyne-Stokes respiration. Proc Am Thorac Soc. 2008;15:226–36.

Hypersomnia Disorders

M. Schredl

B. A. Stuck et al., *Practice of Sleep Medicine*, https://doi.org/10.1007/978-3-030-17412-5_5

An increased likelihood to fall asleep during the daytime is a frequent symptom in a series of widespread sleep disorders, for example, sleep-related breathing disorders. Hypersomnias, such as narcolepsy, and idiopathic (primary) hypersomnia as independent disorders are rarely observed. The symptom of excessive daytime sleepiness, however, is a great burden for these patients. Adequate and often long-term treatment is a challenge for sleep specialists.

Hypersomnias are characterized by an increased *daytime sleepiness* that cannot be explained by disturbed night sleep alone, such as disorders of initiating and maintaining sleep or nonrestorative sleep. Thus, sleep apnea syndrome or periodic limb movements during sleep as the cause of the symptom of hypersomnia have to be excluded before the independent diagnosis of hypersomnia can be made (differential diagnosis of narcolepsy, ► Sect. 5.1.7; differential diagnosis of idiopathic hypersomnia, ► Sect. 5.2.7).

Daytime sleepiness has to be differentiated from *daytime tiredness*. In contrast to daytime tiredness, daytime sleepiness is defined as an increased propensity to fall asleep, mostly in monotonous situations (reading, watching TV, lectures/presentations, meetings, driving) and, thus, not primarily reflecting the sensation of being tired (see ► Table 2.1; ► Sect. 2.1.3; ► Chap. 7).

Classification of Hypersomnias According to the AASM

- Narcolepsy type 1 (with cataplexy)
- Narcolepsy type 2 (without cataplexy)
- Idiopathic hypersomnia
- Kleine-Levin syndrome
- Insufficient sleep syndrome
- Hypersomnia caused by or associated with somatic and mental disorder or resulting from medication or substance abuse

The most important hypersomnias are narcolepsy (type 1 and type 2) and idiopathic hypersomnias. Furthermore, the Kleine-Levin syndrome is a rare but frequently underdiagnosed disease. In the following, these disorders are described with their subtypes. For differential diagnostics, the insufficient sleep syndrome is relevant in practice.

5.1 Narcolepsy

5.1.1 Definitions

Narcolepsy is a chronic disorder that usually has its onset between the 15th and 25th year of life. A second peak is found in the fourth decade. The disorder is characterized by these events:

- An increased propensity to fall asleep during the day, and also in unlikely situations (when eating or talking)
- Cataplexy (sudden loss of muscle tone in the context of emotional excitement)
- Often sleep paralysis and hypnagogic hallucinations occur

The symptoms of narcolepsy are categorized into two groups: rapid eye movement (REM) sleep-associated symptoms and symptoms that are not associated with REM sleep (in particular, daytime sleepiness).

REM sleep-associated symptoms include these:

- Cataplexy
- Sleep paralysis
- Hypnagogic hallucinations

Increased dream recall and the occurrence of negative dreams and nightmares are often reported by narcolepsy patients.

5.1.2 Etiology and Pathophysiology

For REM sleep-associated symptoms (cataplexy, sleep paralysis, hypnagogic hallucinations) in narcolepsy patients to occur, hyperactivity of the *system controlling the REM sleep* is considered responsible. This system becomes active in situations in which it should not be active. An example of such a case is emotional excitement that triggers the REM sleep system, leading to cataplexy.

The REM sleep system serves to reduce the muscle tone of the entire body with its centers located in the brainstem (locus coeruleus, Raphé, and tuberomammillary nuclei) in addition to the increased brain activation (intensive dreaming). In healthy individuals, this ensures that the body does not move during REM sleep despite the motor cortex activation associated with dreamed movements. In cataplexy, however, the system is activated nonphysiologically, which leads to an emotionally induced loss of muscle tone during wakefulness. In sleep paralysis, the individual awakens, but the REM sleep system do not switch to "awake," that is, despite full consciousness the muscle blockade of REM sleep still persists. Only the eyes, which are not blocked during REM sleep, can be moved. Vivid imagination (hypnagogic hallucinations) during sleep onset can probably also be explained by an activated REM sleep system. Narcolepsy patients often show so-called sleep-onset REM phases (SOREM phases; ▶ Chap. 2) as an expression of the increased REM pressure—as in healthy individuals the first REM sleep episode occurs after about 90 minutes.

The association of narcolepsy with gene polymorphism of the HLA system (human leukocyte antigen) indicates that *genetic factors* are involved. However, the typical alleles of HLA-DR15 (former term, DR2) that are found in 85% to 95% of all narcolepsy patients are also frequently observed in the normal population (12–38%), so that the higher familial aggregation of narcolepsy indicates that further genes might contribute. Possibly, the described hypocretin-1 (synonym: orexin) deficiency in the cerebrospinal fluid (CSF) that is found in nearly all narcolepsy patients may be a direction for further research. The reduction of hypocretin-1 levels is caused by a decrease of hypocretin neurons in the hypothalamus. It is hypothesized that autoimmune processes destroy hypocretin cells during the onset of narcolepsy.

Interestingly narcolepsy incidence is increased in subjects who are born in March. This observation supports the idea that *environmental factors* might play a role within narcolepsy etiology that is not yet fully understood, including events such as influenza or rhinovirus infection in the second trimester of pregnancy.

Secondary types of narcolepsy have been described after severe traumatic brain injuries, tumors of the hypothalamus, multiple sclerosis, Parkinson's disease, and multiple system atrophy.

5.1.3 Epidemiology

In Western Europe and the US, the prevalence rate of narcolepsy is estimated to be 0.026% to 0.035%, so narcolepsy is a very rare disease. In Japan, the prevalence rate is significantly higher, 0.16% to 0.59%, whereas in Israel it is lower, 0.002%, compared to Western Europe. If a first degree relative (parents, children, siblings) suffers from narcolepsy, the risk to develop the disease increases for the individual to 1%. This information may be highly relevant if a narcolepsy patient desires to have a child because the risk of narcolepsy is increased.

5.1.4 Clinical Presentation

The following symptoms, also called the narcoleptic tetrad, can be seen in narcolepsy patients with different frequencies:

- Daytime sleepiness (about 95%)
- Cataplexy (70–90%)
- Sleep paralysis (about 50%)
- Hypnagogic hallucinations (about 50%)

Only about one third of the patients suffer from all four symptoms.

In most cases, the disorder starts with *daytime sleepiness*, which is the key symptom of narcolepsy. Although in many healthy individuals sleep deprivation can result in falling a sleep in monotonous situations (watching TV, reading, presentations, etc.), this symptom is present in narcolepsy patients even with sufficient night sleep and can occur in uncommon situations, for example, during a conversation or while eating. The propensity to fall asleep can be perceived beforehand, but from a certain point on, the patients are no longer able to resist (irrepressible urge to sleep). Generally, a brief nap (5–10 min) helps the person to be efficient again, usually for the next 1 to 2 h; then, falling asleep is again possible (▶ Sect. 5.1.8).

In many patients *cataplexies* occur in the course of months or years after the initial symptoms of daytime sleepiness, but the classification differentiates between narcolepsy with cataplexy versus narcolepsy without cataplexy. Although it was assumed that 90% of all narcolepsy patients also experience cataplexies, now the diagnosis of narcolepsy without cataplexy is given to about 30% of the patients.

A cataplexy occurs if emotional excitement (laughing, joy, anger, fear) leads to sudden loss of muscle tone in at least some parts of the body. This tonus loss may be very severe, i.e., patients can actually collapse. Less severe types include the feeling of weak knees or dropping of the lower jaw. Usually, cataplexies persist only several seconds to minutes; consciousness is not impaired. In cases of severe cataplexies, injuries (e.g., head) may occur because the patients cannot counteract the fall. In many cases, cataplexy occurs suddenly and cannot be predicted, so many patients try to avoid situations in which intensive emotions may arise. The cataplexy often ends as suddenly as it had started. Afterward, the patients are generally fit again.

In contrast to epileptic seizures, spasms are not observed, so that cataplexies can be well differentiated from grand mal or minor epileptic seizures. Furthermore, the typical fatigue that appears post-ictally in epilepsy patients is not seen after cataplexy.

Sleep paralysis is found in about half the patients. Most often the complete paralysis of the body muscles occurs after awakening in adults. Only the eye muscles are excluded from the paralysis. This condition also persists only for a few minutes, but is often experienced with panic. Often also images are perceived, for example, a person standing at the bedside.

Hypnagogic hallucinations are vivid images that occur during sleep onset and are often experienced as negative. These hallucinations can be differentiated from normal sleep-onset dreams because they include the real environment and they are more intensive than sleep-onset dreams. Bizarre thoughts or neutral dream images occur during sleep onset, but these are often forgotten except the process of falling asleep is interrupted suddenly.

Another symptom of narcolepsy is disturbed night sleep; narcolepsy patients generally fall asleep easily, but they wake up more frequently at night compared to healthy individuals; and they often have a very fractionated sleep. In some patients, so-called automatic behavior during daytime is observed. In the context of automatic behavior during sleep onset, the patients continue with the activity they had been performing, such as writing or knitting, without being consciously awake. Depending on the activity, this may have severe consequences, such as burn injuries when cooking or smoking.

Polysomnographic studies show that *sleep-related breathing disorders* or *periodic limb movements during sleep* occur more frequently in narcolepsy patients than in healthy subjects, in addition to the aforementioned symptoms. Adequate diagnostics of these co-morbid sleep disorders are essential for maximizing the therapy effect for the patients.

Dreams occurring during the night and not only sleep-onset images, are generally negatively toned in narcolepsy patients. Overall, they are able to recall their dreams more often than healthy individuals. This ability provides important clues for differential diagnostics that can be elicited during history taking because the presence of *high dream recall* and *predominantly negative dreams* in patients with daytime sleepiness point to narcolepsy. About 30% of all narcolepsy patients suffer from nightmare disorder, so that the intervention described in ► Sect. 7.3.8 might be applied beneficially.

Typically, the onset of narcolepsy is observed between the 15th and 25th year of life. Very rarely, the symptoms start before the age of 15. If narcolepsy first manifests at the age of 25 years or later, it might be narcolepsy of the secondary type (► Sect. 5.1.2).

Practical Tip

The course of narcolepsy is chronic and requires lifelong treatment.

5.1.5 Diagnostic Procedures

In the context of history taking, it is important to accurately assess the four key symptoms of narcolepsy. Above all, daytime sleepiness has to be clearly differentiated from complaints of fatigue or tiredness (see ► Sect. 2.1.3).

Practical Tip

Narcolepsy patients often do not spontaneously report the symptoms of cataplexy, in particular when the cataplexies are only minor and occur only in single muscle groups. In cases of mild cataplexy, only facial and neck muscles may be involved. Hence, the symptoms of cataplexy should be evaluated directly in patients with daytime sleepiness.

Weakness in the knees co-occurring with pronounced anger is also known to healthy subjects so that the patients should be asked to give detailed descriptions of the events to clearly evaluate whether muscle tone loss did occur. Vivid images at sleep onset can also experienced by healthy subjects so that this criterion does not lead to a clear diagnosis. Even the presence of sleep paralysis does not always confirm the diagnosis of narcolepsy because it also can occur as an isolated symptom. In addition, patients may report that they have problems getting up in the morning because they feel tired and exhausted and misinterpret this experience as sleep paralysis. In these cases, the patients have to be asked directly if the entire body (except the eyes) is completely paralyzed. About 40% of healthy subjects have reported sleep paralysis at least once in their lives. Isolated sleep paralysis can be a diagnosis on its own (▶ Sect. 7.5).

Frequently, clinical interviews are complemented with questionnaires to assess daytime sleepiness, predominantly the *Epworth Sleepiness Scale* (see ▶ Sect. 2.8.1.5). This self-assessment of the propensity to fall asleep in eight typical everyday situations, for example, reading, sitting, watching TV, and talking, which provides valuable information.

Laboratory examinations such as the determination of hypocretin-1 in the CSF and HLA II geno typing may be performed in the diagnostic process to complete anamnestic data and polysomnographic findings - if necessary. In the context of genotyping of HLA DR15, nearly all narcolepsy patients have the haplotypes DQB1∗0602 and DQA1∗0102. However, these haplotypes are also frequently observed in the normal population (12–38%). Only negative findings would increase the diagnostic certainty for excluding narcolepsy.

Many narcolepsy patients with cataplexies have hypocretin-1 concentrations of less than 110 pg/ml in the CSF. The percentage in narcolepsy type 2 patients without cataplexy is clearly lower; only 10% to 20% of these patients have reduced hypocretin-1 values in the CSF. Because most narcolepsy patients without cataplexy present a diagnostic challenge, lumbar puncture may help to increase the diagnostic certainty in some cases.

Practical Tip

The HLA haplotypes that are typical for narcolepsy are also found quite frequently in the normal population; accordingly, genotyping may support the exclusion of narcolepsy. Positive findings, however, only poorly contribute to the diagnosis.

Not all patients suffering from narcolepsy have reduced hypocretin levels in the CSF, but findings of a very low levels are specific for narcolepsy. Because of the invasiveness, lumbar puncture should be reserved to exceptional cases.

A comprehensive *neurological examination* including imaging of the head is recommended in patients with atypically late onset (after the age of 25) of narcoleptic complaints.

5.1.6 Sleep Diagnostics

In the context of narcolepsy, history taking and clinical examination do not suffice for valid diagnoses in. Polysomnographic examination over two nights and a multiple sleep latency test (MSLT) during the daytime are mandatory. The MSLT must be performed after a night with polysomnography (see below).

Special attention should be paid to the early occurrence of REM sleep in the *polysomnography* (*PSG*; ◘ Fig. 5.1).

The first REM phase, occurred before the first non-REM sleep stage 2. The early occurrence of REM is also called SOREM (sleep-onset REM). It is defined as REM latency less than 15 min and is indicative for narcolepsy. Some authors define SOREMs with a latency of 10 or 20 min.

The number of periods of wakefulness after sleep onset was relatively low; however, many body movements (BM) were present. ◘ Figure 5.2 shows the *multiple sleep latency test (MSLT)* of the same patient conducted after the night shown in ◘ Fig. 5.1.

Usually, five tests are scheduled within the protocol of the clinical MSLT (9 AM, 11 AM, 1 PM, 3 PM, and 5 PM) (▶ Sect. 2.7.1). For the present patient, the diagnosis was already clear after four naps. It can be seen that the patient fell asleep

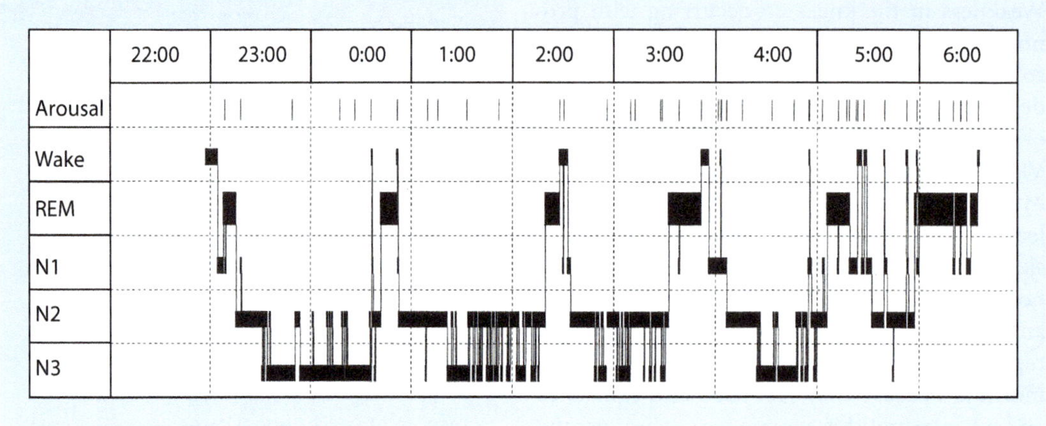

Fig. 5.1 Night sleep profile of a narcolepsy patient

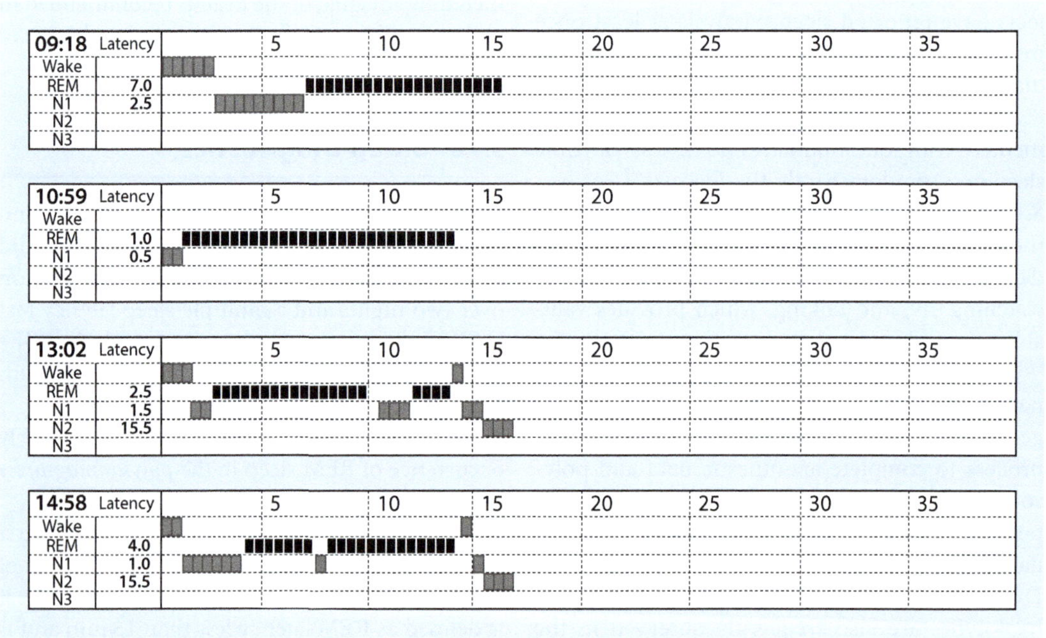

Fig. 5.2 Multiple sleep latency test of a narcolepsy patient

in every test, the longest sleep latency was only 2.5 min. In all naps, a SOREM phase occurred. Large studies revealed that narcolepsy patients need an average of about 3.1 min to fall asleep (standard deviation: 2.9 min) and show REM sleep in at least two of five naps. For this patient (Figs. 5.1 and 5.2), the diagnosis of narcolepsy was confirmed after the stay in the sleep lab.

In practice, primarily all five tests (9 AM, 11 AM, 1 PM, 3 PM, 5 PM) have to be planned and performed, in particular when the staff performing the recording is not fully sure about the occurrence of SOREM phases and further evaluations by somnologists or sleep physicians are required.

For the diagnosis of narcolepsy, at least two identified SOREM phases have to be present in the MSLT or in one of two polysomnographic night recordings so that the MSLT may be shortened in single cases (see earlier example). The diagnostic validity, however, typically increases with the number of tests. The upper limit for sleep latency average over the five daytime naps should be 8 min or less. This second criterion (in addition to the two SOREMs), however, is not specific for narcolepsy because such values might also be measured occasionally in healthy sleepers. In order to demonstrate that night sleep before the MSLT was sufficient, the MSLT has to be performed after a night with polysomnographically documented sleep duration of at least 6 h.

Sleep lab diagnostics are also necessary to differentiate between other possible origins of daytime sleepiness, in particular when the sleep history does not provide clear hints regarding the presence of cataplexies. For example, sleep apnea syndrome or periodic limb movements during sleep have to be excluded. However, narcolepsy patients may suffer from co-morbid mild to moderate sleep apnea syndromes or periodic limb movements during sleep. Measuring night sleep to detect probable SOREM phases and carrying out a MSLT are always indicated in cases of clinically suspected narcolepsy even if relevant findings regarding sleep-related breathing disorders and leg movements during sleep have been made. In cases of severe sleep apnea syndrome, treatment of this sleep-related breathing disorder is recommended before further narcolepsy diagnostics are initiated.

For technical guidelines and general instructions of the MSLT, see ▶ Sect. 2.7.1.

Diagnostic Criteria of Narcolepsy Type 1 (with Cataplexy), Based on the Criteria of the American Academy of Sleep Medicine (AASM)

- The patient has daily phases with an irrepressible urge to sleep or "sleep attacks" during the daytime over a period of at least 3 months.
- One or both of the following conditions must be fulfilled:
  1. Presence of cataplexies (episodes of usually bilateral, symmetrical loss of muscle tone with full consciousness), triggered by strong emotions (laughing is a frequently observed trigger), and an average sleep-onset latency of less than 8 min and two or more SOREM phases in a MSLT performed according to standard methods. One SOREM phase occurring in the previous night in the sleep lab may replace a SOREM phase of the MSLT.
  2. The hypocretin-1 concentration in the CSF (measured by immune reactivity) is either less than 110 pg/ml or lower than one third of the average values of healthy subjects examined with the same method.

For the diagnosis of *narcolepsy type 2 (without cataplexy)*, nearly identical rules are applied, without the symptom of cataplexy, however. Subjects with low hypocretin-1 levels are included in the type 1 also without cataplexy; that is, for patients with type 2 narcolepsy, the hypocretin-1 concentrations are not reduced (or not measured). If cataplexies in patients with narcolepsy type 2, the diagnosis is changed to narcolepsy type 1.

5.1.7 Differential Diagnostics

It has to be clarified by differential diagnostics whether other sleep disorders might be causing increased daytime sleepiness. Besides *sleep-related breathing disorders* (▶ Chap. 4), this includes *limb movements during sleep* (▶ Chap. 8). It is important to perform polysomnography over two nights with measurement of the nocturnal breathing activity and periodic leg movements during sleep in addition to the MSLT. It must be taken into account, however, that both disorders are frequently found in narcolepsy patients as co-morbidity.

The differentiation between narcolepsy without cataplexies and *idiopathic hypersomnia* is only possible by means of a well-performed MSLT. It is crucial that the night sleep before daytime sleep examinations has a minimum 6 hours so that sleep deficit or selective sleep deficit (less REM sleep than usual) does not bias the result. Generally, patients with idiopathic hypersomnia fall asleep also very quickly; however, they never or only once show SOREM sleep episodes in the MSLT.

The insufficient *sleep syndrome* also may be a differential diagnosis of narcolepsy without cataplexies because the chronic sleep deficit causes an increased propensity to fall asleep during the day; and often one or two of the short daytime sleep episodes may contain REM sleep. These REM sleep phases in the MSLT may be a result of the REM sleep deprivation when sleep duration is too short because REM sleep is mostly found in the second half of the night.

In the context of excessive daytime sleepiness, secondary sleep disorders with hypersomnia complaints have to be ruled out by differential diagnostics (▶ Chap. 10). Those disorders are, in addition to mental disorders (e.g., depressive syndrome or treatment with neuroleptics for schizophrenia), also secondary sleep disorders in the context of organic diseases (e.g., metabolic or cardiovascular diseases, thyroid diseases).

5.1.8 Therapy

Therapy of Narcolepsy

- Non-drug therapy
  - Psychoeducation
  - Structuring of the day
  - Behavioral therapy
- Drug therapy
  - Treatment of the REM sleep-associated symptoms
  - Treatment of the non-REM sleep-associated symptoms
- Treatment of comorbid sleep disorders
  - Treatment of a sleep-related breathing disorder
  - Treatment of periodic limb movements during sleep

5.1.8.1 Non-drug Therapy

First, *information* and psychoeducation about the disorder and its consequences is top priority; also, the chronic course must be discussed with the patients. In single cases, especially for adolescents in their personality development, psychotherapeutic measures may be indicated to impart coping strategies.

This information are not only important for the patients themselves but also for the environment because these patients are often considered as "sleepyheads" or "lazy bums." It has to be discussed with the patients that certain jobs are not suitable for them and also that sports with high accident risks should be avoided. Driving a car, especially in the context of drug intake, has to be openly discussed, because an endangerment of self and others may occur (▶ Chap. 12). In many cases, no or only a limited fitness to drive must be certified.

An appropriate *daytime structure* is very important for narcolepsy patients. First, sufficient time for night sleep has to be planned. Sleep deprivation might aggravate symptoms greatly. For many patients, it is helpful to include two or three short naps (maximum, 30 min; better: only 10 min) during the daytime to reduce the sleepiness during the rest of the day.

Coffee, tea, and caffeinated soft drinks (e.g., coke) may improve the general condition; however, the effect varies from patient to patient. Alcohol should be avoided, because symptoms such as the propensity to fall asleep are enhanced and the already disturbed night sleep is further deteriorated.

5.1.8.2 Drug Therapy

For the treatment of narcolepsy, different groups of substances are available. With few exceptions, the substances aim at isolated symptoms such as daytime sleepiness, cataplexies, or disturbed night sleep. With this background, combined treatment approaches are often necessary. Possible interactions between the different drugs must be taken into consideration. ◘ Table 5.1 summarizes the drugs with regard to REM sleep-associated and non-REM sleep-associated symptoms (daytime sleepiness). Sodium oxybate for the treatment of cataplexies as well as pitolisant for the treatment of daytime sleepiness may have a positive effect on the group of other symptoms.

Because of their etiology (hyperactivity of the REM sleep system), *REM sleep-associated symptoms* (cataplexy, sleep paralysis, hypnagogic hallucinations) may be treated with substances suppressing REM sleep. The level of cataplexy suppression is directly correlated with the noradrenergic reuptake inhibition of the compound.

The drug of first choice is the *tricyclic antidepressant* clomipramine. Its side effects (weight gain, xerostomia, increased sweating, obstipation, and disturbed libido/potency) limit its application. With this background, *selective serotonin reuptake inhibitors*, for example, fluoxetine, citalo-

■ **Table 5.1** Drug therapy of narcolepsy

Substance	Dosage
REM sleep-associated symptoms	
Clomipramine	bis 200 mg/day
Imipramine	bis 200 mg/day
Desipramine	bis 200 mg/day
Fluoxetine	20–60 mg/day
Citalopram	20–60 mg/day
Venlafaxine	Up to 300 mg/day
Duloxetine	Up to 60 mg/day
Sodium oxybate	4.5–9 g/divided into two doses
Daytime sleepiness	
Modafinil (vigil)	Up to 400 mg/day
Methylphenidate	Up to 60 mg/day
Atomoxetine	up to 25 mg/day
Dextroamphetamine	up to 60 mg/day
Methamphetamine	up to 25 mg/day
Pitolisant	9–36 mg/day

pram, and noradrenalin reuptake inhibitors (e.g., venlafaxine), are administered. Stimulating antidepressants such as venlafaxine may also have a positive effect on daytime sleepiness in addition to the positive effect on cataplexies. In single cases, further treatment of daytime sleepiness might not be necessary. It is important to balance the effect and the side effects of the different substances for each individual patient, because long-term medication is often required for patients suffering from frequent cataplexies.

MAO inhibitors, such as tranylcypromine, that have a strong REM sleep suppressive effect are only applied very rarely in practice because a strict diet has to be maintained (avoiding certain cheese varieties, chocolate and nougat ice cream, instant soups, industrially manufactured sauces, yeast extracts, beer, wine, sparkling wine, champagne, bananas, overripe pears and avocados, nectar from citrus fruits).

Practical Tip

It must be taken into account that the discontinuation of REM sleep suppressive compounds may lead to a massive rebound of the cataplexies.

Sodium oxybate is approved for the treatment of cataplexies. Because of its properties as a former narcotic, it also has a positive effect on night sleep. Even daytime sleepiness may be positively influenced so that some patients do not require further medication. It must be observed that because of its short half-life, sodium oxybate has to be taken immediately prior to sleep onset and the second dose after a scheduled awakening after about 3 h. The intake should be 2 h after eating (risk of vomiting because of nausea). Alcohol should be avoided.

Practical Tip

Patients with an addiction history should not receive sodium oxybate because the substance may be abused as a party and date rape drug.

For treating daytime sleepiness the following substances were used: modafinil, methylphenidate, and pitolisant. Also, atomoxetine and dextroamphetamines or methamphetamines have a vigilance-increasing effect.

In dosages of 100–400 mg, *modafinil* is highly effective for the treatment of daytime sleepiness in narcolepsy. In severe cases, a maximum dosage up to 600 mg per day may be applied. Typically, 400 mg is administered in the morning and a further 200 mg at noon. Later intakes increase the risk of disturbed sleep at night.

In dosages between 10 and 60 mg, *methylphenidate* also has a positive effect on daytime sleepiness. In cases of severe daytime sleepiness, modafinil and methylphenidate may be combined. Furthermore, the combination of sodium oxybate with modafinil or methylphenidate shows an additive effect on the symptom of daytime sleepiness. Tolerance effects are frequently observed, so that switching medications are recommended in the course of treatment. If possible, "drug holidays" on weekends or during a vacation should be scheduled as this may avoid tolerance.

Pitolisant has an effective mechanism as a histamine H3 receptor antagonist that enhances the activity of histaminergic neurons, representing an important arousal system with far-reaching projections into the whole brain, by means of blocking the histamine autoreceptors. The great advantage of pitolisant is probably the new mode of action. In a dosage up to 36 mg, the effect on daytime sleepiness is comparable to that of modafinil. Moreover, it could reduce cataplexies in 64% of the cases as shown in clinical studies. Data and experiences regarding the long-term effect on daytime sleepiness and the incidence of cataplexies beyond a period of 8 weeks do currently not exist because of relatively short availability of pitolisant on the market. Whether patients might develop tolerance to the effects is also not known.

The addictive potential of modafinil, methylphenidate, and pitolisant has to be estimated as rather low. In clinical practice, the adequate treatment of daytime sleepiness is a big challenge. Supportive measures for structuring daily activities and sleep pattern are particularly important, e.g., regular bedtimes with sufficient night sleep and structured naps during the daytime.

Case reports are available in the literature showing that treatment with immunoglobulins in the early stage of the disorder (≤9 months) has a positive effect on the course of the disorder. The assumption is that the destruction hypocretin cells in the hypothalamus by autoimmune reaction can be modulated.

5.1.8.3 Treatment of Comorbid Sleep Disorders

So far the effectiveness long-term drug treatment for disturbed night sleep, for example, with triazolam, clonazepam, zolpidem, zopiclone, or eszopiclone is still under debate. The effect on the daytime symptoms of narcolepsy patients by treating comorbid sleep disorders, such as sleep-related breathing disorders or periodic limb movements during sleep, is still not studied. Because both disorders impair the restoring function sleep, treatment seems to be recommended, even in less severe cases as daytime sleepiness might improve.

5.2 Idiopathic Hypersomnia

5.2.1 Definitions

Idiopathic hypersomnia, also called primary hypersomnia, is characterized by increased daytime sleepiness, even though night sleep is undisturbed and may be very long. Some patients have normal sleep duration (<10 h) and some a very long sleep duration (>10 h). In analogy to narcolepsy, it is not the symptom of daytime tiredness but the increased likelihood of falling asleep during the daytime (daytime sleepiness). For basic diagnostic criteria of measuring daytime sleepiness by means of the multiple sleep latency test (MSLT), see ▶ Sect. 5.2.6.

5.2.2 Etiology and Pathophysiology

In contrast to narcolepsy, no increased activity of the REM sleep system is observed in idiopathic hypersomnia. The etiological model postulates a shift of the sleep–wake regulation in the direction of more non-REM sleep.

A high familial incidence of the disorder has been found, but specific gene loci have not yet been identified. An association with gene polymorphisms of the HLA system seems to exist. Viral infections (e.g., mononucleosis, pneumonia) might trigger idiopathic hypersomnia. Hypersomnia can also be observed as a sequela of organic brain damage (inflammations, tumors, cerebral insult). Furthermore, the chronic abuse of substances and stimulants is discussed as a possible trigger of hypersomnia; after abstinence, the hypersomnia complaints can persist.

Finally, from what is known so far, the etiology of idiopathic hypersomnia has not yet been clarified.

5.2.3 Epidemiology

Reliable data on the prevalence of idiopathic hypersomnia are currently not available. Many sleep centers state that the diagnosis of patients seeking help for daytime sleepiness is rarer by a factor of 10 compared to narcolepsy. Converted to the prevalence, this would be a minor percentage of 0.01%.

The prevalence of patients with idiopathic hypersomnia in the sleep laboratory of the Central Institute for Mental Health in Mannheim, Germany, is higher, about twice as high, compared to narcolepsy. However, this sleep center has a psychiatric focus. For young patients with long sleep durations and/or daytime sleepiness atypical depression is an important differential diagnosis to hypersomnia. Thus, epidemiological surveys are needed to determine whether the prevalence of primary hypersomnia is in the same range as narcolepsy.

Similar to narcolepsy, the main onset of the disorder is between the ages of 15 and 25 years. Typically, the course of the disorder is chronic.

5.2.4 Clinical Presentation

Similar to narcolepsy, the major symptom in idiopathic hypersomnia is not feeling tired during the day but the increased likelihood to fall asleep during the daytime (daytime sleepiness).

In contrast to narcolepsy, naps during the day are typically not restorative for those patients and do not have a positive effect on daytime sleepiness. In some of the patients, sleep drunkenness can occur after night sleep or even after short naps.

Frequently, patients report that it is difficult to awaken in the morning. One patient of our sleep center told us that he often came too late to work despite a scheduled sleep duration of 8 h and three alarm clocks positioned in different locations, because he switched off the alarm clocks, still half-asleep, and continued sleeping.

In a subgroup of idiopathic hypersomnia patients, vegetative symptoms (cold hands and feet), orthostatic hypotonia, and headaches have been observed. As in narcolepsy, automated behavior occurs rarely, that is, activities that are continued in a semiconscious way without being able to recall them afterward.

5.2.5 Diagnostics

Diagnosing idiopathic hypersomnia is mostly a process of exclusion. Other causes for increased daytime sleepiness must be excluded. If idiopathic hypersomnia is suspected, a polysomnographic examination over two nights with a multiple sleep latency test on day 1 or 2 after the polysomnography night is indicated (see following section).

Sleep history taking must differentiate between daytime tiredness and daytime sleepiness. Hypersomnia patients show daytime sleepiness, that is, an increased likelihood to fall asleep in monotonous situations. Severe problems with waking-up in the morning and sleep drunkenness should be assessed very precisely.

For diagnostics, it is helpful to ask the patient to write a *sleep diary* for at least 1 week. The recorded times of going to bed, sleep-onset duration, nightly wake phases, and times of getting up allow estimating if a normal sleep duration (about 7–9 h) or a prolonged sleep duration (>10 h) is observed. This method may be completed by wrist actigraphy.

It is furthermore essential to perform *psychiatric history taking* because an atypical depression may be present as an important differential diagnosis: it is called atypical because about 90% of depressive patients complain about insomnia disorders. However, some of them, especially younger patients and those with seasonal depression, have an increased need of sleep as seen in idiopathic hypersomnia. If history taking reveals depressive symptoms (depression, negative thoughts, loss of interest), it is recommended to refer the patients to a psychiatrist.

Because organic origins such as hypothyroidism or chronic renal insufficiency may also cause hypersomnia complaints, somatic history taking must be performed comprehensively. Viral diseases and organic brain damage have to be clarified as well as the consumption of stimulants and substances. Respective lab diagnostics (▶ Sect. 2.2) and physical examination are included in the routine diagnostics of idiopathic hypersomnia. If the aforementioned causes are suspected, further diagnostics by a specialist are recommended.

5.2.6 Sleep Diagnostics

As already described, sleep examination must consist of two nightly *polysomnographies* combined with a *multiple sleep latency test* (▶ Chap. 2) for diagnosing idiopathic hypersomnia.

Despite brief periods of wakefulness during the night, the sleep profile regarding the cycle of REM and non-REM phases has to be considered as regular (◘ Fig. 5.3). The time awake after sleep onset is also short; sleep efficiency amounted to 89%, comparable to the figures found in healthy sleepers.

In ◘ Fig. 5.4 the multiple sleep latency test of the same patient is depicted.

In all five sleep episodes, the patient fell asleep rapidly. On average, she needed 2 min, i.e., the subjectively reported daytime sleepiness could be confirmed. In the first test, a REM phase occurred, however, after the first appearance of non-REM stage 2.

According to the diagnostic criteria of the AASM, the averaged sleep-onset latency over all five tests has to be less than 8 min. As mean sleep-

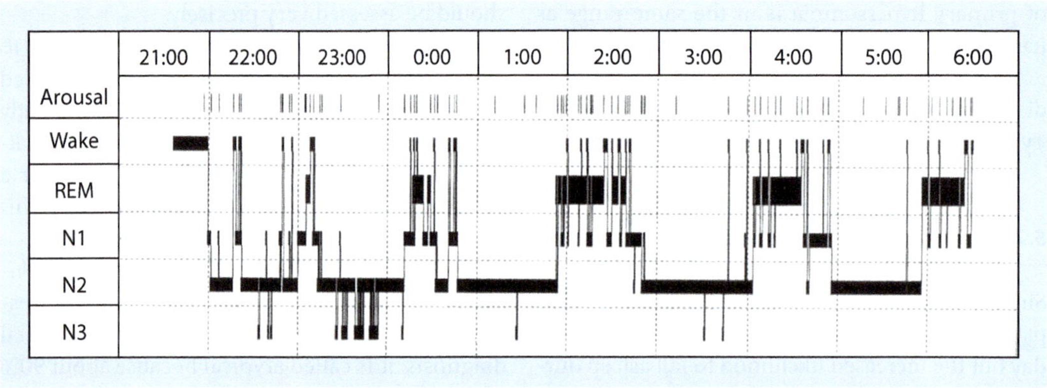

◘ **Fig. 5.3** Night sleep profile of a 36-year-old female patient with idiopathic hypersomnia

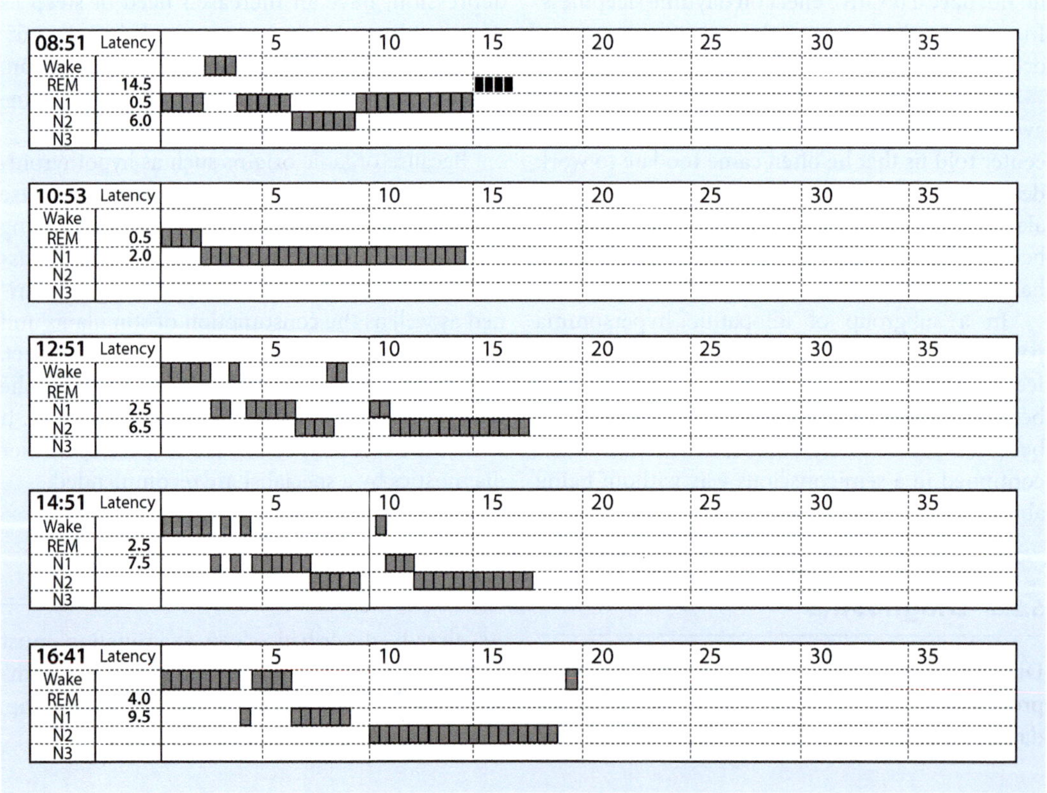

◘ **Fig. 5.4** Multiple sleep latency test of a female patient with idiopathic hypersomnia

onset duration for this disorder, a duration of 6.2 min is reported. However, it must be considered that such mean sleep-onset durations can also be observed in up to 30% of healthy sleepers, that is, good anamnestic data on an increased daytime sleepiness in everyday-life are important for the correct diagnosis. To differentiate from narcolepsy, a REM phase must only occur once in all five tests.

The MSLT should always be performed after a normal and polysomnographically recorded night (sleep duration, 6 h to a maximum of 10 h). In this polysomnography, it can be clarified if a clinically relevant sleep-related breathing disorder and/or periodic limb movements during sleep are present. The diagnosis of idiopathic hypersomnia cannot be made, if another sleep disorder explains the daytime sleepiness and an appropriate treatment of the sleep disorder(s) has to be initiated.

Diagnostic Criteria of Idiopathic Hypersomnia, According to the AASM

- The patients have daily phases with an irrepressible need to sleep or sleep-onset attacks during daytime for at least 3 months (sleep drunkenness and nonrestorative naps during daytime are frequently observed complaints).
- Cataplexies do not occur.
- The adequately performed multiple sleep latency test (MSLT) shows less than two SOREM phases or no SOREM phase in the MSLT when the REM latency in the night before the MSLT was under 15 min.
- One of the two following criteria has to be fulfilled:
  - The MSLT shows an averaged sleep latency of 8 min or less.
  - The overall sleep duration over a 24-h polysomnography (after correction of possible chronic sleep deprivation) is longer than 660 min (typically, 12–14 h) *or* an actigraphic measurement at the wrist including a sleep protocol averaged over at least 7 days of unrestricted sleep.
- Insufficient sleep syndrome is excluded (if daytime sleepiness does not improve despite extending the nightly bedtimes; actigraphy over at least 7 days is desirable).
- Hypersomnia complaints and/or MSLT findings cannot be explained by any other sleep disorder, medical, or psychiatric disorder, or use of drugs or medications.

5.2.7 Differential Diagnostics

Other sleep disorders that can cause daytime sleepiness have to be excluded, e.g., *periodic limb movements during sleep* (▶ Chap. 8) and *sleep-related breathing disorders* (▶ Chap. 4). In particular *mild sleep apnea syndromes*, formerly called upper airway resistance syndromes, are discussed as possible differential diagnosis because these patients are usually of normal weight and do not report snoring.

The differential diagnostics for *narcolepsy* is based on performing two polysomnographic recordings and a multiple sleep latency test under controlled conditions in the sleep lab. The average sleep latency of narcolepsy patients is typically shorter than that of patients with idiopathic hypersomnia. REM sleep phases occur in at least two sleep episodes of the MSLT. However, this criterion is not always clear-cut because at the onset of narcolepsy daytime sleepiness is the first symptom and the hyperactivity of the REM sleep system is not always fully developed. Sometimes, it is necessary to give the preliminary diagnosis of idiopathic hypersomnia until the first symptoms that are typical for narcolepsy such as cataplexies, sleep paralysis, or hypnagogic hallucinations or SOREMs in the MSLT occur. Typically, a reexamination of the patient after 1 to 2 years provides clarification.

Practical Tip

Because narcolepsy has daytime sleepiness as its first symptom comparable to hypersomnia and as initially REM sleep hyperactivity is often not fully developed, it is possible that patients who do not have MSLT with two SOREM phases develop narcolepsy in the further course. In cases of uncertainty, reexamination after 1 to 2 years is recommended.

It must also be clarified if *insufficient sleep syndrome* might be present. For this purpose a sleep diary assessing the sleep durations at home or (in single cases) actigraphy is useful. If the average sleep durations amount to clearly less than 7.5 to 8 h, a sleep deprivation syndrome (▶ Sect. 5.3.1) might be diagnosed.

The differentiation between idiopathic hypersomnia and *atypical depression* is not always easy. Extensive psychiatric history taking regarding psychopathological moods, sleep-related thoughts, and motivation is essential. In particular, the two disorders widely overlap in regard to reduced motivation. Also in this context, the MSLT may be helpful because depressive patients may spend much time in bed during the daytime, although they do not sleep as much as the patients with idiopathic hypersomnia.

Hypersomnia can also observed in *seasonal depression*. In addition to the association with seasons (fall and winter), other characteristics like craving for carbohydrates, mood swings have to be elicited.

Also, *posttraumatic stress disorder* may be accompanied by hypersomnia symptoms so that the trauma history should be included in the anamnesis.

Another disorder that has to be differentiated from idiopathic hypersomnia is the *chronic fatigue syndrome* (CFS). The most obvious difference is sleepiness. Although CFS patients always feel tired, a frequent and rapid falling asleep under controlled conditions of the multiple sleep latency test is only rarely observed in this patient group. These differential diagnoses highlight the significance of examination of these patients (probable idiopathic hypersomnia) in a specialized sleep medical center.

5.2.8 Therapy

Only a very few solid clinical data are available about the therapeutic options for treatment of idiopathic hypersomnia. *Sufficient night sleep* is certainly recommended because sleep deprivation may lead to enhanced daytime sleepiness. In contrast to narcolepsy patients, daytime naps are not considered as beneficial as they increase the dizziness during daytime because of sleep drunkenness.

Not much experience is available regarding drug therapy. The first choice treatment is *modafinil* (vigil) because positive effects are reported, at least in small studies. Side effects such as headaches and tachycardia, however, are a frequent problem in these patients. Furthermore, tolerance development is often observed and, thus, a sufficient long-term treatment of these patients with modafinil is not always possible.

In clinical practice, also stimulants such as methylphenidate, pitolisant, dextroamphetamines, or stimulating antidepressants such as fluoxetine, citalopram, or venlafaxine have been applied for symptomatic treatment. Few clinical experiences have been reported in individual cases using MAO inhibitors or levodopa.

5.3 Other Hypersomnias

In this chapter, two other types of hypersomnia are described:

- Insufficient sleep syndrome
- Kleine-Levin syndrome

5.3.1 Insufficient Sleep Syndrome

As in other hypersomnias, *daytime sleepiness* is the key symptom in the context of insufficient sleep syndrome. Problems with *concentration and attention* are often additional complaints.

The reason for this daytime sleepiness is a permanently too short sleep duration. The patients have become accustomed to short sleep periods because they thought that they did not need much sleep and wanted to spend more time on work and leisure activities. This strategy may work without any complaints for months or even years. In this way, the sleep behavior becomes a habit and the patients are not aware that the hypersomnia symptoms are due to too short sleep because the reduced sleep duration has worked well for a long time.

Often, the insufficient sleep syndrome is observed in adolescents and young adults. Prevalence rates, however, are not yet available. It is also unknown whether predisposing factors can increase the risk for developing these symptoms.

For diagnostics, a *sleep diary* kept over 1 week is useful, possibly complemented by actigraphic measurement. Information about the patient's sleep duration on weekends or on vacation is also important to estimate the sleep need. For an average sleep duration of about 6 h, there are certainly people who do not show hypersomnia complaints (healthy short sleepers). However, if daytime sleepiness is observed, then this subject most likely needs to sleep more than 6 h per night.

Because insufficient sleep syndrome is an important differential diagnosis of idiopathic hypersomnia, assessment of the sleep duration in the home setting is very important, in particular because insufficient sleep syndrome patients show similar findings compared to patients with idiopathic hypersomnia with regard to polysomnographically measured night sleep (short sleep-onset latency, high sleep efficiency) and in the multiple sleep latency test (average duration to fall asleep less than 8 min).

Of course, the therapeutic options have to be discussed with the patient, e.g., how a new daytime structure may be found that allows sufficient sleep.

5.3.2 Recurrent Hypersomnias

The prevalence rates of recurrent hypersomnias are very low.

Only about 1000 cases of *Kleine-Levin syndrome* (KLS) with periodically recurring hypersomnia phases have been described in the literature.

The KLS is a rare disease with recurrent episodes of severe hypersomnia associated with cognitive disorders, behavioral problems, mood disorders, hyperphagia (eating high-calorie food), and hypersexuality (obscene language, being naked in public). The recurrent phases with 15–21 h of sleep per 24 h may last for some days to several weeks.

Based on the phasic occurrences which can be clearly differentiated from the typical behavior of the patient and that include very long sleep periods and the aforementioned accompanying symptoms, the diagnosis can be based on clinical judgement; an evaluation in a sleep laboratory is in most cases not necessary.

According to a review article published by Arnulf (2008), the prevalence amounts to 1 or 2 cases in 1,000,000 persons. The patients are mostly male (68–78%) and adolescent (81%). In 72% of the cases, the first episode is triggered by infection. The average age at onset is about 15 years; the patients have between 7 and 19 episodes with an average duration between 10 and 13 days that repeat every 3.5 months on average. The overall duration of disorder is between 8 and 14 years.

Even if some studies indicate genetic influences (high familial incidence, higher prevalence in people with Jewish origin), the origin of the disorder is unknown; the HLA genes (see narcolepsy), however, might be involved. Physiologically, the symptoms are likely to be caused by functional problems in the hypothalamus. Complications at birth and development disorders were more frequently observed in patients with Kleine-Levin syndrome compared to matched control groups, which may suggest that environmental factors are also of relevance. In addition, autoimmune processes are discussed as the possible origin of the dysfunction in the hypothalamus.

In chronic cases the phase prophylacticum of lithium has positive effects (reducing the number of hypersomnia phases). During hypersomnia phases, stimulants such as modafinil or methylphenidate may be helpful for patients. Positive experiences are also available with amantadine.

Also, hypersomnia phases lasting for about 1 week that are associated with *menstruation* and occur for the first time in the first months after menarche are very rare. A hormonal dysregulation is probably responsible for the complaints because the intake of oral contraceptives can alleviate the symptoms.

5.4 Questions

? 1. What are the four key symptoms of narcolepsy?

? 2. Which examination method is essential for diagnosing narcolepsy?

? 3. What are the leading symptoms of idiopathic hypersomnia?

? 4. Please list the most important differential diagnoses of idiopathic hypersomnia.

Further Reading

1. American Academy of Sleep Medicine. The international classification of sleep disorders. ICSD-3. Darien: American Academy of Sleep Medicine; 2014.
2. Arnulf I, Lecendreux M, Franco P, Dauvilliers Y. Kleine-Levin syndrome: state of the art. Rev Neurol. 2008;164(8-9):658–68.
3. Kryger MH, Roth T, Dement WC. Principles and practice of sleep medicine, Sixth edition, Philadelphia: Elsevier/Saunders; 2017.
4. Goswami M, Pandi-Perumal SR, Thorpy MJ. (Eds.), Narcolepsy: a clinical guide. New York: Springer.
5. Billiard M, Mignot E, Bassetti C. Narcolepsy and Hypersomnia. New York: Taylor & Francis; 2007.

Circadian Rhythm Sleep–Wake Disorders

J. T. Maurer

B. A. Stuck et al., *Practice of Sleep Medicine*, https://doi.org/10.1007/978-3-030-17412-5_6

This group of diseases is characterized by a lack of synchronization of the intrinsic circadian rhythms with light-dark alternation. Either the intrinsic pacemaker itself is disturbed or the sleep-wake rhythm deviates from a normal intrinsic circadian rhythm because of external factors. Insomnia or hypersomnia complaints, or both, are the consequence. If the patient is able to adapt the sleep times to the inner rhythm, sleep duration and quality as well as the performance in the awake phase are normal. Sleep-wake disorders occur most frequently in shift workers, with negative effects on health and impaired performance at work. Sleep diaries are the basis for diagnosis, and the strict adherence to defined bedtimes in combination with light therapy are the basis for therapy.

6.1 Basics and Diagnosis

A disorder of the circadian sleep–wake rhythm is diagnosed when the intrinsic circadian rhythm of an individual cannot be synchronized with the light–dark alternation or social zeitgebers. This lack of synchronization may be caused by a disorder of the intrinsic pacemaker itself or may be a mostly behavior-related deviation of the sleep–wake rhythm of a normally working circadian rhythm.

The complaints may be of an insomnia (see ▸ Chap. 3) as well as a hypersomnia (see ▸ Chap. 5) nature, often even occurring in phases in the same individual, and they have to prevail for at least 3 months. Performance at work, social contacts, and the person's private activities are severely impaired. If the patient can choose his sleeping times according to his intrinsic rhythm, his sleep is restorative, and performance during the wake times is normal.

In most cases, the affected individuals may clearly name behavioral deviations of the day–night rhythm when they are asked directly. By means of a sleep diary that is generally required (see ▸ Sect. 2.3) for at least 1 week, or better 2 weeks, a suspected diagnosis can be made that has to be confirmed by actigraphy (see ▸ Sect. 2.4) for at least 1 week eventually. An assessment with and without social contacts (e.g., work, school) may be helpful. Morning- and evening-chrono type individuals can be evaluated by means of a publicly available and validated morningness/eveningness questionnaire (MEQ) according to Horne and Östberg. In doubtful cases, measurement of the core body temperature and melatonin profile may be required. In those cases, it is important to avoid social time givers during measurement. Polysomnography (PSG) is useful in unclear cases when other diseases, for example, sleep-related breathing disorders (see ▸ Chap. 4), are assumed.

For therapy of circadian rhythm sleep disorders, see ▸ Sect. 6.7.

Practical Tip

The most important diagnostic procedure in the context of suspected circadian rhythm sleep–wake disorders is a sleep diary for at least 1 week, or better, for 2 or more weeks.

6.2 Sleep–Wake Phase Disorders

This family of rhythm sleep–wake disorders is characterized by a significantly shifted sleep phase compared to the socially common circumstance that makes it difficult or even impossible to fall asleep or wake up at desired times. If the affected individuals are allowed to sleep according to their needs, they reveal a time-shifted but stable sleep–wake rhythm with normal sleep duration and quality. The shift is usually longer than 2 h. The shifted sleep phase has to be confirmed for at least 1 week in the sleep diary, completed by actigraphy if needed. This shift also manifests in the core body temperature graph and melatonin concentration.

6.2.1 Delayed Sleep–Wake Phase Disorder

The leading symptom of those patients is most commonly *insomnia*, because they go to bed at the usual times but are unable to fall asleep. Some patients can only fall asleep in the early morning hours so that they have to arise after only a short time asleep. Many patients complain of sleep inertia and drowsiness in the morning and greatly impaired performance during the day. Characteristically, a performance peak is reported in the evening. If the biological clock is not considered, about half the patients show psychosomatic symptoms such as flushing, headache, or orthostatic or gastrointestinal disorders; about one third have neurotic conspicuities. Frequently, alcohol or sleeping aids are applied in the evening and stimulant drugs during the daytime to cope with the disorder. Because their sleep deficit accumulates during the workweek, many patients sleep for the whole day on weekends or vacations, which leads to further cementing of the delayed sleep phase.

Typically, the first signs of the disease appear in *adolescence*, which often leads to poor school performance. The differentiation to behavior-related late bedtimes with consecutive sleep deficit may be difficult in those cases. In early adulthood, the complaints may disappear when a regular sleep–wake rhythm is entrained by the onset of the working life. If this training is not successful, the disorder remains lifelong. However, with increasing age, the affected individuals have less difficulty, in particular with getting up in the morning.

Delayed sleep phase disorders are observed in about 0.5% of the population; in cohorts of insomnia patients and during adolescence, an incidence of about 10% was reported. In approximately 40% of the cases, the family history is positive; a genetic component may be considered. So far, the pathogenesis of the disease remains unclear.

6.2.2 Advanced Sleep–Wake Phase Disorder

For diagnosis, an advanced sleep phase compared to the desired time of sleep onset is crucial, with high sleep pressure in the early evening and waking up early in the morning without being able to fall asleep again.

Nearly all affected patients are *morning-chrono type individuals*. They complain typically about extreme sleepiness between 6:00 PM and 9:00 PM and most often wake up between 2:00 AM and 5:00 AM. Even if they go to bed later, they cannot sleep longer, so that often a sleep deficit accumulates that patients try to overcome with stimulants, such as coffee. Because these individuals have their performance peak mostly in the morning, difficulties at work occur only rarely, but social life is impaired by the difficulty of participating in evening activities. Because of the wish to sleep as late as others in the morning, a psychophysiological insomnia may be conditioned. Regarding differential diagnosis, early bedtimes in older people because of the lack of social contacts and early awakening in the context of insomnia (see ▶ Chap. 3) or a depressive disorder (see ▶ Chap. 10) especially have to be differentiated.

A prevalence of 1% is assumed for middle and older age groups. The disorder manifests in most cases in the middle-aged group, rarely in childhood. With increasing age, it more often increases and is considered as a chronic disease. Both genders are affected with equal incidence. Often a family predisposition is seen that allows suspecting an autosomal-dominant inheritance. Mutations in the circadian clock gene hPer2 have been discussed. The pathogenesis of the disease has not yet been clarified.

6.3 Irregular Sleep–Wake Rhythm Disorder

Patients with irregular sleep–wake rhythm disorder complain about excessive daytime sleepiness, disorders of initiating and maintaining sleep, or even both. The diagnosis can be based on ICSD-3, when at least three irregular and unpredictable shorter sleep periods during the 24 h are revealed in the sleep diary or actigraphy over an interval of 7 days. The total sleep time per 24 h corresponds to the age.

The disorder is mainly found in individuals who lack *social schedules*. With increasing age and increasingly rare outdoor activities, reduced light during the daytime also leads to flattening of the endogenous circadian rhythm, which is seen in an amplitude reduction of the core body temperature. An irregular sleep–wake pattern occurs frequently in cases of bed confinement, mental retardation, and neurodegenerative diseases. In cases of demented patients, the term sundowning is used when they show increased activity at the time of sundown.

The disorder has to be differentiated from an arbitrarily irregular sleep–wake pattern resulting from a lack of sleep hygiene.

6.4 Non-24-Hour Sleep–Wake Rhythm Disorder

When the internal clock shows a constant duration that, however, cannot be synchronized with the 24-h rhythm, intermittent insomnia or hypersomnia complaints occur. Thus, the disease is also called free-running sleep-wake rhythm disorder. Sleep diaries or actigraphy over at least 14 days show how the sleep period shifts every day at a constant interval. This shift, which mostly amounts to 1 to 2 h, can be objectified by measuring the core body temperature or determining the dim light melatonin onset.

6

Patients observe a regularly changing complaint pattern when they try to entrain the 24-h cycle. If the endogenous sleep phase is in the morning or in the afternoon, patients present symptoms comparable to delayed or advanced sleep–wake phase disorder. When the light–dark rhythm and the endogenous rhythm are synchronized for some days, the affected individuals are free of complaints. Some patients adapt their daily routine to their internal rhythm to avoid the consequences of nonrestorative sleep.

About half of all *blind people* suffer from this disorder (see ▶ Sect. 1.5). However, the onset cannot be correlated with the date of loss of sight. People who are blind from birth can be affected throughout their whole lives. Sighted individuals are only rarely affected, and when they are, this is often preceded by a longer isolation from zeitgebers or a chronotherapy (see ▶ Sect. 6.7) because of delayed sleep–wake phase disorder. Also, fluid transitions to delayed sleep–wake phase disorders are observed, which is seen in changing appearances of the disorder over longer periods.

6.5 Sleep Disorders in Cases of Jetlag or Shift Work

6.5.1 Sleep Disorder in Cases of Jetlag

When insomnia or hypersomnia complaints with impaired alertness during the day occur after a flight of at least two time zones, this is called jetlag. Additionally, somatic symptoms are reported such as gastrointestinal complaints or general discomfort.

The endogenous rhythm can shift about 60 to 90 min per day, but not all body functions are able to adapt to the new time zone with the same pace. The heart rate and sodium concentration, for example, adapt rapidly. Sleep structure, body temperature, and adrenalin secretion adapt more slowly and cortisol and potassium concentration extremely slowly. This internal dissociation of the endogenous rhythms is not noticed by many people, but it can impede maximum performance.

After flights to the east, disorders of initiating sleep occur, whereas with flights to the west rather disorders of maintaining sleep are observed. The problems mostly become apparent in the second night in the new time zone because in the first night the sleep deficit that developed during the flight is reduced. In addition, daytime sleepiness and reduced performance as well as urination at night, disturbed appetite, constipation, or diarrhea are observed. Because of frequently recurring changes of time zones, the flying staff of intercontinental flights is particularly affected.

The complaints are the more pronounced the more time zones are passed, the more often this happens, and the less the individual concerned is able to adapt to the new time zone. Evening-chrono type individuals, young people, and people with a rhythm with low daytime amplitudes find it easier to adapt. The complaints, however, are always self-limiting and thus have a primarily benign character.

It is easier to cope with flights to the west than with flights in the eastward direction because most people have an endogenous sleep–wake rhythm that is slightly longer than 24 h (see ▶ Sect. 1.5). In flights to the west, it is necessary to stay awake longer relative to the inner clock. With the increased sleep pressure, falling asleep is then easier, but according to the inner clock, at the destination one wakes up in the early morning hours. This longer waking phase is generally associated with increased sleepiness. In severe cases, one or two shorter sleep periods are recommended to compensate for the increased sleep pressure.

In the context of flights to the east, often difficulties of initiating sleep develop because, in relationship to the inner clock, at the destination one needs to fall asleep earlier, that is, without sufficient sleep pressure. In those cases, it may be reasonable to transitorily apply a hypnotic agent or to refuse to sleep in the first night at the destination.

In this way, the sleep pressure is increased for the following night, and acclimatization to the new light–dark rhythm at the destination is facilitated. For compensation of the sleep pressure that is increased by the prolonged waking phase, short sleep periods also may be recommended.

6.5.2 Sleep Disorder in Cases of Shift Work

When shift workers complain about insomnia or hypersomnia that recurs in timely association with night shifts, a shift work sleep disorder may be diagnosed. To confirm such an assumption, the complaints have to be present for at least 3 months, and the timely correlation to shift work has to be proven by a sleep diary (for at least 14 days), possibly combined with actigraphy.

In the European Union, 18.5% of employees are shift workers; night work is performed by 7.8%. Up to 32% of these shift workers with night shifts complain about sleep disorders that persist in about three fourths of the affected people even after ceasing shift work. A prevalence of shift work sleep disorders is assumed for 1% to 4% of the overall population. The present data on the impact of shift work on sleep and daytime alertness, but also the general health condition, are either based on small case numbers or studies with low evidence or the results are contradictory. Thus, no clear answers can be given on most of the specific questions.

There are different working time models of shift work. Under sleep medical aspects, in particular night work and alternating shift systems with night work are relevant. Alternating shifts can rotate forward (i.e., from early shift via late shift to night shift) or backward, as well as changing rapidly or slowly. Permanent night shifts seem to be associated with fewer sleep disorders than alternating shift systems with night shifts. Rapidly rotating shift systems seem to favor a changed sleep duration. After night shifts, shorter times of sleep are found; after late shifts they are rather prolonged in comparison to those of people with regular night sleep. There are suggestions that the percentages of light and REM sleep are reduced, although the deep sleep remains the same. Complaints in the context of shift work are generally similar to those of jetlag, and affected people may even lose their jobs. This problem is caused by the accumulated sleep deficit as well as the recurring need to adapt the inner rhythm. People who are able to relax easily more rarely suffer from sleep disorders in the context of shift work. Especially during night shifts, mental performance is severely impaired at times, and thus also the risk of mistakes and accidents is increased. During night shifts, morning-type individuals accumulate a particularly large sleep deficit because they wake up too early. Evening-type individuals reveal increased sleepiness and impaired performance during early shifts because they cannot advance their sleep pattern.

In the context of severe insomnia, incapability to perform shift work of particular shifts may exist partly until the complaints are sufficiently treated, which also applies for cases of restless legs syndrome that are difficult to treat. In case of sleep-related breathing disorders, generally no incapability to perform shift work is observed; however, in single cases severe insomnia may develop as consequence of device-related therapy, which may also lead to partial shift incapability until satisfactory treatment is achieved. Typically, people suffering from narcolepsy are not capable of performing shift work.

Long-term shift work per se seems to contribute to the genesis of a metabolic syndrome but less to cardiovascular or gastrointestinal diseases. The concern that even breast cancer may be associated with shift work could not be confirmed by a meta-analysis.

6.6 Circadian Sleep–Wake Disorders Not Otherwise Specified

If a circadian rhythm sleep disorder with insomnia or hypersomnia complaints (see ▶ Sects. 6.2, 6.3, and 6.4) cannot be allocated to one of the aforementioned diagnoses, it is classified in this group. The complaints are mostly associated with organic or psychiatric diseases. In the diagnosis, this aspect has to be mentioned specifically. Typical examples are dementia that in some cases shows an inverse sleep–wake behavior with sleep phases during the day and nighttime wandering as well as hepatic encephalopathy, where often a pattern similar to the delayed sleep–wake phase syndrome is found. In the context of Parkinson's disease, all these various disorders may be observed.

6

6.7 Therapy

The observation of *strict bedtimes* combined with *light therapy* is meanwhile an established therapy of rhythm sleep–wake disorders in sighted individuals.

Light is applied in the morning immediately after getting up. Only in cases of advanced sleep–wake disorders light therapy is applied in the evening. The exposure to daylight suppresses the melatonin discharge and thus synchronizes the inner clock. At least 2,000 lux are applied for a duration of 2 h; with 10,000 lux, the duration can be reduced to 45 min. Patients have to turn their face to the light source and maintain a distance of approximately 1 m.

Melatonin is applied at a dosage of 3–5 mg at a time that assures the overlapping of the endogenous and exogenous melatonin maximum.

- In cases of delayed sleep phase disorders, irregular sleep–wake patterns, and free-running rhythm, melatonin is applied about 4 h before turning off the light.
- In cases of advanced sleep phase disorders, melatonin is not indicated.
- In cases of jetlag, 4 days before arrival melatonin may be administered at the time that corresponds to the sleeping time at the place of destination.

Tasimelteon, which is a melatonin receptor agonist, received FDA approval in 2013 and EU approval in 2015 for the treatment of completely blind patients with non-24-h sleep–wake rhythm disorder.

Two clinical trials with 104 participants revealed that treatment with tasimelteon led to longer night sleep duration and shorter daytime sleep duration in comparison to placebo treatment. Most frequently reported side effects were headaches, increased hepatic enzymes (alanine aminotransferase) in the blood, nightmares or strange dreams, disturbed night sleep, infections of the upper airways or the urinary tract, and sleepiness.

The agent tasimelteon may impair activities that require complete mental alertness. So, tasimelteon should be taken every night at the same time, about 30 min before going to sleep. After intake of the drug, activities should be limited.

Also, 1.5–3 mg *activated vitamin* B_{12} (methyl cobalamin) has shown good success in the context of delayed sleep–wake phase syndrome, irregular sleep–wake rhythm disorder and non-24-h sleep–wake rhythm disorder because it increases the sensitivity to light.

Generally, the intake of hypnotics is not recommended because in many cases these attenuate the amplitude of the endogenous rhythm and thus have rather negative consequences. Because of an unfavorable benefit–risk assessment, modafinil has not been approved for shift work sleep disorder by the European Drug Agency since 2011.

Chronotherapy means delaying the daily sleep phase of 2 to 3 h in certain intervals until the desired sleep time is achieved. It is applied to treat delayed sleep phase disorder, and usually it is accepted by patients as pleasant because it concurs with their long endogenous rhythm. However, it should only be applied in exceptional cases because this therapy may trigger a free-running disorder that is then very difficult to treat.

Simple *behavioral measures* may be helpful to support therapy. In this context, on one hand sports and exercise, as well as abstinence from alcohol in the wake phases, must be mentioned. On the other hand, noise should be minimized during sleep after night shifts. If this is not possible, quiet music or radio programs may improve sleep quality. It also seems helpful to plan one third of the individually usual sleep time before working and two thirds after a night shift.

In cases of *shift work*, the work schedule should take into consideration the phase situation of the workers. Morning-type individuals are not suitable for night shifts, and evening-type individuals are not suitable for early shifts. For most people, late shifts do not represent a problematic issue. Generally, older people have more difficulties adapting to shift work than younger ones. In many cases, diabetes mellitus, chronic gastritis, ulcer, thyroid, liver, cardiac, circulatory, pulmonary, and neuropsychiatric diseases including addiction, as well as preexisting sleep disorders are contraindications for employment in shift work. In the context of shift work, not more than three subsequent night shifts should be worked to avoid a modification of the endogenous rhythm of the affected individuals. Taking into consideration all effects on sleep and daytime sleepiness in the context of an overall assessment, rapid forward rotation is recommended. Accordingly, adapted shift schedules with sufficiently long rest periods between the shifts should reduce the morbidity of shift work as well as increase the performance and satisfaction of the workers.

During the night shifts, bright light in the working locations may help to improve the alertness of the workers. In the morning after the night shift, the retina should be protected against too much light by wearing sunglasses and having a dark bedroom to keep the rhythm displacement as low as possible.

In the US and in some other countries, although not in the European Union, modafinil is approved for treatment of sleep disorder in cases of shift work. One hundred milligrams (100 mg) modafinil is taken about 1 h before beginning the night shift to reduce sleepiness during the working time. The subsequent day sleep in the morning after the night shift is not additionally impaired.

Sleep disorders in cases of shift work are frequently associated with psychophysiological insomnia, which has to be treated as well (see ► Chap. 3), because in this way a significant attenuation of the complaints can be achieved in many cases. Recent studies with, however, only small case numbers could show the benefit of psychoeducative and behavioral therapy-oriented interventions for sleep disorders as a consequence of shift work.

Practical Tip

The basis of the treatment of rhythm sleep–wake disorders is the adherence to strict bedtimes in combination with light therapy.

6.8 Questions

1. Please list the characteristics of rhythm sleep–wake disorders.
2. Which diagnostic and therapeutic principles for rhythm sleep disorders do you know?
3. Please define the different rhythm sleep–wake disorders.

Further Reading

1. American Academy of Sleep Medicine. International classification of sleep disorders, 3. Aufl. Darien: American Academy of Sleep Medicine; 2014.
2. Berry RB, Brooks R, Gamaldo CE, Harding SM, Lloyd RM, Marcus CL, Vaughn BV for the American Academy of Sleep Medicine. The AASM manual for the scoring of sleep and associated events: rules, terminology and technical specifications, version 2.6. http://www.aasmnet.org: Darien: American Academy of Sleep Medicine; 2016.
3. Eurostat. Statistiken. 2017. http://appsso.eurostat.ec.europa.eu/nui/show.do?dataset=lfsa_ewpshi&lamg=de. Zugriff 30.03.2017.
4. Folkard S. Do permanent night workers show circadian adjustment? A review based on the endogenous melatonin rhythm. Chronobiol Int. 2008;25:215–24.
5. Griefahn B. Zur Validität der deutschen Übersetzung des Morningness-Eveningness-Questinonaires von Horne und Östberg. Somnologie. 2001;5:71–80.
6. Pandi-Perumal SR, Trakht I, Spence DW, Srinivasan V, Dagan Y, Cardinali DP. The roles of melatonin and light in the pathophysiology and treatment of circadian rhythm sleep disorders. Nat Clin Pract Neurol. 2008;4:436–47.
7. Paridon H, Ernst S, Harth V, Nickel P, Nold A, Pallapies D (2012) Deutsche Gesetzliche Unfallversicherung, Hrsg. Schichtarbeit – Rechtslage, gesundheitliche Risiken und Präventionsmöglichkeiten (= DGUV Report 1/2012). Berlin. ISBN 978-3-86423-022-6.
8. Sack RL, Auckley D, Auger RR, Carskadon MA, Wright KP Jr, Vitiello MV, Zhdanova IV, American Academy of Sleep Medicine. Circadian rhythm sleep disorders: part I, basic principles, shift work and jet lag disorders. An American Academy of Sleep Medicine review. Sleep. 2007a;30:1460–83.
9. Sack RL, Auckley D, Auger RR, Carskadon MA, Wright KP Jr, Vitiello MV, Zhdanova IV, American Academy of Sleep Medicine. Circadian rhythm sleep disorders: part II, advanced sleep phase disorder, delayed sleep phase disorder, free-running disorder, and irregular sleep-wake rhythm. An American Academy of Sleep Medicine review. Sleep. 2007b;30:1484–501.
10. Toh KL. Basic science review on circadian rhythm biology and circadian sleep disorders. Ann Acad Med Singap. 2008;37:662–8.
11. Travis RC, Balkwill A, Fensom GK, Appleby PN, Reeves GK, Wang XS, Roddam AW, Gathani T, Peto R, Green J, Key TJ, Beral V. Night shift work and breast cancer incidence: three prospective studies and meta-analysis of published studies. J Natl Cancer Inst. 2016;108(12):djw169.

Parasomnias

M. Schredl

B. A. Stuck et al., *Practice of Sleep Medicine*, https://doi.org/10.1007/978-3-030-17412-5_7

Even if parasomnias do not directly impair the quality of sleep and recovery due to sleep, they may represent an major burden for the affected individuals. Nightmares may have a negative impact on the daytime mood; pavor nocturnus and sleepwalking are often experienced as embarrassing by adults, and furthermore even injuries may occur. It is in particular the fact that actions are carried out about which the individual has no control and cannot even recall in the morning that is perceived as distressful. Parasomnias are found more frequently in children, but they may also be observed in adults or persist until adulthood. About 5% of all adults report that they suffer from nightmares. Sleepwalking and night terrors (pavor nocturnus), however, are rather rarely found in adults (less than 1%).

The term parasomnia defines sleep disorders that occur "besides, parallel to" (para) "sleep" (somno), which means that these phenomena are observed during sleep but they do not directly impair the quality of sleep and recovery due to sleep.

In practice, however, this distinction is sometimes difficult to make. For example, female patients suffering from nightmares often report impaired quality of sleep and recovery due to sleep. This problem can be explained on one hand by waking up from negative dreams (impaired sleep continuity), and on the other hand by fear of again having a stressful nightmare after falling asleep. On the other hand, organic factors should never be dismissed in the context of changed subjective experiences such as dreaming. Hence, dream activity that is subjectively perceived as exhausting might also be associated with a REM-sleep associated sleep-related breathing disorder. The arousal occurring at the end of apneic phases in REM sleep may result in recalling the dream events very well and, thus, the person attibuted the nonrestorative sleep to exhausting dreams. However, actually the sleep-related breathing disorder is responsible for the reduced recovery, and thus it is the correct diagnosis in this context. This example illustrates that diagnosing parasomnias should include comprehensive sleep differential diagnostics.

In this chapter, the most important types of parasomnia are presented, including non-REM parasomnias such as night terrors (pavor nocturnus) and sleepwalking, as well as such REM parasomnias as nightmares and REM sleep behavior disorder. Other parasomnias are only rarely observed in adults; for these topics the authors refer to a short summary of those disorders listed at the end of this chapter.

Classification of Parasomnias

- Disorders of arousal (associated with non-REM sleep)
  - Night terror (pavor nocturnus)
  - Sleepwalking (somnambulism)
  - Sleep drunkenness
- REM sleep parasomnias
  - Nightmares
  - REM sleep behavior disorders
  - Isolated recurrent sleep paralysis
- Other parasomnias
  - Enuresis
  - Sleep-related eating disorders

7.1 Pavor Nocturnus

7.1.1 Definitions

Night terrors (pavor nocturnus) are associated with sudden awakenings from slow wave sleep, i.e., from non-REM sleep. These episodes often start with a loud cry, sitting up in bed with eyes wide open. In about 30% to 50% of the cases of pavor nocturnus, sleepwalking may occur after the event; the two disorders are etiologically closely related. If the person calms again and continues sleeping, he/she usually does not recall the nightly event. Therefore, pavor nocturnus and also sleepwalking are termed disorders of arousal. Even if awakened, people cannot give comprehensive dream reports during or shortly after their arousal, even though the actions observed by others, for example, a man who wants to protect his wife during a pavor nocturnus event, clearly show that the person experiences a story during the episode (in this example, a threat to his wife). Mostly, only single images are recalled, for example, something threatening, an assailant, a fire in one's home, or a wall that tumbles down.

7.1.2 Etiology and Pathophysiology

The marked decrease of pavor nocturnus frequency between about 4 and 7 years of age suggests that cerebral maturation processes contribute to their development. The exact mechanisms of those maturation processes, however, are not yet clarified.

In some adult patients, a very high portion of slow wave sleep is observed, which indicates a component of predisposition. *Genetic influences* have been confirmed by twin and family studies.

Stressors such as school enrolment for children or professional or private stress in adults increase the probability of the occurrence of pavor nocturnus episodes. However, it has been shown that not only does extraordinarily severe stress influence the frequency but also that the usual daily stress may lead to nightly attacks when the person has the predisposition. Traumas that often lead to nightmares may also increase the incidence of pavor nocturnus episodes.

Practical Tip

Overall, a diathesis stress model explains the etiology of pavor nocturnus.

Besides stress, some behaviors that lead to slow wave sleep rebound may increase the probability that pavor nocturnus episodes will occur (e.g., a sleepless night, irregular sleep–wake rhythm, alcohol consumption). After a short or sleepless night, the sleep of the following night is characterized by more slow wave sleep (rebound), which increases the probability of night terror episodes. Also, elevated body temperature (fever) may increase the frequency of pavor nocturnus episodes in cases of predisposition.

In sleep practice, cases have also been reported in which sleep-related breathing disorders triggered pavor nocturnus episodes due to micro-arousals at the end of an apneic phase. Thus, in adults with pavor nocturnus comprehensive diagnostics seem to be appropriate with regard to sleep-related breathing disorders (see ▶ Chap. 4).

7.1.3 Epidemiology

About 20% of all children have experienced pavor nocturnus episodes at least once in their lives. The peak of their occurrence is observed between the ages of 4 and 7 years. The prevalence of pavor nocturnus episodes in adults that reach sufficient severity to require treatment is estimated at less than 1%.

7.1.4 Clinical Presentation

Because pavor nocturnus consists of a sudden *arousal* from slow wave sleep, the episodes mostly occur about 1 h after sleep onset due to the distribution of the sleep stages over the course of the night (see ▶ Chap. 1). Only very rarely does more than one attack occur per night.

From a clinical point of view, it must be mentioned that adult patients present with the desire to be treated even when the incidence of the pavor nocturnus episodes amounts to only once or twice per month. These patients are, for example, afraid of spending a night away from home because they fear that such an attack might occur. A young woman, for example, reported that she was afraid of participating in a course in a training center for 1 week because she might have screamed at night and disturbed the whole group. At home, her family was accustomed to this event.

A loud yell at the beginning of pavor nocturnus is often reported. Even if the physiological *anxiety reaction* that can be clearly seen by observers is generally great (heart rate increases from 60 to 180 beats per minute are frequently observed), the person is not fully awake and not oriented with regard to the surroundings even if the eyes are open. The brain is in a state between sleeping and waking. After the pavor nocturnus episode, *sleepwalking* may occur. This hybrid state allows simple actions such as orienting within the room, but more complex performances such as recognizing another person are not possible. The event is generally not recalled, in particular when the person falls asleep again.

Because of the subjectively perceived severe panic, hazardous actions may sometimes occur. The author knows of a case in which a patient jumped out of the window in the context of an episode (fortunately only from the low height of a first floor into the front garden) because he thought his apartment was on fire. There are reports about two other patients who choked their partners because they erroneously considered them as attackers. These examples make clear that even a low incidence of pavor nocturnus episodes, for example, once per month, may justify treatment.

7.1.5 Diagnostics

In the context of diagnosing pavor nocturnus, a comprehensive *sleep history* is very important. One question is clarifying if other sleep disorders might induce the episodes. It is not always easy to distinguish pavor nocturnus from other parasomnias, for example, nightmares or REM sleep behavior disorders. In addition to asking the patients themselves, reports by their partners may be required because the affected persons often do not recall the nocturnal events.

First, it is important to ask about the typical time of night terror attack. In contrast to nightmares, the occurrence about 1 h after sleep onset is characteristic for pavor nocturnus. It is also relevant to know which behavior patterns are observed at night (screaming, subsequent sleepwalking). In addition, it is interesting to know if damage or injury had occurred in the context of the episodes and if the person awakening from such an episode may recall a vivid dream.

Practical Tip

According to the distribution of the sleep stages over the night, disorders of arousal (pavor nocturnus, sleepwalking) typically occur in the first half of the night, whereas REM-related parasomnias (in particular nightmares) are found mainly in the second half. This fact is relevant in the context of differential diagnostics.

The maximum *incidence of episodes* per night provides further important diagnostic hints. Even if single patients have been observed to have several sleep terror episodes per night, ten episodes or more indicate a possible epilepsy (see ▶ Sect. 7.1.7). So, it should be asked if epileptic seizures have already occurred during the daytime. In this context, it must be considered that some epilepsies are characterized by the fact that they are observed exclusively at night. Therefore, history taking alone cannot definitely exclude epilepsy. If simple, stereotype behaviors are observed with always the same procedure, epilepsy might be the correct diagnosis.

The question of restorative sleep may provide important hints. If recovery is impaired, questions about symptoms of sleep-related disorders (snoring, etc.) and restless legs disorder (mostly associated with periodic limb movements during sleep) should be asked, and if needed further examination should be induced (see ▶ Chaps. 4 and 8).

Diagnostic Criteria of Pavor Nocturnus, According to the AASM

First, all diagnostic criteria of disorders of arousal have to be fulfilled.

- Recurrent episodes with incomplete awaking from sleep (mostly during the first third of night sleep).
- Inappropriate or missing response to efforts of other people who want to intervene or lead the person experiencing the episode into another direction. The affected person may appear disoriented or confused, even several minutes afterward.
- Limited experience (e.g., one single visual scene) or no thoughts or dream images in the context of the episode.
- Partly or complete amnesia regarding the episode.
- The disorder cannot be better explained by any other sleep disorder, mental disorders, medical conditions, neurological diseases, psychological diseases, or drug intake or substance abuse.

In addition, there are specific criteria for pavor nocturnus.

- The disorder meets all criteria for disorders of arousal (see foregoing list).
- The episodes are characterized by sudden panic typically with alarming vocalizations such as a cry of fear.
- Intensive fear and heightened autonomous activity are seen that consists of mydriasis, tachycardia, rapid breathing, and sweating.

7.1.6 Sleep Diagnostics

Because one important differential diagnosis of pavor nocturnus is epileptic seizures at night, examination in a *sleep laboratory* is recommended for all adult patients for two nights. In children, a sleep deprivation electroencephalogram (EEG) is performed in the morning only when epilepsy is strongly suspected (observation of stereotype movements). However, it must be taken into account that severe pavor nocturnus episodes occur more rarely in a sleep lab than at home because of the unfamiliar environment (presence of medical staff; unfamiliar sleeping conditions that may lead to lighter sleep).

7

However, behavioral patterns may be observed such as sitting up in bed, picking at the blanket, or similar actions. To evaluate the nocturnal behaviors, continuous video monitoring and recording of the video signal are obligatory. For differential diagnostics, it applies that movements during pavor nocturnus are less stereotype and repetitive compared to nocturnal epileptic seizures. When cardiorespiratory *polysomnography* (PSG, in combination with video recording and history taking) does not allow the clear diagnosis of pavor nocturnus, *long-term epilepsy diagnostics* are recommended for at least 24 h (i.e., including one day and one night) with at least 12 electrodes placed on the patient's scalp. Sometimes it makes sense to perform the measurements after sleep deprivation.

To distinguish pavor nocturnus from REM sleep behavior disorders, it must be documented in the sleep lab from which sleep stage the behavior patterns occur. In this context it is optimal to have a *polysomnographic machine* that records the EEG and other channels synchronized to the video. Intact suppression of the muscle tone during REM sleep also contradicts REM sleep behavior disorder.

Because other sleep disorders such as sleep-related breathing disorders, as already mentioned, may trigger pavor nocturnus episodes, history taking is recommended with subsequent device-assisted diagnostics if relevant symptoms are found (see ▶ Chap. 4).

7.1.7 Differential Diagnostics

In practice it is not easy to distinguish pavor nocturnus from *other parasomnias* because several studies demonstrate that parasomnias, in particular pavor nocturnus, sleepwalking, and nightmares, frequently co-occur. Thus, in the context of comprehensive history taking and sleep lab examinations, it is not the question of either/or but of diagnosing all types of parasomnia that may be present.

Another differential diagnosis from the field of parasomnias is the *REM sleep behavior disorder*. In nearly all cases, sleep lab diagnostics is able to provide clear evidence (non-REM sleep associated versus REM sleep associated) due to the heightened muscle tone in REM sleep behavior disorder, especially when the patient's history does not allow drawing clear conclusions on the time of pavor nocturnus occurrence (typically at the beginning of the night sleep).

Furthermore, nocturnal *epileptic seizures* must be distinguished. Based on the history (number of the episodes per night), PSG, and video recordings (stereotype, repetitive movements), generally epilepsy can be excluded with high probability so that comprehensive examination with the entire set of EEG electrodes is required only in exceptional cases.

7.1.8 Therapy

Even if adults experience pavor nocturnus with low frequency of only one to two events per month, therapeutic intervention might be indicated because the episodes are perceived as very distressing by many people and their partners, and also as embarrassing when the individuals have to sleep somewhere else. If children suffer (or also the parents as a consquence of caring for the child) from pavor nocturnus, information given to the parents is of high significance because they consider the nocturnal events (severe physiological fear reaction, unresponsiveness) as much more dramatic than does the child, who usually cannot recall the episode in the morning.

Because imagery rehearsal therapy that is very effective in cases of nightmares (see ▶ Sect. 7.3.8) cannot be applied to pavor nocturnus, an exact diagnostic differentiation is crucial. However, this is not always easy because these disorders may co-occur.

Therapeutic Steps in Cases of Pavor Nocturnus

- Information
- Create a safe sleep environment
- Information about the handling of pavor nocturnus episodes by bed partners or parents
- Sleep hygiene
- Relaxation exercises before going to bed
- Psychotherapeutic measures

First of all, the adults should be informed about the symtomatology and etiology of the disorder. Often they are very worried because they do something at nighttime they cannot control. These concerns are much more important in adults than in children because adults typically do not sleep in such a well-protected environment. Most patients, or the parents in cases of affected children, are already reassured when they know that pavor nocturnus is a disorder itself and not a symptom of a major psychiatric disease. That these extraordinary nocturnal activities can be described by a specific term and are known to specialists often implies some form of relief.

The descriptive explanation of the *diathesis stress model* also helps in particular when it is emphasized that normal daily stress may lead to pavor nocturnus in persons with a predisposition. Parents can be reassured because they often think that something went wrong in their upbringing. Also the influence of organic factors such as fever, sleep deprivation, or alcohol should be mentioned because many patients have already observed this correlation.

The proverbial *somnambulistic confidence*, however, is a myth. Many adults suffering from pavor nocturnus or sleepwalking have already experienced injury. Nonetheless, injuries to children are only very rarely reported. On the one hand, the brain is not fully functional, and in the dark the people cannot see everything even if their eyes are open. If the individual tends to leave the apartment, it is usually sufficient to lock the door and to put the key somewhere else. During the sleepwalking that often occurs after pavor nocturnus, patients are generally not able to perform complex searching activities (see ▶ Sect. 7.2).

It also appears to be useful to inform the people around the affected person about the occurrence of pavor nocturnus episodes. In this way, embarrassing situations at night may be avoided, and that knowledge that there is someone that could help (calming the person, guiding him/her back to bed) might already reduce the probability of pavor nocturnus episodes with loud screaming and walking around.

Another important factor concerns *sleep hygiene* when dealing with pavor nocturnus. Because pavor nocturnus is linked to slow wave sleep, a slow wave sleep rebound (caused by previous sleep deprivation) leads to an increased probability of occurrence. Regular bedtimes are recommended for those patients, and spending sleepless nights is discouraged. Furthermore, only moderate alcohol consumption, or even abstinence from alcohol, is recommended. One patient from the author's own practice reported increased pavor nocturnus episodes in the second and third night after alcohol consumption; in this context it was probably also triggered via a slow wave sleep rebound.

Practical Tip

If a child or an adult wakes up all of a sudden and sits upright in bed or walks around, it is recommended to talk quietly and calmingly to the person and to guide him/her back to the bed.

Excepting emergency cases that represent a risk for the affected person, serious attempts to awaken the person should be avoided because this might even reinforce the fear. Generally the individual is not able to recognize the helper, which means that the close person may be considered strange or menacing.

In accordance with the diathesis stress model, it is important to *reduce stress*. Adults are recommended to learn *relaxation techniques*, for example, autogenic training or progressive muscle relaxation according to Jacobson.

Especially in the context of autogenic training, it is important that the exercises are performed in a sitting position before going to bed to achieve the full effect of relaxation. Otherwise, the patient risks falling asleep before the end of the exercise. Regular exercises result in a reduction of the impact of normal daily stress on sleep. In this way the frequency of pavor nocturnus episodes can be significantly reduced. Even for children as young as 6 years in age, relaxation techniques are available that are based on autogenic training.

In cases in which those approaches cannot be successfully applied, *cognitive behavioral therapy* is recommended in particular for adults. The aim is developing coping strategies for stressful situations including associated thoughts and emotions. Furthermore, specific strategies are taught about coping with stress situations. Although positive outcomes could be achieved by means of psychotherapeutic therapy of pavor nocturnus, controlled trials are not yet available.

The data base with regard to *drug therapy* of pavor nocturnus is also unsatisfactory. Even if positive effects could be shown in single cases with the application of benzodiazepines (clonazepam, diazepam) or antidepressants such as imipramine and paroxetine, randomized placebo-controlled trials are completely lacking. Only in extreme cases with several pavor nocturnus episodes per night does a long-term medication seem to be appropriate.

7.2 Sleepwalking

7.2.1 Definitions

Sleepwalking is an activity that a person performs at night out of non-REM sleep stage 2 or slow wave sleep without being fully awake. After about 30% or 50% of pavor nocturnus episodes (see ▶ Sect. 7.1), sleepwalking may occur; the two disorders are etiologically closely related.

Many of these activities termed sleepwalking take place in bed. If the person actually leaves the bed, mostly well-automatized activities are performed. The person's eyes are open; however, he/she is not in full possession of his/her mental power and usually cannot recall the episode when subsequently returning to bed and continuing to sleep.

7.2.2 Etiology and Pathophysiology

Sleepwalking and pavor nocturnus are closely related and are termed disorders of arousal. It is assumed that an awakening stimulus (from the outside or the inside) does not lead to complete awakening but the brain remains in an intermediate state between wakefulness and sleep. That is to say, parts of the brain are awake and other parts are asleep, which may explain the loss of memory of the nocturnal event in the morning, as well as the impaired responsiveness and the activities that sometimes appear rather meaningless.

Formerly, the *gravity force of the moon* was considered responsible for sleepwalking. Many pictures exist showing so-called lunatics who walk in the direction of the moon. From a current point of view, the explanation is rather simple. The sleepwalking person who has his/her eyes open just walks in the direction of the greatest brightness to see better.

Furthermore, the opinion once prevailed that the person was *acting out dreams* during sleepwalking. This explanation could also be disproved as it is well known today that the muscle tone is actively inhibited by the sleep centers during REM sleep (when intensive dreaming takes place) to impede this kind of acting out. Sleepwalking occurs from non-REM sleep, that is, of sleep phases without active inhibition of the skeletal muscles. However, reports are available where projects, for example, a task that has not been finished in the evening before, were accomplished during an episode of sleepwalking, suggesting that sleepwalking is also associated with subjective experiences. This explanation seems plausible because in non-REM sleep dreaming also takes place that is mostly less intensive or pictorial. In the context of REM sleep behavior disorder, which is the most important differential diagnosis of sleepwalking, however, exactly this acting out of dreams occurs (see ▶ Sect. 7.4). The most significant difference is that the person suffering from REM sleep behavior disorder mainly follows dream images, whereas the sleepwalker perceives the environment (in a limited way) and associates it with their own concepts and ideas, for example, of doing something.

The current status regarding the etiology of sleepwalking is a *diathesis stress model*. As in other parasomnias (pavor nocturnus, nightmares), an increased family incidence is observed. Normal stressors such as school enrolment of children, spending the night elsewhere, and occupational stress or stress at home may increase the incidence of sleepwalking episodes. Also, physiological stressors such as fever, previous sleep deprivation, or significant alcohol consumption may trigger sleepwalking. Furthermore, a sleep disorder may lead to a fragmented sleep profile (sleep apnea syndrome, periodic limb movements during sleep) that may increase the incidence of sleepwalking. Environmental noise that would cause other people to awaken might induce episodes of sleepwalking in affected individuals.

7.2.3 Epidemiology

About 30% of all children have sleepwalked at least once in their lives. The occurrence peak, comparable to pavor nocturnus, is between the ages of 4 and 7 years.

In adults, the prevalence of sleepwalking is estimated to be less than 1%. The burden of adult patients, however, may also be clinically relevant when the incidence of sleepwalking episodes is rather low (about once or twice per month). Adults experience those episodes as very embarrassing when they perform activities during the night that they cannot control and cannot recall in the morning. Marked fear arises when the person wants to sleep elsewhere, not in the familiar home setting.

7.2.4 Clinical Presentation

Sleepwalking episodes typically last for some seconds up to several minutes, rarely longer. Mostly, the activities occur in the middle and/or at the end of the night. In practice, cases have also been described wherein sleepwalking has occurred in the first half of the night.

Many of these activities take place in bed, for example, sitting up and looking around, pulling at the blanket, or examining the wall near the bed. If the person leaves the bed, mostly well-automatized activities are performed, for example, dressing, walking into another room, or opening the windows. The person's eyes are open, and simple visual-motor coordination works well; however, the individual is not in full possession of their mental powers and usually cannot recall the event when returning to bed and continuing to sleep. The responsiveness to external stimuli, as in addressing the person, is reduced.

Frequently, the person who addresses the sleepwalker is not recognized so that sometimes violent counterreactions (beating, etc.) may be observed. In the US, one patient who was assessed by a portable monitoring unit had driven his car during a sleepwalking episode. The situation becomes dangerous when the person leaves her or his home.

Amnesia for sleepwalking is very often observed; sometimes single dream-like memories are reported, and the persons have a sensation in the morning that something might have happened at night.

For the discipline of forensics, the topic of sleepwalking is of great interest because every now and again people claim that they have committed a crime in a state of sleepwalking. The German law includes a paragraph that states that a person cannot be guilty when unable during the commission of an act to understand the criminal character of this act because of a pathological mental disorder, deeply disturbed consciousness, mental deficiency, or any other severe mental disorder. In such a context, independent experts face the difficulty of determining whether the person was sleepwalking at the time of committing the crime, as no EEG electrodes have been attached that might confirm the state of sleepwalking; and so it is only possible in individual cases to judge based on the person's history, on polysomnographies performed in the further course (if needed with awakening provocations), and on the action itself.

Case Reports

One patient reported that he wanted to go to the toilet. He opened the door, urinated, and went back to bed. The next morning, however, he found that it wasn't the toilet that he had been using during the sleepwalking episode but his wardrobe.

One patient reported that she had woken up from a sleepwalking episode when she was already in the kitchen and wanted to prepare a sandwich. She was very scared because she was holding a sharp bread knife in her hands, and for this reason she sought advice at the sleep clinic.

In contradiction to the proverbial somnambulistic certainty, sometimes injuries occur. Another patient reported fracturing his ankle after a sleepwalking episode during which he caught his foot on a shelf (even if the eyes are open, it might be difficult to orient oneself when the room is dark).

Another patient reported massive bruises that had developed when she tried to open the skylight of her bedroom.

7.2.5 Diagnostics

Regarding the diagnostics of sleepwalking, comprehensive *case history taking including bedpartner/relatives* is essential. On one hand it should be assessed exactly at what time of night the sleepwalking episodes occur and if they are observed as being caused by current stressors. On the other hand, it is essential to clarify if the person responds and if amnesia regarding the nocturnal events is observed. A detailed description of which behaviors and actions are performed may provide relevant information to distinguish sleepwalking from epileptic seizures. In the same way, questions should be asked about intensive dream experience at the beginning and during sleepwalking episodes so that a differentiation from REM sleep behavior disorder is possible.

Diagnostic Criteria of Sleepwalking According to the AASM

First, all diagnostic criteria of disorders of arousal have to be met.

- Recurrent episodes with incomplete awaking from sleep.
- Inappropriate or lacking responsiveness toward efforts of other people to intervene or to guide the person experiencing the episode to another direction. The affected person may be disoriented and confused even several minutes after the event.
- Limited experiences of (e.g., single visual scenes) or no ideas or dream images in relation to the episode.
- Part or complete amnesia for the episode.
- The disorder cannot be explained by any other sleep disorder, mental disorders, medical conditions, neurological disease, psychological disease, or drug intake or substance abuse.

In addition, there are the specific criteria of sleepwalking.

- The disorder meets all criteria of disorders of arousal.
- The episodes are characterized by walking around or other complex behaviors that are performed outside the bed.

7.2.6 Sleep Diagnostics

To complete history taking, generally an *examination in a sleep lab* over two nights is recommended because some disorders may be confounded with sleepwalking.

Because of the "well-protected" sleep environment, severe sleepwalking episodes with leaving the bed only rarely occur in sleep labs, but behaviors such as sitting up in bed, pulling up the blankets, or other actions like looking around may be observed. If typical polysomnography equipment is used (no telemetry system but electrode wires that are firmly connected with the device), attention must be paid that the staff attentively monitors the patient to quickly awaken him/her when he/she starts to leave the bed. In those cases, awakening is not only done to avoid tearing off the electrodes but also to conduct an interview with the patients to assess if the person is easily oriented and knows where he/she actually is. At the same time, video monitoring that is synchronized with the EEG is essential.

Sleep lab diagnostics also serve to exclude other sleep disorders such as sleep-related breathing disorders or periodic limb movements during sleep as the origin or at least a triggering factor of sleepwalking.

7.2.7 Differential Diagnostics

The most important differential diagnosis that has to be taken into consideration is *REM sleep behavior disorder*. It is not always easy to differentiate these disorders if based only on the history of the affected person, so in adults comprehensive diagnostics in a sleep lab are nearly always indicated. Generally, it becomes obvious that the person with a REM sleep behavior disorder rapidly bumps into an obstacle because he/she has a dream vision, whereas the sleepwalker recognizes the environment and walks around almost safely (attention: limited sight in the dark). If the person awakens the sleepwalker is not able to report about the episode with the exception of single images, whereas generally a vivid dream is reported by persons with REM sleep behavior disorder, mostly with strong emotions and/or marked body movements as part of the dream action.

Another differential diagnosis of sleepwalking (such as pavor nocturnus) is the occurrence of nocturnal *epileptic seizures*. Generally, the movements in cases of epileptic seizures are stereotypic and may be observed frequently in one night (ten times or even more often). Because the epileptic event is not always visible in scalp EEG in the context of focal seizures, video documentation is of highest significance in these patients.

In older people, nocturnal *states of confusion*, for example, in the context of dementia or hypnotics consumption (benzodiazepines), may be confounded with sleepwalking. In the sleep history taking in elderly people, the assessment of medications and the question about possible dementia symptoms must not be forgotten.

In recent times, also *sleep-related eating disorder* came into the focus of discussion. It is partly different from sleepwalking. Some of the patients perform this kind of eating in a somnambulistic way, being not fully awake. Another group of patients with sleep-related eating disorder generally completely wake up, can recall the nocturnal event, and are only able to fall asleep again when they have eaten a snack (biscuits, bread, etc.). Similar to insomnia, it is the question of conditioning processes (eating has a calming effect and promotes falling asleep).

Another disorder that can be categorized to sleepwalking is the so-called sexsomnia, that is, the sleepwalking person performs sexual actions on himself or herself or harasses the bed partner. This behavior is very embarrassing for the affected persons because they cannot control it, and additionally, it might enormously stress the relationship.

7.2.8 Therapy

Because pavor nocturnus and sleepwalking are etiologically closely related, the treatment strategies are also very similar. In the context of adult sleepwalking, consultation/treatment is also indicated when the episodes of sleepwalking occur rarely or only under stress because the affected persons feel extremely embarrassed. Furthermore, there is the risk of injury of the sleepwalker. For children who sleepwalk frequently, it is recommended to initiate further therapeutic interventions in addition to comprehensive information about the disorder given to the parents.

Therapeutic Steps in the Context of Sleepwalking

- Information
- Securing of environment
- Information of bedpartner/relatives about how to handle sleepwalking episodes
- Sleep hygiene rules
- Relaxation exercises before going to bed
- Intentional formulas
- Psychotherapeutic interventions

First of all, the affected adults or parents of affected children should be *informed* about the disorder. Adults especially are very worried about doing something at night they cannot control. Most patients are reassured when they learn that sleepwalking (and pavor nocturnus, if they occur together) is an independent disorder and not the symptom of an underlying psychiatric disease. The fact that those extraordinary nocturnal activities have a specific definition and are known to specialists may already lead to relief. The descriptive explanation of the diathesis stress model helps affected persons in particular when it is emphasized that already normal stress may lead to sleepwalking in persons with the predisposition for sleepwalking.

Securing the environment is very important because the proverbial somnambulistic security is a myth. Many adults suffering from sleepwalking (and/or pavor nocturnus) have already experienced injury.

If the person tends to leave the home, it is usually sufficient to lock the door and to store the key in a remote location because the person is not able to perform complex searching actions during sleepwalking. Also, windows and doors to "dangerous" rooms (kitchen, crafts room, boiler room) may be secured in this way. Sharp-edged furniture or objects that may potentially lead to injury should be removed from the bedroom.

The people around the affected person should also be *informed*. In this way, embarrassing scenarios at night may be avoided because those persons know that it is most appropriate coping strategy to calmly address the patient and to guide him/her back to bed. Waking the person up is only recommended when the person endangers himself/herself or others. The knowledge that the sleepwalking person does not fully access the mental abilities is important to understand why, for example, familiar persons are not recognized at night and, as already mentioned, why somnambulistic activities sometimes seem to be bizarre.

It is important when managing sleepwalking as well as pavor nocturnus to observe *sleep hygiene*. Regular bedtimes and avoiding sleep deficits are recommended. Only moderate alcohol consumption, or even abstinence, is advised. A short nap during daytime may decrease the sleep pressure of the following night and in this way reduce the probability for sleepwalking episodes.

With regard to the diathesis stress model, it is important to *reduce stress*. For adults, it is recommended to learn relaxation techniques, for example, autogenic training or progressive muscle relaxation, according to Jacobson. Autogenic training should be exercised in a sitting position to avoid the patient falling asleep before the end of the exercise. The training objective, that is, relaxed sleep, would not be achieved otherwise. By regular exercising, the body learns to start sleeping in a more relaxed way and to reduce the impact of daily stress on sleep. The incidence of sleepwalking can be significantly reduced in this way. Child-appropriate relaxation techniques may also be very helpful for children at about 6 years or older (see ▶ Sect. 7.1.8).

In the context of autogenic training, a technique is available that has already shown effects in single cases: training of *intentional formulas*. Hereby, the affected individual imagines a sentence after the instructions of the relaxation procedure, for example, "When my feet touch the ground, I will fully wake up." This internally spoken sentence is then also supported by vivid imagination. In this way, the body is trained with regard to new behavioral patterns in waking that may terminate sleepwalking at night. However, only a few anecdotal reports are available for the effectiveness of this approach.

Only in cases wherein these approaches are not successful is further *cognitive behavioral therapy* recommended, particularly for adults. Such therapy aims at coping with stress situations and the associated negative thoughts and emotions as well as learning basic strategies to cope with stressful situations.

Data for *drug therapy* are unsatisfactory. Even if the administration of benzodiazepines (clonazepam, diazepam, tricyclic antidepressants) shows positive effects in single cases, evidence-based recommendations are completely lacking. Long-term medication seems to be useful only in exceptional cases.

7.3 Nightmares

7.3.1 Definitions

Nightmares are strongly negative dreams that lead to awakening in most cases. They are distinguished from distressing dreams or anxiety dreams that also show negative emotions but do not directly lead to waking up.

For the dreamer, this difference (being woken up by the dream or not) is not always easy to recognize. Regarding some dream contents, for example, falling dreams, it seems to be obvious because the person wakes up directly before hitting the ground. In more complex dreams (persecution, death of closely related persons), however, it is more difficult to distinguish if awakening occurred independently from the dream action or was induced by the strong emotions that occurred in the dream. Therefore, the diagnostic criteria (see ▶ Sect. 7.3.5) focus more on the stress caused by nightmares than on awakening criterion.

7.3.2 Etiology and Pathophysiology

In the nineteenth century, the assumption prevailed that dyspnea or heavy meals are responsible for nightmares, but today the etiology is based on a *diathesis stress model.*

Factors in Nightmare Etiology

- Genetic factors
- Personality dimension, so-called thin boundaries
- Neuroticism, anxiety
- Stress
- Trauma
- Medication
- Maintaining factors (cognitive avoidance)

A large Finnish twin study confirms a genetic influence for the occurrence of frequent nightmares in adults. Further genetic studies (genome-wide association studies, GWAS) are currently not available.

Also, the findings published by Ernest Hartmann can be categorized into the field of predisposition. He described a personality type with so-called *thin boundaries* in people suffering from frequent nightmares. Persons with thin boundaries have difficulties in distancing from external stimuli; they have extraordinary sensual experiences and intensive and conflictual relationships, but they are also very creative and emphatic.

The correlation with *anxiety* and *neuroticism* (emotional instability) seems to be apparent because the continuity hypothesis of dreaming predicts that waking life is reflected in dreams. Anxiety events and experiencing other negative emotions during daytime lead to more nightmares. This correlation corresponds to the observation that *stress* (occupational or partnership) leads to a significant increase nightmare frequency.

Experiencing a *trauma* such as sexual abuse, war events, violence, or a car accident with severe injuries may lead to the full symptomatology of a posttraumatic stress disorder. In this context, trauma-related nightmares represent one of the key symptoms. However, the frequency of nightmares is also increased in people who do not fully develop posttraumatic stress disorder. These nightmares may contain non-trauma-related dreams as well as trauma-related content (or both).

Another possible origin for nightmares is a *medication* such as L-DOPA (medication for Parkinson's disease), serotonin reuptake inhibitors (antidepressants), donepezil (medication for dementia), and some blood pressure agents.

The etiology of nightmares is based on an interaction of predisposition and current stressors. Especially with regard to the treatment, however, it is important to consider another factor that might perpetuate the disorder: *avoidance*. In many nightmares, anxiety plays a major role, for example, in dreams of being chased in which the dream-self runs away, that is, avoids confrontation. From research on anxiety disorders, for example, arachnophobia, it is well known that the wish to avoid fear contributes to preserving the fear or even aggravates it because a fear of the anxiety develops. Only the confrontation and coping with fears can lead to long-term improvement. In cases of nightmares, this avoidance strategy is often applied, for example, when using the sentence, "It was only a dream." Many people try to forget distressing dreams as quickly as possible. However, in this case no active coping with the anxiety takes place, and reoccurrence of nightmares is very likely.

7.3.3 Epidemiology

Nightmares are a phenomenon that nearly everybody experiences in childhood or adolescence. Nightmares peak between the 6th and 10th year of life. About 5% of all children have nightmares at least once per week or more frequently. Even if nightmares occur more frequently in children, studies show that about 5% of adults also report distressing nightmares, i.e., a nightmare disorder. Women are more frequently affected than men. According to cross-sectional studies, frequency of nightmares decreases with age, so that young adults report nightmares more often than older people.

7.3.4 Clinical Presentation

In practice, three phenomena that are associated with nocturnal awakenings associated fear can be distinguished (▫ Table 7.1).

Table 7.1 Different types of awakenings related to fear

Characteristics	Pavor nocturnus	Nightmares	Posttraumatic re-enactments
Time of waking up	Mostly in the first half of the night	Mainly in the second half of the night	Both
Sleep stage	Slow wave sleep	REM sleep	REM and non-REM sleep
Physiological fear reaction	Very strong	Moderate	Strong to very strong
Dream content	Almost no content, single images	Detailed dream	Relatively direct replay of the trauma
Awareness after waking up	Almost no orientation, impaired responsiveness	Often fully oriented; fear of the dream may persist	Often fully oriented, strong aftereffect
Recall in the morning	Rare recall of the event	Good dream recall	Good dream recall

In the context of pavor nocturnus (see ► Sect. 7.1), that is, in sudden awakening from slow wave sleep, the person is barely oriented and cannot recall the event. Nightmares, however, can be *well recalled* because the patient awakens from a very emotional dream.

The typical *contents* of nightmares in children and adolescents are the following:

- Being chased (50%)
- Own death or injury (20%)
- Death or injury of others (15%)
- Falling into bottomless space (10%)

Although detailed studies on the content of nightmares in adults are scarce, the predominating topics encompass falling, being chased, being paralyzed, being late, and the death of close persons.

Nightmares occur mainly in the second half of the night because at that time the REM sleep phases are longer and the dreams are more intensive than at the beginning of the night.

In comparison to pavor nocturnus, the vegetative *fear reaction* is moderate. Especially in children, the fear that arose during the dream may persist after awakening although the children are generally fully oriented after awakening. This fear may make it difficult for them to reinitiate sleep after the nightmare.

So-called posttraumatic re-enactments should be distinguished from nightmares. The dream contents are very close to experienced trauma (war events, sexual abuse, natural catastrophes, etc.) and may occur at any time during the night independently of the sleep stage. Posttraumatic re-enactments can be compared to flashbacks, that is, trauma-related intrusions that occur during the daytime.

Practical Tip

Nightmares - as typical REM parasomnia - occur more frequently in the second half of the night, whereas the disorders of arousal pavor nocturnus and sleepwalking occur during slow wave sleep, which means that the events mainly occur in the first half of the night. After awakening from a nightmare, the affected person is usually rapidly oriented and recalls the dream content well. In the context of pavor nocturnus or sleepwalking, the person, if awakened, is barely oriented, and the event is hardly recalled.

7.3.5 Diagnostics

Comprehensive *sleep anamnesis* is generally sufficient to diagnose nightmares if no further hints regarding the occurrence of other parasomnias (pavor nocturnus) and acting out of dreams (REM sleep behavior disorder) are mentioned (see ► Sect. 7.3.7). Regarding the etiology, the patient must be asked when nightmares started to occur (predisposition) and if stressors are currently present. Also, exact assessment of the current medications is essential to determine a possible correlation.

Diagnostic Criteria of Nightmare Disorder According to the AASM

A. Recurrence of extended extremely dysphoric, and well-recalled dreams that typically contain threats to survival, security, or physical integrity.
B. After awakening from a distressing dream, the affected person rapidly orients herself and becomes alert.
C. The dream experiences or the sleep interruption caused by nightmares causes clinically relevant distress or impairment in social, occupational, or other important areas of functioning. At least one of the following nightmare effects should be reported:
   - Mood disturbances (e.g., persistence of the nightmare emotion, anxiety, dysphoria)
   - Sleep resistance (e.g., fear of going to bed, fear of falling sleeping because then nightmares might occur)
   - Impaired cognitive performance (e.g., distracted by intrusive nightmare images, impaired concentration, impaired memory)
   - Negative effect on the caregiver or family (e.g., because of sleep disruptions at night)
   - Behavioral problems (e.g., avoiding going to bed, fear of darkness)
   - Daytime sleepiness
   - Fatigue, low energy
   - Impaired performance at work or problems at the place of education
   - Problems with social and interpersonal relationships

7.3.6 Sleep Diagnostics

Sleep diagnostics are usually not indicated for the diagnosis of nightmares. As already mentioned, it is not always easy to differentiate nightmares from other parasomnias (pavor nocturnus, REM sleep behavior disorders), so that in unclear cases sleep lab diagnostics might be appropriate.

However, clinical reports as well as empirical findings suggest that nightmares occur less often in the sleep laboratory than at home, which is again a reason to perform polysomnography only for differential diagnostic purposes. In particular, when posttraumatic nightmares occur, sleep examination should be performed in cases of possible sleep-related breathing disorders or periodic limb movements during sleep, because some studies reported that those two disorders occur more frequently in patients with posttraumatic stress disorder than in the normal population.

7.3.7 Differential Diagnostics

Nightmares must be distinguished from *pavor nocturnus*, which occurs predominantly in the first half of the night and is rarely recalled (Table 7.1). The differentiation is important not only from an etiological point of view but also regarding the treatment; the approach for nightmares described next is not effective for non-REM parasomnias such as pavor nocturnus.

Usually it is very simple to distinguish nocturnal *panic attacks* that may also develop from a nightmare, as the anxiety or panic reaches its peak only in wakefulness and is accompanied by panic-related thoughts (fear of death, etc.). Even if most patients suffering from panic disorders develop panic attacks during the daytime as well as at night, sometimes cases are reported in which patients only have panic attacks at night. Those persons should undergo cognitive behavioral therapy as the treatment of choice.

If the patient or the patient's bedpartner reports that severe acting out occurs in the context of nightmares, a *REM sleep behavior disorder* may be probable, and polysomnography (PSG) including video documentation should be initiated. In REM sleep behavior disorder, muscle tone during REM sleep does not decrease (see Sect. 7.4).

If nightmares occur regularly, in particular when they have replicative content, the differential diagnosis of *posttraumatic stress disorder* has to be considered. It is not always easy to differentiate these two disorders (nightmare disorder and posttraumatic stress disorder) because severe traumas do not always lead to the full picture of posttraumatic stress disorder. In those cases, nightmares may represent the most relevant after-effect of the trauma. The additional symptoms of posttraumatic stress disorder are:

- Occurrence of intrusions during daytime (thoughts, flashbacks)
- Consciously avoiding activities, places, and persons that might lead to recalling the trauma
- Limited spectrum of affect (e.g., inability to have tender feelings)
- Impression of a limited future

7

In many psychiatric and/or psychosomatic clinics specialized wards have been established for persons suffering from traumatic experiences. If such a clinical department is not available in the individual's area, the affected person may be referred to a psychiatrist or psychotherapist for further diagnostics and treatment.

The therapeutic approach (see ▶ Sect. 7.3.8) can be applied to idiopathic as well as posttraumatic nightmares. In posttraumatic stress disorder the nightmare intervention should be used as add-on to standard psychotherapeutic treatment.

7.3.8 Therapy

Nightmares require treatment when they occur once per week or even more often, especially when the disstress caused by nightmares becomes manifest in the form of fear of falling asleep or daytime functioning is impaired by nightmares, i.e., presence of a nightmare disorder.

Controlled trials are available on the effectiveness of *systematic desensitization* (within the context of behavioral therapy). The patient is confronted with the fear of the nightmare in his/her imagination (in wakefulness) after having learned relaxation procedures with increasing intensities. It is the objective of this intervention to imagine the fear of the nightmare without losing the physical sensation of relaxation.

The most effective and simplest method for treating nightmares was developed by Barry Krakow and colleagues and tested in many trials. The approach is termed *imagery rehearsal treatment* and consists of three steps.

- *Confrontation*: writing down the nightmare or drawing the dream situation.
- *Coping with the nightmare situation*: writing a new end of the dream or finalizing the drawing in such a way that fear is reduced.
- *Training of coping strategies*: the new "dream" is repeated in sensu once per day for about 5 to 10 min during the next 2 weeks.

With a rather low expenditure of one to two sessions that may be conducted in small groups, the therapeutic principle can be taught and practiced based on a recent nightmare. After the person has described the dream, he/she is invited to imagine a new end for this dream.

For children, drawing the most important dream picture is the method of choice. Then, the question is raised as to what the child may add to the picture so that he/she feels less afraid. For the therapist it is important not to make suggestions because the aim is to encourage and stimulate the child's potential to find solutions. Only when this coping strategy is not active or constructive should the child be asked to find other coping strategies for the nightmare situation. If the person suggests, for example, hiding or flying away, the person is asked if there are any other options because those avoiding behaviors like hiding and flying away only lead to short-term attenuation of the fear and the anxiety can reoccur (the pursuer is finally able to find the person or can also fly). Therefore, constructive approaches such as "looking the danger in the eye" or "asking somebody for help" are more effective in the long term.

Having developed a coping strategy for the nightmare situation, the affected individual is asked to write down the new "dream" and to go through it once per day for about 5 to 10 min during the next 2 weeks. In this context, the person should imagine the new behavior as concretely and vividly as possible; for example, not running away but confronting the threatening figure. If the nightmares still persist after 2 weeks, another dream can be chosen and worked on.

Interestingly, the clinical experience with this therapy shows that not only do the nightmares that have been selected for this intervention change but also dreams with other stressful content. It is plausible that the general principle of "facing a fearful situation is equated with searching for coping strategies" has been learned so that the dream-self is also more self-confident in other situations.

Case Report

A 22-year-old woman consulted the sleep clinic because of nightmares that had occurred almost every night for several months.

History taking also revealed singular pavor nocturnus attacks. The patient reported that she often did not sleep well in unfamiliar environments. Diagnostics performed in the sleep lab, however, were unremarkable except for low sleep efficiency. Nightmares or pavor nocturnus did not occur during the two nights in the sleep lab. A questionnaire indicated that the subjective quality of sleep and the feeling of being refreshed in the morning were only slightly reduced, but the patient suffered from a relevant increase in daytime tiredness. In the first session, the patient reported a current conflict in her core family that had led to a discontinuation of contact with her parents.

We explained the therapeutic principles of confrontation and coping with the nightmare situation and compared this treatment with the typically applied intervention for anxiety disorders and phobias. This was well understood by the patient.

During the nightmare the night before the consultation, the patient was in the changing room of a fitness center. First, the whole family was present; then her mother was in the foreground and insulted and criticized her. She felt completely helpless with regard to those accusations.

Being asked how she could change such a dream, the patient had several suggestions such as ignoring the mother's accusations but also being proactive by firmly stating her own needs. The new "dream" contained an active confrontation and the sentence: "I am very well able to handle my life."

In the next session 2 weeks later, the patient reported that she had regularly trained the "new" dream for 1 week. Although dreams containing her mother had not reoccurred since the first session, several other negative dreams had occurred, including a recurrent dream she has had for many years. The dreamer was sitting in her grandmother's kitchen. First the atmosphere was pleasant, but then she sensed a threat from outside, something threatening that might come into the house. Then the scene changed, and the dreamer was in a white room with friendly mythical creatures. Two of those creatures encouraged her to face the threat on her own. At about 5 AM, the patient awakened from the nightmare and still clearly felt the fear of the dream.

After a conversation about the elements of the dream (e.g., the relationship with her grandmother), the patient was again asked to imagine a new end of the dream. The patient imagined how she decided to face the threat with the support of the friendly mythical creatures.

In the final session another 2 weeks later, the patient reported that she had not had any nightmares and that the dreams she had recalled contained new behavioral patterns. Being confronted with other dream persons, the dreamer felt much more self-confident and was able to express her own needs. At the same time, she reported improvement of her daytime tiredness.

Despite the fact that the current stressor (problems with core family) did not change, the intervention was able to reduce the nightmares by strengthening the dream-self. The negative impact of the stress on dreaming and sleep was significantly reduced.

The team of Barry Krakow showed in several controlled trials that this simple treatment approach is effective in persons who had been suffering from nightmares for many years and who had undergone many different and unsuccessful psychotherapeutic or pharmacological treatment attempts. This treatment approach was also effective in a group of female patients who suffered from nightmares as a consequence of sexual assault. Because the therapeutic principle of confrontation and coping strategies is well understood by many patients, the imagery rehearsal method can be well implemented in sleep medical practice.

The effectiveness of these approaches based on cognitive behavioral therapy is well documented, whereas *medication* that suppresses REM sleep (e.g., tricyclic antidepressants) or benzodiazepines has been shown to be less effective for the treatment of nightmares. One exception are the positive effects of prazosin or similar substances such as doxazosin and terazosin on the frequency of posttraumatic nightmares that occur in the context of a posttraumatic stress disorder.

7.4 REM Sleep Behavior Disorder

7.4.1 Definitions

In REM sleep behavior disorder, dreams are acted out, mostly intensive dreams with marked body movements. Many movements occur in bed, but leaving the bed is also possible. The risk of injury is high because the person sees the dream situations in his/her mind and only barely recognizes the real sleep environment.

7.4.2 Etiology and Pathophysiology

The REM sleep behavior disorder is strongly linked to neurodegenerative diseases such as Parkinson's disease or dementia with Lewy bodies, which means that patients with REM sleep behavior disorder are likely to develop neurodegenerative disease 10 to 15 years later. Therefore, it is assumed that it is a particular course of a neurodegenerative disease showing the decline of muscle tone-inhibiting areas in the brainstem as the first symptom.

7.4.3 Epidemiology

The prevalence of this disorder is very low less than 1% of the overall population. Men at the age of 50 years or older are most frequently affected. In cases of Parkinson's disease, REM sleep behavior disorder occurs in at least one third of patients; in cases of other degenerative diseases such as multiple system atrophy, the percentage is even higher. Also, patients suffering from narcolepsy reveal an increased incidence of REM sleep behavior disorder. Nearly all patients with REM sleep behavior disorder develop a neurodegenerative disease in the further course (within 13 years on average).

7.4.4 Clinical Presentation

The following examples illustrate the problems that are associated with REM sleep behavior disorder.

Case Reports

A 67-year-old man reported the following dream: "I was playing football as halfback. And they all expected me to run forward. But there was this 140-kg opponent and according to the rules I tackled him with my shoulder. When I woke up, I stood in front of the chest of drawers and I had thrown everything, lamps, mirror, off the top, hit my head on the wall and my knees on the chest of drawers."

Another patient from our consultation reported about a dream in which his wife drove their car. During the trip she lost control, and the patient tried to regain control of the steering wheel by moving his arm to that direction. When he woke up, he had hit his wife, who was lying calmly beside him, in the face.

Dream-associated movements are explained by the loss of the muscle tone blockade that is active in healthy sleepers during REM sleep. Even though laboratory studies could show that minimal muscle potentials in the extremities may occur in accordance with the dream experience, the efferent neural signals of the motor cortex of the brainstem are strongly inhibited to avoid movements along with the dream images. In the 1960s and 1970s, the French sleep researcher Michel Jouvet studied cats during their sleep that had undergone surgery destroying the centers that are responsible for this inhibition. Those cats showed behaviors such as licking, hunting, and defending during REM sleep. i.e., they had artificially induced REM sleep behavior disorder.

The dream contents of those patients are often described as being aggressive or intensive (body movements). However, until now no studies have been available that examine normal dreams of those persons, that is, dreams that are not acted out. It seems obvious that dreams with intensive movements that are most likely to overcome the weakened muscle tone inhibition represent only the tip of the iceberg, whereas normal dreams can still be well inhibited and thus are not accompanied by extensive movements. Because awakenings due to acting out dream scenes or injuries does not occur in these cases, these normal dreams are not recalled.

7.4.5 Diagnostics

First of all, *history taking* must clarify if intensive dream contents are acted out by movements (see ▶ Sect. 7.4.4, case reports). This step is important to distinguish this phenomenon from sleepwalking, during which single thoughts and images are reported but no intensive dream experience is recalled.

Because REM sleep behavior disorder can occur in narcolepsy patients, narcoleptic symptoms (tendency to fall asleep, cataplexy, sleep paralyses) should be asked about in the interview, and if needed suitable diagnostics should be conducted (e.g., multiple sleep latency test).

For further diagnostics, it has to be clarified if REM sleep behavior disorder is part of an already manifest neurodegenerative disease such as Parkinson's disease, dementia with Lewy bodies, or multiple system atrophy.

A comprehensive *neurological examination* is required; regular follow-up in the further course of the disease should be performed by a specialized neurologist.

Diagnostic Criteria of REM Sleep Behavior Disorder According to the AASM

- Repetitive episodes of sleep-related vocalizations or complex motor behavior; these are linked to dream experiences occurring simultaneously so that this phenomenon is termed "acting out one's dreams."
- These behaviors occur during REM sleep documented by polysomnography or most probably occur during REM sleep based on the clinical history.
- The polysomnographic recording confirms the presence of REM sleep without atonia (according to the current version of the scoring manual of the American Association of Sleep Medicine).
- The disorder cannot be better explained by any other sleep disorder, mental disorder, or medication or substance abuse.

Annotations:
If the patient's history allows the most probable conclusion of REM sleep behavior disorder but the criteria of atonia during REM sleep (see ▶ Chap. 2) are only partly fulfilled, a preliminary diagnosis can be made. As medication may unmask an existing REM sleep behavior disorder, the diagnosis is generally also made when the REM sleep behavior disorder occurs in the context of medication.

7.4.6 Sleep-Related Diagnostics

In addition to history taking, an *examination in a sleep lab* must be performed over two nights because polysomnography is mandatory (documenting REM sleep atonia), as some disorders (see ▶ Sect. 7.4.7) may be confused with REM sleep behavior disorder. As with nightmares and non-REM parasomnias, the probability of measuring an active episode with acted-out dreams in the sleep lab is rather low, first because the incidence of acted-out dreams is also quite low in the home setting, and in the protected environment intensive dreams that are typically accompanied by movements (the tip of the iceberg) occur rarely.

Nevertheless, these patients show relevant characteristics in the PSG. The *muscle tone* (chin electromyogram (EMG)) is significantly increased during REM sleep (in healthy individuals, the minimum is reached during REM sleep). The minimal muscle tone during non-REM sleep serves as reference; thus, the disorder can be diagnosed with high certainty without actual acting out of a dream in the sleep lab.

In sleep diagnostics, special attention must be paid to the occurrence of *periodic limb movements during sleep* because they occur more frequently in patients with REM sleep behavior disorder compared to healthy sleepers. The extreme form of leg movements (with hitting and kicking the bed partner) in patients with periodic limb movements during sleep can be misinterpreted as possible REM sleep behavior disorder, so that in these cases the polysomnographic examination of the leg movements is important.

7.4.7 Differential Diagnostics

Sleepwalking has to be taken into consideration as an important differential diagnosis. Sleepwalking occurs out of non-REM sleep and can be differentiated by overnight polysomnography. Based on the anamnesis it might be sometimes difficult to differentiate, but generally the patients suffering from REM sleep behavior disorder are not able to walk around for a longer time like sleepwalkers but bump into things because they see dream images and are usually not aware of the actual environment in their bedrooms. Furthermore, good recall of dream images is characteristic of REM sleep behavior disorder.

7.4.8 Therapy

Some case reports are available showing that application of *melatonin* may improve the symptoms of REM sleep behavior disorder.

However, the most effective therapy consists of administering 0.5–2.0 mg *clonazepam*. Clinical experience shows that up to 90% of patients benefit from this treatment. The effect is mostly seen already in the first night: acting out of dreams disappears. Even after longer treatment periods, the drug tolerance for this benzodiazepine is generally not problematic. After several years, the effect of this medication can still be seen even if smaller movements during REM sleep may reappear after initial suppression.

7.5 Other Parasomnias

In this chapter, parasomnias are presented that are observed very rarely in sleep medicine.

7.5.1 Sleep Drunkenness

Sleep drunkenness is classified as non-REM parasomnia and also termed a disorder of arousal comparable to sleepwalking and pavor nocturnus. The diagnostic criteria of disorders of arousal are described in the context of pavor nocturnus (see ▶ Sect. 7.1.5) and sleepwalking (see ▶ Sect. 7.2.5). The person in these cases is dizzy and not fully oriented. Confused actions may even be performed.

Polysomnographic studies revealed that extreme sleep drunkenness is observed after awakening from slow wave sleep. For some persons it is particularly stressful because they have difficulties waking up in the morning. In our sleep medical clinic, a considerable number of individuals have presented who had overslept in the morning despite having set several alarms because they had not heard them or turned them off and continued sleeping. The solution was that they were woken up by another person in order to get to work on time.

The etiology of sleep drunkenness and difficulties of waking up is mostly unclear; treatment approaches are unknown.

7.5.2 Isolated Sleep Paralysis

Isolated sleep paralysis is defined by waking from REM sleep with complete paralysis of the voluntary movable muscles except the eye muscles. The episodes may last for several minutes. Frequently, bizarre perceptions are described in this condition, for example, a stranger standing beside the bed. The affected individuals are often in panic, in particular during first occurrence because of the complete paralysis. Sleep paralyses are mostly observed after waking up in the morning; in rare cases they are also reported during sleep onset.

Sleep paralysis may be a symptom of *narcolepsy* (see ▶ Sect. 5.1), so that patients who report frequent sleep paralysis episodes should undergo PSG evaluation. While taking the sleep history it should be asked if the extremities are really paralyzed because some patients confound extreme tiredness resulting in the difficulty to immediately getting up with this condition.

The incidence of persons who experience such sleep paralysis once in their lifetime is estimated to be as high as 40%. Repeated occurrences of this symptom outside the diagnosis of narcolepsy, however, are very rare (less than 0.1% in the general population).

In the course of the disorder, patients try to move one part of their body, such as an arm or leg, by concentrating on this movement to rapidly end the paralysis quicker. So far, the effectiveness of REM-suppressing antidepressants that are also applied for the treatment of REM sleep-related symptoms of narcolepsy has not been demonstrated.

7.5.3 Enuresis

Bedwetting (enuresis) is subdivided into two types:
- *Primary enuresis*: children who have never been successfully trained to control urination
- *Secondary enuresis*: children who have been dry for at least 6 months but revert to bedwetting

The incidence of enuresis is estimated to be about 5% in 10-year-old children. In adults, enuresis is extremely rare.

In the etiology, organic factors such as disorders of the bladder function or an underlying disease such as diabetes mellitus may be involved, and further diagnostics by a specialized urologist are recommended. In some cases, the development of a sleep apnea syndrome in childhood may cause enuresis, so that the clinical hints (see ► Sect. 11.1) should be followed up by a comprehensive sleep anamnesis (if needed, with polygrahic or polysomnographic evaluation of the nocturnal respiratory function).

In addition, psychosocial stressors (parents' divorce, birth of a sibling, abuse, neglect) may result in the development of bedwetting. In clinical practice, behavioral therapy has turned out to be effective, for example, positive feedback after dry nights and awaking schedules in which the affected child is awakened twice per night and taken to the toilet. Those awakenings are first applied after the first and second third of the night sleep and then successively pre- and postponed so that finally no more awakenings are required.

7.5.4 Sleep-Related Eating Disorders

Sleep-related eating disorders may manifest in different ways.

In cases of *night-eating syndrome*, patients consume at least 20% of their daily calories after dinner. This late food intake frequently causes problems with initiating sleep. The disorder, however, has not been investigated in detail and requires behavioral therapy.

In the context of *sleep-related eating disorder*, the difference is made between a condition comparable to sleepwalking in which the patients are not completely awake and only barely or not at all recall their nighttime activities and a second type in which where the patient completely wakes up but has the impression that he/she is only able to reinitiate sleep after eating (in most cases, a snack such as a biscuit or toast suffices).

In cases of eating during sleepwalking, some studies could show an association to the restless legs syndrome. For these patients, treatment with dopamine agonists such as pramipexole can be beneficial. Furthermore, clonazepam and topiramate have been successfully applied. Simple behavioral measures such as locking away all food does not seem to work appropriately according to clinical experience because the affected person may react very angrily if food is not available. In addition, the hypothesis has been developed that eating problems that occur during daytime reappear in the sleepwalking episodes. In these cases, therapeutic measures as described in ► Sect. 7.2.8, that is, physiological relaxation before going to bed, should be applied. If the patient is completely waking up and has problems of reinitiating sleep without eating something, this can be interpreted as learning processes that are also observed in the etiology of primary insomnia (see ► Chap. 3). Therefore, methods of behavioral therapy regarding sleep training are probably effective.

7.6 Questions

1. What is the difference between pavor nocturnus and nightmares?
2. What is the difference between sleepwalking and REM sleep behavior disorder?
3. Which are the most important treatment strategies of sleepwalking?
4. What must be taken into account in the further time course of REM sleep behavior disorder?

Further Reading

1. American Academy of Sleep Medicine. The international classification of sleep disorders. ICSD-3. Darien: American Academy of Sleep Medicine; 2014.
2. Schenck C. Paradox lost: midnight in the battleground of sleep and dreams: violent moving nightmares (REM sleep behavior disorder). Minneapolis: Extreme-Nights; 2005.

Sleep-Related Movement Disorders

H.-G. Weeß

B. A. Stuck et al., *Practice of Sleep Medicine*, https://doi.org/10.1007/978-3-030-17412-5_8

Several sleep-related movement disorders may cause insomnia complaints and daytime sleepiness; however, patients are not always aware of these disorders. They are characterized by simple, often stereotyped movements that can interfere with the restorative function of sleep by inducing vegetative and/or EEG arousals. The restless legs syndrome (RLS) is also grouped into the sleep-related movement disorders; not because of its clinical symptoms but due to its high association with periodic limb movements in sleep. Even if RLS is one of the most important neurological diseases and reduces the quality of life of patients considerably (even early retirement has been reported) it is often not recognized and/or correctly diagnosed.

The regulation of motor function during sleep is controlled by a complex neurochemical and neurophysiological mechanism that matures with childhood development. Thus, it is plausible that many sleep-associated motor disorders occur during childhood, and again with increasing age or in the context of neurological diseases (increasing chances of dysfunctioning) (▶ Chap. 11).

In this chapter, the most relevant sleep-related movement disorders occurring in adult patients are described. Nighttime epileptic seizures that are also associated with motor disorders during sleep are not included, but they are discussed in the context of possible differential diagnoses. The characteristics of sleep-related movement disorders in childhood are summarized in ▶ Sect. 11.1.

According to the ICSD-3, the following sleep-related movement disorders are differentiated:

- Restless legs syndrome
- Periodic limb movement disorder
- Sleep-related leg cramps
- Sleep-related bruxism
- Sleep-related rhythmic movement disorders
- Sleep-related myoclonus of infancy
- Propriospinal myoclonus at sleep onset
- Sleep-related movement disorder resulting from a medical disorder
- Sleep-related movement disorder caused by a medication or substance
- Sleep-related movement disorder, unspecified

8.1 Restless Legs Syndrome

8.1.1 Definition

The restless legs syndrome (RLS) is also called Ekbom syndrome, discomfort in the legs, or focal akathisia of the legs. Currently, American patient groups would welcome the use of Willis-Ekbom disease as the official term because they perceive "restless leg syndrome" as disparaging.

RLS is characterized by mostly circadian paresthesia (discomfort) in the lower, more rarely upper, extremities, associated with the urge to move, and sleep disorders. During sleep, periodic limb movements occur in about 80% of patients (▶ Sect. 8.2).

8.1.2 Etiology and Pathophysiology

The pathophysiology of RLS is still not fully understood. Dopamine, iron, and genetic predisposition seem to play a major role.

Recently, genome-wide association studies discovered *RLS genes*. Carriers of high-risk variations in these genes have an increased risk of developing RLS. Based on the function of the identified genes, RLS might be partly explained by an early development disorder of the central nervous system.

Iron deficiency also seems to be a crucial factor, at least in all secondary forms, because an increase of the iron reservoirs in the body reduces RLS complaints in patients with low iron values even if clinically no other symptoms of iron deficiency are observed. Investigations of the cerebrospinal fluid indicate a possible iron deficiency in the central nervous system. Postmortem studies in patients with early onset of RLS showed alterations in the substantia nigra. Reduced ferritin and reduced iron transportation in these areas are very likely.

The dysfunctional iron metabolism could subsequently interfere with the *dopamine system*. This hypothesis is supported by pharmacological studies as dopamine agonists reduce RLS symptoms whereas dopamine antagonists may enhance them. The positive effect of opiates on

RLS symptoms indicate that opioid systems in the central nervous system are also involved.

In secondary RLS, *hormone inbalances* or *renal failure* seems to be involved in addition to iron deficiency. Patients undergoing dialysis show a high risk of RLS. The co-occurrence with peripheral polyneuropathy indicates that a modified peripheral neural perception possibly induces the motor and sensor symptoms of RLS.

Drug-induced RLS as a side-effect can occur in dopamine antagonists, metoclopramide, atypical neuroleptics, antidepressants, and lithium. In particular, tricyclic antidepressants may induce RLS quite often but, for example, mirtazapine, a noradrenergic and specifically serotonergic antidepressant (NaSSA), can also trigger significant RLS complaints.

8.1.3 Epidemiology

Prevalence rates of RLS depend on methodological aspects of the studies and the severity criteria. The prevalence ranges between 1% and 15% in the general population. RLS seems more prevalent in European than in Asian populations. In Europe, and in particular in Germany, about 1.7% to 3% of the population report RLS that requires treatment. RLS symptomes typically start in the middle and older ages. About 10% of individuals between 65 and 83 years of age suffer from RLS and require therapy. Children might be affected by RLS, and there might be a differential diagnosis of attention-deficit/hyperactivity syndrome (ADHS) (▶ Chap. 11). Up to 15% of the general population show symptoms and complaints of RLS on and off; however, if the severity is mild to moderate, treatment is typically not indicated. Whereas several studies did not show gender differences, others indicate a 1.5- to 2-fold higher prevalence of RLS in women. In addition, the risk of developing RLS seems to increase with the number of pregnancies.

The percentage of *idiopathic* RLS ranges between 45% and 57%, depending on the study. In cases of idiopathic or primary RLS, an early onset is typically observed. In about 40% of patients with primary RLS, the first symptoms emerge before the age of 20. In cases of idiopathic RLS, more than 50% of patients have a positive family history. Prevalence among first-degree relatives of RLS patients increases three- to fivefold.

Secondary RLS, is often associated with the following factors:

- RLS symptoms occur in 15% to 40% of dialysis patients.
- Among pregnant women, 12% to 20% show temporary RLS, with remission after delivery.
- Of patients with rheumatoid arthritis, 30% report RLS.
- Among patients with iron deficiency, 25% report RLS. Thus, it must be taken into consideration that the low to normal values of these patients may also benefit from iron substitution.
- RLS is found in 20% to 25% of the patients with polyneuropathy even though the differentiation between these two entities is not easy.
- Twenty percent of patients with uremia suffer from RLS symptoms.
- RLS can also occur in rheumatoid and neurodegenerative diseases such as ataxia, multisystem atrophies, Parkinson's disease, diseases of the spinal cord (multiple sclerosis, syringomyelia, paraplegia, etc.), after stroke, folic acid deficiency/vitamin B_{12} deficiency, chronic obstructive pulmonary disease, and cancer.

8.1.4 Clinical Presentation

Patients complain about distressing *discomfort* (tingling, crawling, itching) in the lower legs, and more rarely the thighs or arms. In some cases, discomfort is also experienced over the entire body. Frequently, additional pain in the extremities is reported. Consequently, sleep onset or going back to sleep during the night may be disturbed. The symptoms occur in the evening, at rest, in a lying position, and sometimes during longer resting periods during daytime (e.g., in front of the TV, sitting in a car as passenger, in airplanes). Relief is often achieved by moving the legs, sometimes also by physical stimulation (rubbing, cold water). In bed, patients often stretch their legs out from under the blankets or get up at night to put cold water on their legs.

Case Report

"In the late afternoon, it is difficult for me to sit quietly because my legs are tingling. Meetings at work can become a torture. Watching a movie in the evening (TV) has not been possible for a long time. I always have to get up and walk around. Meeting friends or going to the cinema is also impossible. Later in bed, I am really tired, I want to sleep but my restless legs urge me to get up. At nighttime I walk around for hours, only walking provides relief for the uncomfortable pains and cramps in the lower legs."

In this or similar ways, RLS patients report their complaints emerging in resting phases during nigh-time or sometimes during daytime. For many affected people, the disturbed sleep rhythm with the associated consequences during the daytime, e.g., tiredness is distressful both for professional and family life.

8.1.5 Diagnostic Procedures

RLS is a clinical diagnosis that can generally be made based solely on the patient's history.

Diagnostic Criteria According to the International Restless Legs Study Group (IRLSSG)

- An urge to move the legs usually but not always accompanied by or felt to be caused by uncomfortable and unpleasant sensations in the legs.
- The urge to move the legs and any accompanying unpleasant sensations begin or worsen during periods of rest or inactivity such as lying down or sitting.
- The urge to move the legs and any accompanying unpleasant sensations are partially or totally relieved by movement, such as walking or stretching, at least as long as the activity continues.
- The urge to move the legs and any accompanying unpleasant sensations during rest or inactivity only occur or are worse in the evening or night than during the day.
- Nonessential criteria:
  - Positive family history: more than 50% of the patients with primary RLS have at least one first-degree relative suffering from RLS.
  - Response to L-DOPA test: 90% of the patients show an improvement application of small doses of L-DOPA (100 mg). A negative test, however, does not exclude RLS.
  - Periodic movements during sleep (PLMS) occur in about 80% of the patients, often associated with arousals.
  - Disorders initiating and maintaining sleep, daytime sleepiness, and impaired performance.
  - Neurological examinations often yield negative results in idiopathic RLS.

The clinical diagnosis may be complemented by using *questionnaires* measuring RLS symptoms (see ▶ Chap. 2). Questionnaires are also used to assess RLS severity in a standardized fashion.

Practical Tip

Sleep disorders such as insomnia due to RLS have to be actively elicited.

Drug and substance history is necessary to exclude substance-induced RLS. Special attention has to be paid to dopamine antagonistic compounds, e.g., classic and atypical neuroleptics, metoclopramide, tri- and tetracyclic antidepressants, and serotonin reuptake inhibitors. Among antidepressants, mirtazapine is considered to be a drug with RLS as a quite common side effect. Based on Stiasny-Kolster [7], paroxetine, sertraline, escitalopram, venlafaxine, duloxetine, fluoxetine, and citalopram may also cause RLS symptoms.

General *physical examination including laboratory parameters* (◻ Table 8.1) and bilateral nerve conduction studies (ENG) of the anterior tibialis nerve, if necessary also of the sural nerve and the median nerve, should be included in the basic diagnostic procedures (▶ Chap. 2).

The physical examination in primary RLS is often without specific findings. However, it is useful for identifying secondary RLS, to assess possible underlying diseases.

Table 8.1 Laboratory parameters for exclusion of secondary restless legs syndrome (RLS)

Group	Single parameter
Blood analysis	Full blood count (erythrocytes indices)
Iron metabolism	Serum iron, ferritin, transferrin
Vitamins	B_{12}, folic acid
Kidney values	Creatinine, urea
Glucose metabolism	Serum glucose, HbA1c if needed
Thyroid parameters	fT3, fT4, TSH
Parathyroid parameter	Parathormone (facultative)

8

The response to L-*DOPA* (L-DOPA test) is sometimes applied for diagnostic confirmation of RLS, in particular when a dopaminergic therapy had not yet been performed or the initial therapeutic effect of the dopaminergic therapy cannot be clearly evaluated. A single dose of 100 mg L-DOPA should be applied after the onset of RLS complaints; the response is then measured via severity scales; an improvement of 50% in the severity index is defined as responder. This test can confirm the diagnosis of RLS in about 90% of untreated patients. Not responding to the L-Dopa test (i.e., improvement of less than 50% with L-DOPA), however, does not exclude a possible RLS.

8.1.6 Sleep Diagnostics

Sleep diagnostic procedures should include a *sleep history* to rule out other disorders that may be associated with insomnia complaints. Sleep-related history taking also helps to assess impaired performance during daytime and the risk of daytime sleepiness in dangerous situations like driving a car or supervising heavy machinery.

A *sleep diary* may provide data about RLS severity and frequency. For assessing severity as well as for therapy evaluation, ambulatory measurement of periodic leg and arm movements during sleep in the home situation may be beneficial, for example, using *actigraphy*. In diagnostically unclear cases, an *immobilization test* (systematic assessment of the complaints during immobilization of the legs) and *polysomnography* (*PSG*) may provide further evidence regarding the presence of PLMS (periodic leg movements in sleep) (see ▶ Chap. 2).

Especially in the following cases of RLS, PSG is indicated (▶ Sect. 2.6.4):

- Cases with unclear diagnosis
- Children and adolescents with RLS
- Therapy-refractory RLS
- Persisting daytime sleepiness or sleep disorders under dopaminergic therapy (or other therapeutic options)
- Complex RLS needing pharmaceutical strategies including opiates, anticonvulsants, or other treatment approaches

PSG provides data about the severity of the sleep complaints and can exclude other sleep disorders that might be responsible for hypersomnia or insomnia symptoms. Typically, a fragmentary sleep profile with slow wave and REM sleep suppression and increased light sleep stages (N1) is a consequence of arousals associated with periodic arm and/or leg movements during sleep. Sleep latency is generally increased because of the urge to move the extremities while trying to fall asleep (▶ Sect. 2.13).

Periodic arm and/or leg movements are not essential criteria of RLS; about 20% of the RLS patients do not show these symptoms. The assessing of period limb movements associated with arousals is only possible via polysomnography. A maintenance of wakefulness test (MWT) or other procedures to assess the propensity to fall asleep in monotonous situations and impaired performance during daytime might be required (▶ Chap. 2).

Practical Tip

In the context of high-risk patients, medical reports, or severe RLS, neuropsychological tests are necessary to assess sleepiness- and fatigue-related impairments of the patient's daytime performance.

The IRLSSG (▶ Sect. 8.1.5) and the AASM formulated diagnostic criteria for RLS. The IRLSSG criteria are highly significant for the diagnostic process;

the AASM criteria represent the international consensus.

Diagnostic Criteria of RLS (Subjects Older Than 12 Years) Based on ICSD-3

- The patient reports an urge to move the legs, usually accompanied by or thought to be caused by uncomfortable and unpleasant sensations in the legs.
- This urge begins or worsens during periods of rest or inactivity, such as lying down or sitting.
- The urge to move is partially or completely relieved by movement such as walking or stretching, at least so long as the activity continues.
- The urge to move occurs or worsens exclusively or predominantly in the evening or at night.
- The condition cannot be explained by other sleep disorders, medical condition (leg cramps, myalgia, venous stasis, arthritis, etc.), or a behavioral disorder (e.g., agitated depression), drug intake, or substance abuse.
- The symptoms of RLS cause concern, distress, sleep disturbance, or impairment in the mental, physical, social, occupational, educational, and behavioral aspects of life or in important areas of functioning.

8.1.7 Differential Diagnoses

One of the most important differential diagnoses of RLS is *peripheral polyneuropathy*, with symptoms like painful legs and moving toes, and *venous malperfusion*. Also *irritable nerve roots* and *spinal syndromes* often are accompanied by complaints that are similar to RLS symptoms. On occasion, RLS is misdiagnosed as a *psychosomatic disorder with restlessness* or an *agitated depression*.

In chronic pain syndromes affecting the legs, careful differential diagnostics have to be carried out. Small-fiber neuropathy, (sleep-related) muscle cramps, peripheral vascular disease, akathisia due to neuroleptics, and myelopathy are possible differential diagnoses. On the other hand, RLS might be the underlying cause of insomnia complaints.

Practical Tip

All differential diagnoses did not show the circadian rhythm of symptom severity that is typical for RLS.

8.1.8 Therapy

Pharmaceutical therapy is symptomatic. The treatment of RLS is focused on the individual patient and is often characterized by complications if long-term application is necessary. Lack of effectiveness, tolerance, and side effects can be a challenge for the sleep specialist. In severe cases, combination therapies with different compounds might be necessary, thus, requiring knowledge about their pharmacology and interactions with each other. Finally, the circadian rhythm of the symptoms and the associated sleep disorders also require from therapists to suggest a drug schedule based on the individual rhythms of the patients.

8.1.8.1 General Therapeutic Principles

The individual treatment stategy is adapted to the complaints of the patient. The burden of RLS is due to reduced quality of life and massive daytime sleepiness and fatigue as well as the disrupted sleep. The primary therapeutic target is the improvement of sleep. For the majority of affected subjects with severe symptoms a permanent drug treatment has to be carried out.

In secondary RLS, the underlying disease has to be treated - if possible. Measuring ferritin levels to assess the iron status is one of the diagnostic procedures that should be part of the routine. Iron substitution is recommended in cases with regular but low ferritin values. According to clinical experience, at least 50 μg/l should be reached.

The treatment of RLS during *pregnancy*, however, may be difficult and should be limited to conservative measures without resorting to pharmaceuticals.

In cases where monotherapy is not sufficient even after long-term application, the physician may prescribe combination therapies (e.g., dopamine agonist plus L-DOPA).

The following compounds are recommended for the treatment of RLS. L-DOPA and dopamine agonists are considered as first-line drugs.

8.1.8.2 L-DOPA

In Germany, L-DOPA is approved in combination with benserazide for treatment of RLS, and clinical trials have demonstrated its effectiveness in doses up to 300 mg per day.

For the treatment of sleep disorders caused by RLS, a combination with immediate release (effect duration, 3–5 h) and retarded (maximum plasma level after 3 h) levodopa may be beneficial. Tolerance developments requiring dosage increase and an "end-of-dose" rebound are quite common (◘ Table 8.2).

◘ Table 8.2 Therapy of RLS with L-DOPA and dopamine agonists

Substance	Half-life in hours	Dosage in mg
Levodopa with benserazide	3–5	50–300
Levodopa with benserazide (retard)	Maximum plasma level after 3 h	50–400
Pramipexole	8–12	0.088–0.54
Ropinirole	5–7	0.25–2
Rotigotine	2–3	1–3 per 24 h

Practical Tip

It is recommended to adapt the time of intake to the occurrence of the complaints in the individual patient and to establish an exact intake scheme together with the patient (based on a sleep protocol). L-DOPA is effective in mild or episodic RLS. In contrast to dopamine agonists, the dosage has not to be slowly increased, so that it can be applied in situations with severe complaints, such as traveling by bus or airplane with lack of movement opportunities. It can also be used in combination with dopamine agonists as an add-on in cases of severe complaints.

Augmentation under L-DOPA medication is a frequently observed phenomenon (it can also occur in dopamine agonists) and, according to clinical studies, can occur in up to 70% of the patients.

Augmentation is defined as:

- An earlier onset of the symptoms within the 24-h cycle, e.g., midday or morning
- A more rapid onset of the complaints when the patients are at rest
- Complaints in other body parts that have not been affected prior to therapy

A dose-dependent risk for augmentation has been described for levodopa/benserazide. Dosages above 200 g per 24 h may lead to augmentation. In severe cases, switching to another drug is recomomended. If augmentation under L-DOPA occurs, the treatment should be switched to dopamine agonists, if possible with low doses.

Practical Tip

Augmentation is considered as the most significant complication of dopaminergic therapy. It has been described most frequently for L-DOPA but also for dopamine agonists.

Increase of the symptom severity is another sign of augmentation. In addition, decreasing effectiveness of the current drug dosage (tolerance) is also a problem.

Diagnostic Criteria of Augmentation According to IRLSSG 2007

(a) Basic features (all of which need to be met)

- The increase in symptom severity was experienced on five out of seven days during the previous week
- The increase in symptom severity is not accounted for by other factors such as a change in medical status, lifestyle, or the natural progression of the disorder
- It is assumed that there has been a prior positive response to treatment

(b) Persisting (although not immediate) paradoxical response to treatment: RLS symptom severity increases sometime after a dose increase, and improves sometime after a dose decrease
(c) Earlier onset of the symptoms by at least 4 h or by 2 to 4 h, whereby in the latter (2 to 4 h) the following criteria also have to be met:
  - Shorter occurrence latency while at rest
  - Extension of the symptoms to other parts of the body
  - Higher intensity of the symptoms
  - Duration of the relief is reduced because of the therapy

Augmentation is confirmed when the following criteria combinations are met: a + b, a + c, or a + b + c.

8.1.8.3 Dopamine Agonists

Dopamine agonists are classified into ergoline and nonergoline dopamine agonists (◘ Table 8.2). Clinical trials have demonstrated the effectiveness of ropinirole, pramipexole (non-ergoline dopamine agonists), and rotigotine in large patient populations. Generally, daily doses for RLS treatment are smaller than for the treatment of Parkinson's disease. Thus, it is always recommended to test the effectiveness of the smallest dose.

The recommended initial dose of *pramipexole* (half-life, 8–12 h) is 1/2 tablet of 0.18 mg once per day. If the effect is not sufficient, the dose can be increased to 1 tablet of 0.18 mg and every 4th day additional increases of 0.09 mg up to a maximum dose of 0.54 mg per day (◘ Table 8.2). If needed, combination with L-DOPA is possible.

The recommended initial dose of *ropinirole* (half-life, 5–7 h) is 0.25 mg. According to the recommendations from clinical studies, the dose is increased to 0.5 mg on day 3, as of the 2nd week to 1 mg, as of the 3rd week to 1.5 mg, and after the 4th week to 2 mg. To achieve an optimal effect, further dose increase might be necessary (e.g., week 5, 2.5 mg; week 6, 3 mg; week 7, 4 mg). Dosages beyond 4 mg have not been evaluated in the clinical studies for RLS (◘ Table 8.2). If needed, combination therapy with L-DOPA is possible.

The positive effect of *rotigotine* for RLS has been demonstrated by several studies. The half-life of rotigotine is 2 to 3 h. The transdermal application seems to have certain advantages. From the continuous transdermal release, rotigotine patches with doses of 1, 2, or 3 mg for 24 h maintain a stable level that is usually achieved after 2 days. The constant level may reduce the augmentation rate. Because of skin irritations, the patch has to be placed each day on another body location for a cycle of 2 weeks. The recommended initial dose is 1 mg; the dose may be increased by 1 mg every week. If needed, combined therapy with L-DOPA is possible.

The ergoline dopamine agonists such as *cabergoline* and *pergolide* that are also used in treating Parkinson's disease are highly effective for RLS; however, the substances have significant side effects. Among others, there are reports on fibrous cardiac valve pathologies and imperative sleep attacks after higher doses. Hence, they are no longer recommended for the treatment of RLS.

Practical Tip

Because of the side effect of nausea observed at therapy onset with dopamine agonists, the additional intake of a noncentrally effective dopamine antagonist is recommended, if needed, such as domperidone.

8.1.8.4 Opioids

Being the most potent medication, opioids such as *tilidine*, *oxycodone*, or *codeine* are available to treat severe and very severe, especially painful, RLS cases or nonresponders to dopaminergic treatment.

Controlled observational studies and case reports have been published for oxycodone. The approval of oxycodone/naloxone was achieved in Europe as second-line therapy for patients with severe to very severe idiopathic RLS after not responding to dopaminergic therapy. The initial dose amounts is 5/2.5 mg oxycodone hydrochloride/naloxone every 12 h. If the effect is not sufficient, a weekly dose increase may be recommended. The limit is 60/30 mg oxycodone hydrochloride/naloxone per day. Additional therapy with L-DOPA or dopamine agonists can be applied.

The dopaminergic component of opiates influences the extrapyramidal motor mechanisms via an activation of central μ-receptors. Increasing tolerance and a ceiling effect (no further increase in the therapeutical effect after reaching a certain dose) represent a problem so that the application of these substances should be delayed as long as possible. Therapy with apomorphine or methadone might be required in individual cases to achieve the therapeutic objective of maintaining substantial quality of life in the patients with very severe RLS.

Practical Tip

Because RLS may also occur as a withdrawal effect of opiate addiction, opiates have to be reduced very slowly.

8

8.1.8.5 Other Substances and Treatment Modalities of RLS

Among the anticonvulsant drugs, pregabalin and gabapentinenacarbil (a precursor of gabapentin in retarded form) are the drugs that were best investigated in controlled trials. In April 2011, gabapentin enacarbil was FDA approved in the US with the brand name Horizant and is discussed as the first-line therapy of RLS if the classic side effects such as daytime sleepiness, nasopharyngitis, suicidal thoughts, and weight gain are minimal. This substance is not available in Germany. The sedating and anxiolytic effect of pregabalin may have an additional therapeutic advantage if comorbid insomnia disorders are present. Neither pregabalin nor gabapentin is FDA or EMEA approved for the treatment of RLS. Other medications like, clonazepam, carbamazepine, clonidine, and valproic acid are off-label.

An oral iron substitution may be indicated for patients whose ferritin level is below 75 μg/l. Several studies in patients with severe RLS have shown that intravenous application of iron improved RLS complaints in 40% to 60% of cases, sometimes complete remission lasting for several months occurred.

Two studies confirmed a positive effect of high-dose magnesium (12.5 mmol before going to sleep) in mild RLS.

Practical Tip

In cases of mild or intermittent RLS, treatment with high-dose magnesium may be beneficial.

Nonpharmaceutical strategies such as sleep hygiene, sports (gymnastics, stretching, yoga), massages, or showers with cold or hot water may alleviate RLS symptoms in patients.

Contraindicated or ineffective are treatment attempts with hypnotics, antidepressants, neuroleptics, and beta blockers, as well as psychotherapeutic measures. Passive relaxation techniques such as autogenic training, progressive muscle relaxation, or meditation can enhance the symptoms and, thus, have negative effects.

8.2 Periodic Leg Movement Disorders During Sleep

8.2.1 Definition

The periodic limb movement disorders (PLMD) during sleep are also known by these terms:
- Periodic movement disorder of sleep (PMDS)
- Periodic limb movements in sleep (PLM)
- Leg convulsions
- Nocturnal myoclonus syndrome
- Sleep myoclonus syndrome

In particular, the term myoclonus should be avoided because in epileptology it is used for completely different symptoms.

PLMD is characterized by periodic and repeated stereotyped movements of the limbs during sleep. PLMD may cause insomnia symptoms and/or result in nonrestorative sleep and subsequently daytime sleepiness.

8.2.2 Etiology and Pathophysiology

The exact etiology of PLMD is unknown. In addition to genetic factors, a dysfunctional dopaminergic or opioidergic system with suppression of the supraspinal inhibitory pathways or rhythmic fluctuation of reticular activity might be responsible. Furthermore, a disturbed iron metabolism is considered as a potential factor in PLMD because low ferritin values seem to favor the development of PLMD or enhance frequency of PLM. The centrally induced repetitive limb movements can be accompanied by arousals and sleep fragmentation.

These etiological considerations are supported as disorders with dysfunctional dopaminergic systems such as RLS, narcolepsy, and REM behavioral disorder often also show PLMD. The increasing prevalence of PLMD in the elderly might be explained by reduced dopamine levels or the physiological decrease of dopamine receptors.

Periodic movement disorders in sleep are understood as separate entity. As PLMD are frequently associated with RLS, REM behavior disorder, obstructive sleep apnea, and narcolepsy, the additional diagnosis of PLMD is not necessary. PLMDs can also occur in patients with the following diseases:

- Kidney failure
- Congestive heart failure
- Arterial hypertension
- Polyneuropathy
- Multiple sclerosis
- Multisystem atrophy
- Spinal lesions
- Psychiatric disorders such as posttraumatic stress disorder, depression, and sleep-related eating disorder
- Chronic insomnia
- Attention deficit/hyperactivity syndrome
- Parkinson's disease
- Withdrawal of benzodiazepine
- Therapy with anticholinergic substances, for example, tricyclic antidepressants and serotonin reuptake inhibitors

8.2.3 Epidemiology

Periodic limb movements in sleep are quite prevalent and are a nonspecific symptoms related to many sleep disorders and diseases. However, often the PLMs are not directly affect sleep continuity. Sometimes the bed partner experiences sleep problems due to the periodic limb movements of the patient. Movement disorders can occur in children as well as in adults. The prevalence of PLMD with an index higher than 15 movements per hour is about 8% in 18- to 65-year-old individuals and more than 45% in persons older than 65 years. Gender differences in prevalence rates have not been studied.

Regarding the epidemiology of PLMD, the following aspects have to be taken into consideration:

- In about 80% of RLS cases, periodic limb movements during sleep co-occur.
- In 1% to 15% of patients with insomnia, PLMD occurred, varying between studies.
- In REM behavior disorder, PLMD occurs in 70% of the patients and in 45% to 60% of patients with narcolepsy-.

A high incidence of PLMD is described in patients with mental disorders (mood disorders, anxiety disorders, etc.) and neurological diseases (multisystem atrophy, spinal cord lesions) (see ▶ Chap. 2).

The present data regarding the epidemiology of PLMD, however, are limited because the diagnostic criteria vary from study to study and researchers did not always define strict inclusion and exclusion criteria.

8.2.4 Clinical Presentation

In PLMD, the patients complain about nonrestorative sleep (often associated with hypersomnia symptoms) but also quite often PLMD is accompanied by insomnia symptoms. Reduced feelings of being refreshed by sleep, daytime sleepiness, and monotony intolerance as well as depressive symptoms, memory problems and reduced concentration spans may be a consequence of the fragmented sleep.

Sleep continuity is negatively affected by the periodic movements of the legs, sometimes arms are moving too mostly after flexion of the large joints and stretching the big toes. Subsequently, associated arousals impair sleep continuity. The tonic contractions can also occur in wakefulness in many patients, but often they are go unnoticed.

Periodic limb movements are clinically relevant and should be treated if they cause clinically significant insomnia or hypersomnia symptomatology that cannot be explained by other sleep disorders or somatic diseases.

Practical Tip

Generally, patients are not consciously aware of the periodic movements of the extremities. More often, the bed partners observe the restless sleep in the patient with jerky movements of the extremities.

The limb movements are frequently accompanied by fast frequencies in the EEG due to a central nervous activation that triggers PLM, among other events, and not as a consequence of the PLM. The movements may also be associated with autonomous arousals like brief increases in heart rate and blood pressure.

8.2.5 Examination Procedures

The examination includes individual *history taking* as well as *interviewing with the bedpartner* because the patient is often only aware of the daytime symptoms.

Eliciting medication and substance consumption is crucial to rule out medication-induced types of PLMD. The following procedures should be part of diagnostic standards:

- Vitamin B12 levels
- Iron, ferritin levels
- Folic acid level
- Diagnostics of polyneuropathy
- Diabetes mellitus diagnostics

Other (neurological) diseases possibly underlying symptomatic forms of PLMD, but also can cause insomnia disorders, have to carefully evaluated.

Practical Tip

Insomnia complaints are often misattributed to periodic limb movements. In psychopathology of insomnia, periodic limb movements might be considered associated and not does not require treatment.

8.2.6 Sleep Diagnostics

Sleep diagnostics include *sleep anamnesis*, *sleepiness-related anamnesis*, and a *sleep diary*. *Actigraphy* performed in the home setting may be helpful to complete assessment of the severity (► Chap. 2).

PLM are determined according to the current criteria of the AASM (► Chap. 2).

Severe forms of PLMD show as many as 1500 periodic limb movements per sleep period. Depending on the number of PLMs with arousals (index of periodic limb movements in sleep = number of limb movements per hour of sleep; see ► Chap. 2), sleep fragmentation, reduced slow wave sleep and REM sleep can occur.

Practical Tip

To avoid false-negative diagnoses, it has to be kept in mind that PLM indices vary significantly from night to night. Even in severe PLMD, nights with low PLM indices might occur.

In high-risk patients or severe cases, neuropsychological tests are required to assess the sleepiness-related impairments of performance such as MWT, multiple sleep latency test (MSLT), or pupillography measuring the propensity to fall asleep during the day (► Chap. 2).

Diagnostic Criteria of PLMD based on ICSD-3

1. Polysomnography shows PLM as it was defined according to the current version of the AASM manual on the assessment of sleep and associated phenomena (► Chap. 2).
2. The PLM index exceeds 5 per hour in children and 15 per hour in adults. Note: The movement index is interpreted in the context of the patient's sleep-related complaints and not in a normative way. In adults, normative values might be even higher in studies that did not exclude PLMs related to respiratory events or other causes.

3. The PLMs cause clinically significant sleep disturbance and/or impairment in mental, physical, social, occupational, educational, behavioral, or other important areas of functioning. Note: An increased PLM index without clinical symptoms can be documented as polysomnographic finding; however, it does not meet the criteria for diagnosing PLMD.
4. PLMs cannot be explained by other sleep disorders, medical or neurological diseases, mental disorders, or medication or substance abuse. It is recommended not to diagnose PLMD in patients with untreated sleep-related breathing disorders, RLS, narcolepsy, and REM sleep behavior disorder.

8.2.7 Differential Diagnoses

In *sleep-related breathing disorders*, PLM may occur in association with apnea-related arousals. Diagnostic assessment of PLM should be carried out after successful treatment of the sleep-related breathing disorder.

PLM may be observed in the context of nocturnal *cerebral seizures* and of *myoclonic epilepsy*. In these cases, additional epilepsy diagnostics and PSG with more EEG electrodes may be necessary.

If PLM is suspected in the context of neurodegenerative diseases such as Alzheimer's disease, nerve root irritations, or spinal syndromes, further neurological examination is indicated. Benign phenomena like hypnagogic foot tapping and the alternating leg muscle activation (ALMA) can be differentiated by polysomnography.

8.2.8 Therapy

Treatment is only required if PLM *indices* are elevated and associated with clinically relevant to *insomnia* or *hypersomnia* symptomatology.

Other etiological factors explaining the clinical symptoms have to be excluded; if needed, a therapy attempt with L-DOPA may help to identify PLMD. There are no randomized trials on the effectiveness of medication for treating PLMD that does not occur within RLS syndromes. If treatment is required, the therapeutic approach is similar to treating patients with RLS (▶ Sect. 8.1).

In patients with RLS, L-DOPA, dopamine agonists, and second-line medications have a positive effect on RLS symptoms but also on the frequency of periodic limb movements in sleep. If PLMD is symptomatic, causal therapies, e.g., iron substitution, have to be performed first. Adherence to the principles of sleep hygiene may be useful; however, pharmacological strategies are the major focus. The treatment effects can only be evaluated by polysomnography assessing PLM indices.

8.3 Sleep-Related Leg Cramps

8.3.1 Definition

These terms are used synonymously:
- Leg cramps
- Nocturnal leg cramps
- "Charley horse"

The etiology of the idiopathic form has not yet been clarified. In contrast to dystonia, these cramps are not characterized by simultaneous contractions of agonists and antagonists.

8.3.2 Etiology

Most sleep-related muscle cramps seem to be idiopathic. As a transitory phenomenon, nocturnal leg cramps can occur in healthy individuals after intense physical activity whereby microtraumas of the muscles and electrolyte disbalances may be involved. Symptomatic muscle cramps can also occur in magnesium or calcium deficiency, in pregnancy, and in neuromuscular and metabolic diseases. Genetic factors have not been identified yet.

8.3.3 Epidemiology

About 10% to 16% of the population suffers from clinically relevant nocturnal leg cramps, with increased prevalences in the elderly. Thirty-three percent of persons older than 60 years and 50% of persons older than 80 years report nocturnal leg cramps at least once every 2 months. In 6% of individuals older than 60 years, these leg cramps occur at night. The lifetime prevalence for leg cramps is probably near 100%.

8.3.4 Clinical Presentation

The cramps occur spontaneously, mostly during sleep, but sometimes during wakefulness, without any precursor or after short mild pain and are associated with painful hardening of the muscles. In most cases, the calf and foot muscles, rarely the thigh muscles or other muscle groups, are affected. Those cramps may last for a few seconds up to several minutes. They subside spontaneously or after stretching, massaging, movements, or application of heat. Sporadic events may occur, but also series of cramps have been reported. The disorder is more common in older adults. If cramps recur, the frequency might fluctuate over many years. The disstress can be high, but objectifiable lesions do not occur. As a consequence of these mostly painful events, problems of initiating and maintaining sleep can occur.

8.3.5 Diagnostics

During *PSG*, the events usually emerge spontaneously during sleep or awake phases. *Electromyography (EMG)* of the affected muscles, shows a sudden, persisting activity.

Diagnostic Criteria of Nocturnal Muscle Cramps According to ICSD-3

- A painful sensation in the leg or foot with sudden, involuntary muscle hardness or tightness, indicating strong muscle contraction
- Emerging in bed, in either sleep or wakefulness
- Pain relief is achieved by forcefully stretching the affected muscles

8.3.6 Therapy

Intensive and regular stretching, massage, and application of heat may relieve the acute symptoms.

For longer-term prophylaxis or therapy, causal measures (e.g., balancing of electrolytes) should be initiated if possible.

Symptomatically, magnesium, quinine sulfate, verapamil, and theophylline may be applied in off-label use. Contraindications of the medications have to be carefully evaluated, rare occurring but severe side effects have to be evaluated against the expected benefit.

8.4 Bruxism

8.4.1 Definition

Synonymous terms:

- Nocturnal bruxism
- Nocturnal tooth grinding
- Tooth clenching
- Sleep-related bruxism

Bruxism is an involuntary grinding or clenching of the teeth, mostly during sleep but can occur also in wakefulness. This activity causes abrasion of the teeth, and even lesions of the maxillary joints are possible.

8.4.2 Etiology

The etiology of the disorder may include these factors:

- Psychological factors (increased levels of tension, anxiety disorders)
- Central nervous factors (congenital or acquired brain lesions)
- Anatomical factors (malocclusion, malformation)

These factors may be associated with bruxism although pathophysiological mechanisms have not been identified.

Personality traits associated with high achievement need and tension might be associated with bruxism. Bruxism runs in families but genetic associations have not yet been identified.

8.4.3 Epidemiology

Typically, the disorder starts in childhood and prevalence decreases with age. Rhythmic masticatory activity is seen also in almost every healthy sleeper. About 15% to 20% of children show transitory bruxism, the lifetime prevalence is about 50%. In adults, women report bruxism more often than men. The prevalence of clinically relevant bruxism is less than 5%.

8.4.4 Clinical Presentation

Activation of the masticatory muscles during sleep can be accompanied by disturbing grinding sounds that are unpleasant for others and also leads to an intensive abrasion of the teeth's enamels, associated with pain around the teeth and within the masticatory muscles. In severe cases, sleep may be fragmented due to arousals and insomnia complaints are reported. Most often, however, a dentist or a neurologist (because of headaches) is consulted. The contractions of the chewing muscles may be tonic or phasic, the so-called rhythmic masticatory muscle activity (RMMA). The typical event is of a stereotyped nature, starting with autonomous and EEG arousals that are followed by the contraction of the masticatory muscles. Sometimes swallowing can occur at the end of an episode.

8.4.5 Diagnostics

Sleep anamnesis combined with *dental examination* is essential and sufficient in most cases. *PSG* is only required to rule out other disorders. An increased *EMG activity* of the masticatory muscles associated with arousals that occur most often in light sleep are indicative. Masticatory muscle activity is sometimes associated with REM sleep in older people and this might be a symptom of a beginning REM sleep behavior disorder. Movements of the body or the extremities can occur in 25% of arousal reactions associated with bruxism. The EMG activity of the maxillary muscles (masseter and temporal muscles) may be increased phasically in intervals between 0.25 and 2.0 s, tonically of more than 2.0 s, or with a mixed rhythm.

Diagnostic Criteria of Bruxism According to ICSD-3

- Regularly occurring sounds of tooth grinding or tooth clenching during sleep
- At least one of the following clinical symptoms occurs:
  - Abnormal tooth wear associated with tooth grinding during sleep
  - Transitory morning jaw muscle pain or fatigue, and/or temporal headaches; and/or jaw locking upon awakening, consistent with reports of nocturnal tooth grinding.

8.4.6 Therapy

In pediatric patients, it is possible to "wait and see". After maxillary deformities have been diagnostically ruled out spontaneous remissions are frequent. In cases of (threatening) dental damage, occlusal splints should be applied. If the patient is very tense, relaxation techniques, hypnotherapy, biofeedback, and psychotherapy may be helpful. For acute pain relief, physiotherapy and massages are recommended.

Medications such as muscle relaxants are only indicated in very severe cases (short-term benzodiazepines, antidepressants). Before initiating pharmaceutical therapy strategies, a thorough risk to benefit evaluation should be done.

8.5 Sleep-Related Rhythmic Movement Disorder

8.5.1 Definition

Synonymous terms:

- Jactatio capitis nocturna
- Jactatio corporis nocturna
- Rhythmie du sommeil
- Head banging
- Body rocking
- Head rolling
- Body rolling

Sleep-related rhythmic movements are defined as repetitive, stereotyped, and rhythmic motor movements of large muscle groups, occurring mainly during sleep onset and or during sleep. The diagnosis requires that the behavior have clinically significant consequences.

8.5.2 Epidemiology

In infants, stereotyped movements can occur as normal transient phenomenon related to self-stimulation. About 50% to 70% of infants show temporarily such a behavior. In persisting symptomatology or later beginning, sleep-related movement disorders are likely to be associated with psychiatric/neuropsychiatric disorders. The gender ratio of boys to girls varies from 2:1 to 4:1.

8.5.3 Clinical Presentation

The clinical picture is characterized by stereotyped rhythmic head or body movements during sleep onset or light sleep, with these possible variations:

- Head banging from back to forth (anterior–posterior)
- Head rolling in lateral direction
- Body rocking in elbow-knee position
- Body rolling in prone position

Occasionally, the head banging is accompanied by monotonous singing or humming. In some cases, injuries have been reported - caused by hitting the head against a hard surface (hematoma, intracerebral, and retinal bleedings). Very often the rhythmic movements are associated with sleep onset or light sleep. The movements usually begin in infancy; in healthy children, the symptoms disappear spontaneously. In older children, this simple form of self-stimulation, however, has to be considered as a symptom of a more severe mental disorder.

8.5.4 Diagnostics

The diagnostics consist of *history taking* by interviewing parents or bed partners (in adult patients) and assessing developmental aspects. A *pediatric-neurological examination* including EEG to exclude cerebral seizures is recommended. If cerebral lesions are suspected, *developmental diagnostics* including *MRI* or cranial computer tomography CCT are required.

Sleep diagnostics comprise *sleep history* and keeping a *sleep diary* in order to assess the frequency and the severity of the episodes. *PSG with video monitoring* should be performed. Because the symptoms occur before falling sleep, the sleep profile is tpyically in the normal range compared to age-matched healthy sleepers. The rhythmic movements occur when falling asleep, less frequently in light sleep, and very rarely in N3 or REM sleep. Regarding differential diagnosis, cerebral seizures have to be ruled out by carefully analyzing the EEG of PSG.

Diagnostic Criteria of Sleep-Related Rhythmic Movement Disorders Based on ICSD-3

- The patient shows repetitive, stereotyped, and rhythmic motor behaviors involving large muscle groups.
- The movements are predominantly sleep related. They occur near naps or near bedtime, or when the individual appears drowsy or asleep.
- The behavior leads to significant complaints as manifest by at least one of the following aspects:
  - Interference with normal sleep
  - Significant impairment in daytime function
  - Self-inflicted bodily injury or likelihood of injury if preventive measures are not applied
- The rhythmic movement disorder cannot be better explained by another movement disorder or epilepsy.

Note: The diagnosis is only made when the behavior has clinically significant consequences.

8.5.5 Therapy

If infants are affected, it is important to reassure the parents to wait for spontaneous remission. In cases of symptomatic types, causal therapy, in exceptional cases with adjuvant neuroleptics or benzodiazepines, is indicated after elaborate diagnostics. In older children, psychotherapy and relaxation procedures are a promising option.

8.6 Questions

1. Please describe pharmaceutical options of RLS therapy.
2. What are the indications for RLS treatment?
3. Which diseases are likely to be associated with periodic limb movements during sleep?
4. When are periodic limb movement disorders treated?
5. Which approaches are beneficial for treating bruxism?

Further Reading

1. Allen RP, Picchietti D, Hening WA, Trenkwalder C, Walters AS, Montplaisi J. A report from the Restless Legs Syndrome Diagnosis and Epidemiology workshop at the National Institutes of Health, International Restless Legs Syndrome Study Group. Restless legs syndrome: diagnostic criteria, special considerations and epidemiology. Sleep Med. 2003;4:101–19.
2. American Academy of Sleep Medicine. International classification of sleep disorders, 3. Aufl.: diagnostic and coding manual. Westchester: American Academy of Sleep Medicine; 2014.
3. American Academy of Sleep Medicine. The AASM-manual for the scoring of sleep and associated events: rules, terminology and technical specifications. Version 2.3. Darien: American Academy of Sleep Medicine; 2016.
4. Clarenbach P, Benes H. Restless Legs Syndrome. Die unruhigen Beine. Klinik, Diagnose, Therapie. Bremen: Uni-Med; 2006.
5. Happe S, Benes H, Hornyak M, Kotterba S, Mayer G, Stiasny-Kolster K, Mitglieder der Arbeitsgemeinschaft "Motorik und Schlaf" der Deutschen Gesellschaft für Schlafforschung und Schlafmedizin. Begutachtung des Restless Legs Syndroms – Zusammenfassung der Konsensusempfehlung. Somnologie. 2006;10:206–9.
6. Hornyak M, Feige B, Voderholzer U, Riemann D. Spectral analysis of sleep EEG in patients with restless legs syndrome. Clin Neurophysiol. 2005;116:1265–72.
7. Stiasny-Kolster K. Medikamentöse Therapie des RLS. Somnologie. 2013;17:252–8.
8. Trenkwalder C, Beneš H, Grote L, García-Borreguero D, Högl B, Hopp M, Bosse B, Oksche A, Reimer K, Winkelmann J, Allen RP, Kohnen R, RELOXYN Study Group. Prolonged release oxycodone-naloxone for treatment of severe restless legs syndrome after failure of previous treatment: a double-blind, randomised, placebo-controlled trial with an open-label extension. Lancet Neurol. 2013;12(12):1141–50.
9. Wilt T, MacDonald R, Ouellette J, et al. Pharmacologic therapy for primary restless-legs syndrome. A systematic review and meta-analysis. JAMA Intern Med. 2013;173(7):496–505.
10. Winkelmann J, Schormair B, Lichtner P, et al. Genome-wide association study of restless legs syndrome identifies common variants in three genomic regions. Nat Genet. 2007;39:1000–6.
11. Winkelmann J, Armstraong MJ, Allen RP, Chaudhuri KR, Ondo W, Trenwalder C, Zee PC, Gronseth GS, Gloss D, Zesiewicz T. Practice guideline summary: treatment of restless-legs syndrome in adults: report of the guideline development, dissemination and implementation subcommittee of the American Academy of Neurology. Neurology. 2016;87(24):2585–93.

Isolated Symptoms, Normal Variants, and Other Sleep Disorders

J. T. Maurer

B. A. Stuck et al., *Practice of Sleep Medicine*, https://doi.org/10.1007/978-3-030-17412-5_9

Not all phenomena or symptoms that occur between falling asleep and waking up can be clearly assigned to the large group of sleep disorders, even if they have been classified in the ICSD-3 according to their predominant phenomenology. Some of them appear isolated, have no or only marginal illness significance, have been only poorly investigated, or display highly variable symptoms, so that they can neither be allocated to an existing sleep disorder nor defined as a novel sleep disorder. A sleep disorder caused by environmental influences, for example, noise, heat, or the bed partner, has to be included because the objectively present disturbing factor as well as its subjective perception may lead to insomnia, hypersomnia, or nonrestorative sleep.

9.1 Isolated Symptoms, Normal Variants, and Unresolved Issues

9.1.1 Long and Short Sleepers

Individuals who sleep for longer or shorter times than the age-specific average during a 24-h day and who feel restored after this sleep duration are defined as long and short sleepers, respectively. Sleep phases other than the main sleep phase have to be included in this calculation.

- In the context of adults, long sleepers are those who need 10 h of sleep or more during the 24-h day.
- Short sleepers are those who need only 5 h of sleep or less per day.

Both normal variants, long sleepers and short sleepers, who have already manifested in childhood or adolescence, are found in about 2% of the adult population and generally persist lifelong. The affected people feel restored when they can maintain their individual sleep duration. Disorders are only observed when a long sleeper tries to, or is forced to, cope with less sleep over longer periods or if the short sleeper wants to prolong the sleep duration by means of centrally acting substances. The last-mentioned case is often based on the misconception of the affected person or his/her environment regarding the necessary sleep duration. During school or work weeks, many long sleepers consciously accept a sleep deficit that they try to compensate by particularly long sleep phases on weekends. The short sleeper only rarely suffers and very rarely seeks medical advice. Increased morbidity could not be confirmed for either normal variant.

The diagnosis of long and short sleepers can be based on the age of manifestation and the typical *history* regarding the recovery of sleep for individually adequate sleep duration. *Sleep logs* with data on the daytime alertness during the daily routine and during a vacation may facilitate the diagnosis. Generally, device-related diagnostics are not necessary. If long sleepers complain about nonrestorative sleep or report daytime sleepiness because of too little sleep, the differentiation of previously mentioned sleep disorders may be required (see ▶ Chaps. 3, 4, 5, and 8).

For short sleepers, *therapy* is usually not needed. In the context of long sleepers, observation of the individually required sleep duration is the therapy of choice and eliminates possible symptoms.

9.1.2 Sleep-Talking and Sleep-Related Groaning: (Somniloquy and Catathrenia)

About half of all children and as many as 5% of adults talk during their sleep (somniloquy) in a more or less comprehensible way, whereby the content may lead to problems with the bed partner or room partners. Much more rarely, sighing or groaning during sleep is heard (catathrenia). In the context of catathrenia, the duration of expiration is greatly extended so that oxygen desaturation and apnea can occur. The differentiation from sleep apnea is possible by simultaneously monitoring the acoustic phenomenon and the breathing disorder during expiration measured by polysomnography.

The affected individuals are usually not aware of either somniloquy or catathrenia, which may develop during REM as well as non-REM sleep. A high frequency is observed in patients with REM sleep behavioral disorders and those sleepwalking or sleep-related eating disorder. If sleep-talking only manifests in adulthood, often a psychopathology is found.

Regarding differential diagnosis especially in cases of stereotypic vocalization during sleep, epileptic seizures have to be excluded. *Pavor nocturnus* (see ▶ Chap. 7) differs, manifesting as shouting and an anxiety reaction.

If psychological stress is supposed as the origin and if sleep-talking is perceived as stressing, further psychotherapeutic examination may be reasonable, with appropriate therapy if needed.

9.1.3 Sleep-Related Movement Anomalies

In particular during sleep onset, but also during sleep, various movements of the trunk or the extremities may occur.

About two thirds of the population report sudden twitches of single muscle groups or body parts, so-called *sleep-onset myoclonias* or *hypnic jerks* that are frequently associated with hypnagogic sensations (e.g., acoustic, optic, sensation of falling) and lead to short arousal or waking up from light sleep. Taking caffeine or other stimulants, physical activity, or emotional stress may increase the incidence and severity. In rare cases, the sleep-onset twitches are so severe that they prevent people from falling asleep. In those cases, avoiding predisposing factors is most important. Rarely, clonazepam is applied.

In the phase of relaxation before sleep onset, in rare cases movements of the trunk may occur that extend in a peripheral direction to the proximal extremities and the neck. Each mental activation, for example, when the affected person is addressed by the bed partner, reliably interrupts those movements: defined as *propriospinal myoclonias*, these may lead to severe disorders of initiating sleep. Treatment with 1 mg clonazepam before going to bed may reduce the incidence of those myoclonias.

If asymmetrical and asynchronous myoclonias of small muscles or muscle groups (e.g., fingers, toes, corner of the mouth) are observed more than five times per minute over at least 20 min, predominantly in sleep stages N2 and N3, this phenomenon is called an *excessive fragmentary myoclonus*. Myoclonias can often be verified in videometry: they are mostly associated with arousal and lead to disorders of maintaining sleep. Myoclonias are found in approximately 5% to 10% of the patients who undergo examination in sleep centers because of excessive daytime sleepiness, and more often affect males. Often, sleep-related breathing disorders coexist as well as periodic limb movements during sleep (PLMS; see ▶ Chap. 8), narcolepsy (see ▶ Chap. 5), or insomnia (see ▶ Chap. 3).

The treatment is primarily based on the coexisting sleep disorder. In cases of persisting complaints, therapy similar to that for restless legs syndrome/PLMD (see ▶ Chap. 8) is recommended.

During sleep onset, *hypnagogic foot tremor* (see ▶ Sect. 2.6.4) may manifest that typically persists for more than 10 s and in rare cases leads to sleep interruptions. In coincidence with arousals, *alternating activations of the leg muscles* that can be confirmed by polysomnography disappear when falling asleep. In sleep centers, those phenomena are found in about 7.5% and 1.1%, respectively, of adult patients. Their clinical relevance is still unclear.

Very rarely, otherwise completely unremarkable newborns may show intensive bilateral movements of the large trunk muscles and the extremities that occur exclusively during sleep. Those *benign sleep myoclonias in newborns* are considered as a hint to incomplete brain maturation, because on one hand they display spontaneous remission within a few weeks or months and on the other hand are not associated with an increased risk for cerebral seizure disorders.

9.2 Other Sleep Disorders

In particular, *environmental sleep disorders* have high clinical relevance. Until recently, the frequency of sleep disorders caused by environmental factors has not been investigated. However, a high prevalence is assumed. Disturbing factors may be noise, heat, cold, the bedfellow, unfamiliar environment (hospital, hotel, tent), or the attention claimed by an ill person or a newborn. Most affected people are conscious of the responsible disturbing factor and try to meet the condition with suitable measures. Thus, in most cases, the sleep disorders are only transitory, and the origin of the sleep disorder is plausible to the disturbed individual. Affected people typically seek advice only when the subjective perception of the disturbing factor is the focus and when at the same time symptoms of other sleep disorders occur that are believed responsible for their insomnia or hypersomnia complaints.

For the diagnosis of environmental sleep disorders, intensive *history taking* is essential. Sometimes, a *sleep protocol* assessed for 2 weeks may determine the sleep phases with good recovery and the stimulus that is responsible for the disturbance. In particular, insomnia and sleep–

wake rhythm disorders should be excluded in cases of unclear history.

In most cases, intensive counseling is sufficient. If the disturbing factor is psychically overestimated, psychotherapeutic intervention is probably appropriate. In the short term, a hypnotic agent may be applied if the stimulus is transitory and cannot be eliminated. Anamnestic control of the therapeutic success, however, is required.

Case Report

A 25-year-old slim woman presents because of excessive daytime sleepiness and snoring without observed breathing interruptions that is stressful for her husband.

She reliably reports falling asleep in monotonous situations. The quality of her sleep is described as good, without difficulties of initiating and maintaining sleep. The sleep duration amounts to 7 h with regular bedtimes. On holiday or on weekends, the sleepiness does not improve. She cannot think of any origin for her complaints.

In the context of examination, it is possible to exclude organic and psychological origins. The sleep protocol could not reveal any cause for the daytime sleepiness. Outpatient polygraphy does not give any hint of sleep apnea; however, occasional heart rate increases are found. In the subsequent polysomnographic examination over two nights, a regular sleep profile is measured without heart rate changes. Interestingly, the vigilance diagnostics do not show increased daytime sleepiness.

In the context of the final discussion, the patient mentions that she only feels well rested when her husband works night shift and she sleeps alone. Only the nights when they sleep next to each other are stressful. Being asked, the husband confirms that he regularly pushes his wife because of her snoring, which stops the snoring so that he is able to fall asleep again.

After elimination of her snoring by application of a mandibular advancement device, both partners report improved sleep quality and daytime alertness.

Further Reading

1. American Academy of Sleep Medicine. International classification of sleep disorders, vol 3. Aufl. Darien: American Academy of Sleep Medicine; 2014.
2. Berry RB, Brooks R, Gamaldo CE, Harding SM, Lloyd RM, Marcus CL, Vaughn BV, for the American Academy of Sleep Medicine. The AASM manual for the scoring of sleep and associated events: rules, terminology and technical specifications, version 2.6. www.aasmnet.org. Darien: American Academy of Sleep Medicine; 2016.

Secondary Sleep Disorders

B. A. Stuck and M. Schredl

B. A. Stuck et al., *Practice of Sleep Medicine*, https://doi.org/10.1007/978-3-030-17412-5_10

Sleep disorders may be secondary as a symptom of organic or psychic/psychiatric diseases. These disorders can appear as accompanying or temporary symptoms; however, in the context of chronic diseases, they contribute significantly to the morbidity and maintenance of the disease. In those cases, the treatment of the sleep disorder may have a positive effect on the course of the underlying disease. The expertise of the sleep specialist is also required when comorbid sleep disorders need to be treated in patients with organic or psychic/psychiatric diseases. Furthermore, organic or psychic/psychiatric diseases may manifest primarily as a sleep disorder. The sleep specialist is then responsible to discover the basic origin of the sleep disorder and to initiate adequate treatment approaches.

It is clear that not all organic and psychic/psychiatric diseases leading to secondary sleep disorders may be discussed in this chapter. One focus of this chapter is the presentation of the most important secondary sleep disorders that may appear as complaints of insomnia or hypersomnia. The treatment of the underlying diseases however is not included in this chapter.

10.1 Sleep Disorders Caused by Organic Diseases

Sleep disorders and sleep-related symptoms are apparent in numerous organic diseases.

On one hand, organic diseases may be the *origin* of secondary sleep disorders, and on the other hand classic symptoms of sleep disorders such as difficulties of initiating and maintaining sleep or daytime sleepiness may be seen as the *leading symptoms* of an organic disease. Thus, organic diseases have to be considered in the differential diagnosis of insomnia and hypersomnia. Finally, the relevant symptoms can even be the *result* of medical therapy of an underlying organic disease, which emphasizes the necessity of careful history taking regarding medication (► Chap. 2).

The most important organic diseases that should be considered in this context are these:

- Insomnia
  - Endocrine diseases (hyperthyroidism)
  - Chronic pain
  - Neurological diseases (neurodegenerative diseases)
  - Respiratory diseases (bronchial asthma)
- Hypersomnia
  - Endocrine diseases
  - Cardiovascular diseases (cardiac arrhythmia, hypotension, heart failure)
  - Respiratory diseases
  - Renal failure

The aforementioned classification is mainly based on didactic reflections. Many of those diseases may lead to complaints of insomnia as well as hypersomnia, depending on the severity of the disease and the individual patient.

10.1.1 Insomnia as a Symptom of Organic Diseases

10.1.1.1 Endocrine Diseases

Hyperthyroidism is generally associated with symptoms of psychomotor restlessness. In addition to a frequently slight tremor and increased nervousness, in general symptoms of sleeplessness with difficulties in initiating and maintaining sleep are also observed. Other clinical symptoms are goiter, which is encountered in 70% to 90% of the patients, sinus tachycardia with possibly occurring arrhythmia, weight loss, hyperhidrosis, and heat intolerance.

Those symptoms may be seen not only in the context of immunogenic hyperthyroidism (Graves' disease) or thyroid autonomy, but may also be caused by inappropriate dosage of thyroid hormones.

In the daily routine of sleep medicine, patients with the clear manifestation of hyperthyroidism do not present problems of differential diagnosis. In cases of accordingly weak symptoms, however, those patients may primarily complain about disorders of initiating and maintaining sleep as leading symptoms. Regarding the frequent occurrence of thyroid diseases, patients should undergo an appropriate history taking and in suspected cases additional laboratory testing as part of the diagnostic process in cases with insomnia.

10.1.1.2 Chronic Pain

Chronic pain is closely related to sleep disorders and regularly interferes with each other. Chronic pain is often associated with disorders of initiating and maintaining sleep. Approximately two thirds of patients with chronic pain report symptoms of insomnia.

In particular, in the context of *tumor-related pain*, not only does the pain cause sleep disorders, but also the stress caused by the disease contributes to the persisting chronic sleep disorder.

On the other hand, chronic sleep disorders or chronic sleep deprivation may significantly influence the *perception of pain* so that an adequate treatment of the sleep disorder may decisively improve the efficacy of analgesic therapy. In addition to current therapeutic approaches in the treatment of chronic pain, sedating antidepressants are often included in the co-analgesic therapy. Hereby, sedation leads not only to an increased effect of classic analgesics but also to improved sleep.

10.1.1.3 Neurological Diseases

Neurodegenerative diseases such as Parkinson's disease or dementia of Alzheimer's type frequently lead to distinct sleep disorders up to the disintegration of the sleep–wake cycle.

In more than 50% of the cases, *dementia diseases* are associated with sleep disorders. The severity of dementia and the dispersed daytime and nighttime rhythm are closely interrelated. There may be an important discrepancy between the objectively diagnosed sleep disorder and the subjective assessment of sleep. Disorders of the sleep–wake cycle, daytime sleepiness, and daytime sleep episodes are typical symptoms. In up to 50% of the cases, central sleep apnea syndromes occur; furthermore, periodic leg movements are observed.

In those cases, generally a stabilized sleep–wake cycle may be achieved by appropriate sleep hygiene and a stable daytime rhythm that should include regular phases of physical activity. Regarding medical treatment of the difficulties of initiating and maintaining sleep of dementia patients, low-dose, slightly sedating neuroleptics or antidepressants with low anticholinergic components may be applied. Short-acting benzodiazepine receptor agonists are also available.

In the context of *Parkinson's disease*, sleep disorders represent a frequent, non-motor symptom. Neurodegenerative processes, especially in dopaminergic systems, as well as periodic leg movements during sleep, disorder of REM sleep, and secondary sleep-related respiratory disorders seem to be responsible for sleep disturbances frequently associated with Parkinson's disease.

10.1.1.4 Respiratory Diseases

Patients suffering from *bronchial* asthma often report difficulties of initiating and maintaining sleep and present with a reduced percentage of slow wave sleep. Additionally, the application of stimulating bronchodilators at nighttime may have a negative effect on nocturnal sleep.

10.1.2 Hypersomnia as a Symptom of Organic Diseases

10.1.2.1 Endocrine Diseases

In contrast to the aforementioned symptoms of hyperthyroidism, patients suffering from hypothyroid metabolism generally present with a typical activity decrease, lethargy, fatigue, and sleepiness. Other frequently observed clinical symptoms of hypothyroidism are increasing weight (also caused by a generalized myxedema), sensitivity to cold temperatures, and obstipation. In general, those symptoms are not as impressive as in the context of hyperthyroidism. Lethargy and fatigue or sleepiness may be the salient symptoms. Patients with hypersomnia complaints thus should routinely undergo history taking with regard to the described symptoms, to previous surgical interventions of the thyroid, to radioiodine therapy or medical treatment of the thyroid, and finally laboratory testing in suspected cases.

Additionally, hypothyroidism often leads to sleep-related respiratory disorders because of increased weight and tissue edema and thus to hypersomnia in a twofold respect. Even if the percentage of patients with hypothyroidism among all patients suffering from obstructive sleep apnea is rather low (1% to 3% according to the international literature), hypothyroidism seems to be accompanied by obstructive sleep apnea in 50% to 100% of cases.

Case Report

A patient presents in our medical sleep center with complaints of nonrestorative sleep and severe daytime sleepiness (ESS 16).

Besides the predominant complaints of increased tendency to fall asleep, the patient also describes a general lethargy and a clear reduction of physical and mental activity that leads to significant problems at work and in his private life. During the previous year, he has considerably increased in weight although he has not changed his habits of nutrition and life (current BMI, 32 kg/m^2).

Sleep medical diagnosis reveals low-grade obstructive sleep apnea with an AHI of 13. Because of the severe daytime sleepiness with only low-grade sleep apnea and the described complaints, a thyroid-stimulating hormone (TSH) test is initiated that indicates hypothyroid metabolism with a value of 15.3 mU/l. Outpatient diagnostics performed by the general practitioner confirm the diagnosis of hypothyroidism; substitution treatment with thyroid hormones is initiated.

The daytime situation of the patient is significantly improved; the treatment leads to clear weight reduction. A polysomnographic control after 3 months reveals that his respiratory problems have completely disappeared.

Cushing syndrome also may be relevant for differential diagnosis. In general, the affected patients show adynamia and obesity, which is frequently associated with obstructive sleep apnea. Also in this context, the increase of pharyngeal soft tissue related to regularly occurring obesity, is responsible for the development of obstructive breathing disorders. In addition, corticosteroid-induced myopathy is discussed as a possible origin. Some of the patients with high cortisol levels during nighttime also tend to insomnia. This observation is mainly found in patients with adrenal Cushing or ectopic ACTH expression. Both symptoms are not subject to circadian regulation and lead to permanently increased cortisol levels.

In most cases, however, the Cushing syndrome is iatrogenic. In patients who undergo long-term medication with corticosteroids this fact should be included in the diagnostic and therapeutic considerations. Most corticosteroids should be taken in the morning because all preparations cause waking reactions.

Even if it occurs more rarely, *acromegaly* must be mentioned and included in the differential diagnosis. Sleep apnea syndromes are found in about 60% of the patients suffering from acromegaly; obstructive sleep apnea especially is relevant. An increase of the pharyngeal soft tissue seems to be responsible for the development of obstructive sleep apnea in the context of acromegaly. If the typical clinical symptoms of acromegaly become apparent (coarsening of the facial characteristics, increased ring and shoe size, hyperhidrosis, etc.), adequate endocrinological examination has to be performed.

Diabetes mellitus is the most frequent metabolic disease and is associated in a number of ways with sleep-related disorders, in particular with obstructive sleep apnea. Both phenomena frequently occur together in the context of metabolic syndrome. Furthermore, however, obstructive sleep apnea is currently increasingly understood as an independent risk factor for insulin resistance. There are hints that diabetic autonomous neuropathy may lead to an impairment of the breath-synchronized innervation of the muscular dilator muscles of the upper airways.

10.1.2.2 Cardiovascular Diseases

Cardiac arrhythmia may lead to insomnia not only because of tachycardia at nighttime but it can also induce consecutive deterioration of cardiac output: this mainly affects patients suffering from preexisting bradycardial arrhythmia.

An according reduction of the physical activity that may manifest as fatigue or sleepiness with morning waking difficulties is also observed in other diseases accompanied by *hypotension* (e.g., heart failure). Frequently, according symptoms are also found in the context of antihypertensive therapy when undesired low blood pressure results or the patients are not yet adapted to the changed (actually normotensive) blood pressure at the beginning of treatment.

Notwithstanding the foregoing, *heart failure* is regularly associated with sleep-related breathing disorders and may induce central as well as obstructive respiratory disorders. In this context, Cheyne-Stokes respiration represents the classic disorder (see ▶ Chap. 4).

It should be a routinely asked question in sleep-related history taking if the patient suffers from cardiovascular diseases or takes *medication* accordingly. In cases of suspected findings, blood pressure and heart rate should be measured; if necessary, a 24-h record of blood pressure should be initiated.

10.1.2.3 Respiratory Diseases

Chronic respiratory diseases such as *bronchial asthma* or *chronic obstructive pulmonary disease* are often associated with sleep-related breathing disorders. These conditions alone may lead to a sleep-related hypoventilation syndrome (► Sect. 4.1); as comorbidity, however, they frequently aggravate preexisting sleep apnea because of the low pulmonary reserve. In those cases, the diagnosis and treatment of respiratory disorders can be considered as causal therapy of a sleep-related hypoventilation syndrome; also in the context of sleep apnea syndromes, however, a concomitant respiratory disorder should be treated to achieve an optimal therapeutic outcome.

10.1.2.4 Renal Dysfunction

Patients with advanced renal dysfunction often suffer from sleep disorders regularly accompanied by symptoms of daytime sleepiness. In the context of chronic uremia and renal replacement therapy, sleep disorders are reported in as many as 80% of the cases, but they can occur in earlier stages of renal dysfunction.

Besides *disorders of initiating and maintaining sleep*, mainly the following sleep disorders are associated with renal dysfunction:

- *Restless legs syndrome* or *periodic leg movements during sleep*
- Central as well as obstructive *sleep apnea syndrome*

Among others, uremia as well as an associated iron deficiency or associated anemia seem to be responsible for concomitant complaints of restless legs.

The triggering mechanism for the development of central sleep apnea syndromes in this context is not finally clarified; however, disorders of central and peripheral chemosensitivity are increasingly discussed. Furthermore, metabolic disorders are considered responsible for central respiratory regulation disturbances.

Regarding the incidence of obstructive sleep apnea, a narrowing of the upper airway seems also to be responsible.

Concomitant sleep disorders frequently lead to an additional impairment of the patients' quality of life and the clinical course of the underlying disorder. In this context, especially, sleep apnea syndromes are significant, not only because of their incidence but also because of the already described negative effects on cardiovascular morbidity and mortality. Even if concomitant sleep disorders regularly improve after transplantation, the incidence of sleep disorders in transplanted patients remains increased compared to healthy individuals.

Often, associated clinical symptoms such as daytime sleepiness, concentration problems, difficulties of initiating and maintaining sleep, fatigue, and impaired activity are only considered as accompanying symptoms of renal dysfunction. Because effective therapeutic options are available, however, possibly coexisting sleep disorders should be taken into account and adequately diagnosed. Appropriate treatment often improves the quality of life of the affected patients.

10.2 Sleep Disorders and Mental Disorders

In a major portion of the patients, mental disorders such as depression, schizophrenia, or anxiety are associated with sleep disorders. This fact is taken into account in the current version of the *Diagnostic and Statistical Manual of Mental Disorders* of the American Psychiatric Association (DSM-5) by including not only insomnia, circadian rhythm sleep–wake disorders, and hypersomnia in the chapter about sleep disorders but also narcolepsy, sleep apnea syndrome, and restless legs syndrome, explicitly indicating that sleep disorders should be diagnosed in addition to the underlying mental disorder. Because those mental disorders are highly important for the differential diagnosis of insomnia and hypersomnia disorders, they are discussed in this chapter according to their manifestation (insomnia versus hypersomnia complaints).

The close correlation between mental disorders and sleep disorders implies that the question regarding current or previous mental disorders must be included in the sleep history. In particular, the presence of current depressive symptoms and the intake of psychotropic drugs must be clarified. On the other hand, research clearly shows that mood disorders, for example, are more often found in patients with restless legs syndrome and sleep apnea syndrome than in the normal population. Thus, screening with regard to mental disorders is highly important for patients presenting in a sleep center with the main complaint of sleep problems. After therapy of the sleep disorder, those patients should then possibly be referred to an appropriate specialist.

In this context, the following disorders are of major relevance:

- *Insomnia* complaints:
  - Affective disorders
  - Anxiety disorders
  - Posttraumatic stress disorder (PTSD)
- *Hypersomnia* complaints:
  - Atypical or seasonal affective disorder
  - Chronic schizophrenia

It must be taken into account that patients present to sleep centers who might still suffer from significant insomnia or hypersomnia complaints even though the underlying mental disorder has been treated successfully. In those cases, additional diagnostic procedures are required to assess comorbid sleep disorders.

10.2.1 Insomnia Complaints as Symptom of Mental Disorders

10.2.1.1 Affective Disorders

Affective disorders are very common. Depending on the study, the lifetime prevalence of depression amounts to 10% to 25% in females and 5% to 12% in males. Three major subgroups are classified:

- Unipolar depression (episode(s) corresponding to the criteria of major depression)
- Bipolar affective disorder
- Dysthymia

According to the DSM-5 (*Diagnostic and Statistical Manual of Mental Disorders*), an episode of *major depression* is characterized by depressed mood observed on nearly all days and for most of the day as well as a clearly reduced interest or significantly reduced pleasure in all or nearly all activities (also across most situations similar to depressive mood). This criterion of permanence is important for clinical evaluation to clearly differentiate between normal emotional changes or mood swings and depressive symptomatology.

Practical Tip

Important question for history taking: "Do you sometimes experience sad or depressive moods?"

Unipolar depressions are affective disorders wherein the patients do not experience manic phases. They represent the main category of affective disorders.

Patients experiencing depressive and manic phases are classified as *bipolar*. Manic phases are characterized by high moods; often increased activity and a reduced need of sleep are observed. Patients may lose social inhibitions; they have inflated self-esteem or grandiosity and carelessly spend large amounts of money.

Dysthymia is a less severe mood disorder. According to diagnostic criteria, it has to persist for at least 2 years.

The key symptoms of affective disorders, sleeplessness or increased sleep nearly all days/nights, are often explicitly mentioned in the diagnostic criteria of affective disorders. Hypersomnia complaints, which are mainly present in atypical or seasonal affective disorder, are discussed in the following paragraph.

Early morning awakening (at least 2 h before the usual time to get up) is one main sleep problem in depressive patients with melancholia (also show very low mood in the morning). However, depressive patients also suffer from disorders of initiating and maintaining sleep that are comparable to complaints of insomnia patients. Because chronic insomnia may lead to affective disorders for example, dysthymia, it is necessary to evaluate which symptoms had occurred first. Simultaneous occurring of the symptoms indicates that the sleep problems are part of the affective disorder. However, in this context, it should be kept in mind that the sleep disorder may persist after cessation of the depressive complaints.

With regard to the treatment of depression, presenting the symptom of sleep problems is important in selecting the *medication*. Often a combined treatment with an activating medication, for example, a selective serotonin reuptake inhibitor, in the morning and a sedating antidepressant, such as mirtazapine or trimipramine, in the evening is prescribed for patients with severe sleep disorders. In patients with long-term medication, it must be also taken into consideration that many antidepressants can increase periodic leg movements during sleep and cause restless legs complaints. As a consequence, patients might report nonrestorative sleep despite improvement of the depressive symptoms.

10.2.1.2 Anxiety Disorders

Anxiety disorders may also be associated with insomnia complaints. Up to 40% of patients with anxiety disorders also report sleep problems. Anxiety disorders are classified into these diagnostic groups:

- Panic disorder with or without agoraphobia
- Social phobia
- Specific phobias (e.g., arachnophobia)
- Generalized anxiety disorder

With regard to differential diagnosis of sleep disorders, the panic *disorder* must be taken into consideration especially when panic attacks occur solely at night. Although most patients experience panic attacks during the day (with occasional panic attacks at night), some patients only suffer from panic attacks at night during sleep. In this context, it is important to differentiate from the *nightmare* disorder or *night terrors* (pavor nocturnus). It is currently not clear which sleep stage precede those nocturnal panic attacks. Although sleep lab studies indicated that non-REM sleep might precede panic attacks, one study showed that panic attacks in the home setting may also occur after negative dreams, i.e., out of REM sleep.

Practical Tip

The major fear of the panic attack is experienced in the waking stage (dyspnea, sensation of suffocation, nausea, vertigo, or fear to lose control, to go crazy, or to die). In cases of night terror and nightmares, this fear usually ceases rapidly after waking up.

Interestingly, patients with nocturnal panic attacks often show a more severe anxiety disorder than patients who suffer solely from daytime panic attacks.

In general, *therapy of the underlying disorder* is of prime importance. A sedating antidepressant such as mirtazapine or trimipramine may help these patients in addition to psychotherapeutic treatment of the anxiety disorder.

10.2.1.3 Posttraumatic Stress Disorder

Posttraumatic stress disorder is mental disorder that has a strong connection to sleep medicine. Population surveys indicate a lifetime PTSD prevalence of 1% to 14%. For high-risk populations (war veterans, or victims of natural disasters, rape, abuse, or road accidents), the percentages are higher.

It is crucial for the diagnosis of this disorder to assess the occurrence of the traumatic experience(s) with impending death, severe injury, or danger for the physical integrity of oneself or another person. The impact of the trauma is seen in such effects as these:

- Recurring stressful memories
- Avoiding behavior regarding situations that might trigger flashbacks
- Reduced affect
- Negative view of the future

Two common symptoms relate to sleep. First, there are *recurrent dreams*. About 50% of these reflect the traumatic experience more or less exactly. Recent findings indicate show that non-trauma-related nightmares can also cause severe disstress. Although the etiology is different from that of idiopathic nightmares (▶ Sect. 7.3.2), *imagery rehearsal therapy* can be helpful for patients suffering from posttraumatic nightmares (▶ Sect. 7.3.8). Because the dropout rate of women after sexual abuse was very high in a large clinical trial, it is recommended to use nightmare-related interventions as add-ons to standard psychotherapeuty of posttraumatic stress disorder.

Second is the *hyperarousal complex* (e.g., hypervigilance, excessive shock reaction, irritability) includes explicitly disorders of initiating and maintaining sleep. A few studies indicate that sleep-related breathing disorders and periodic leg movements during sleep occur more frequently in patients with posttraumatic stress disorder compared to the general population, i.e., it is recommended that these patients undergo careful sleep anamnesis and if needed also polygraphy and/or polysomnography (PSG).

10.2.2 Hypersomnia Complaints as Symptom of Mental Disorders

10.2.2.1 Atypical or Seasonal Affective Disorder

In cases of *depressive disorders with atypical characteristics*, hypersomnia complaints are often reported. Other symptoms of depressive disorders with atypical characteristics are these:

- Increased appetite or weight gain
- Hypersensitive to rejection

The atypical symptoms (hypersomnia complaints, increased appetite) occur in addition to the symptoms that are typical for depression (mood swings, loss of interest, etc.). Young depressive patients are more often affected by atypical depression than older patients. However, in total, the atypical syndromes are rare, with an incidence of less than 10% of all depressive patients.

The atypical symptoms are quite frequent seasonal affective disorders. Seasonal affective disorders can only be diagnosed if at least two phases occur clearly in relationship to a season (most often fall/winter).

Depression with atypical symptoms is an important differential diagnosis for primary hypersomnia, i.e., patients should be asked about the possible presence of depressive (typical and atypical) symptoms. In addition, the MSLT may provide further diagnostic evidence because patients with atypical depression spend much time in bed but do not sleep much during this time. Long sleep latencies in the MSLT may indicate atypical depression and explain the subjectively hypersomnia complaints of the patient.

With regard to therapy, it must be considered that a significant percentage of patients with seasonal affective depression (between 30% and 60%) respond positively to *light therapy* (30 min in the morning and 30 min in the evening with a light intensity of 10,000 lux).

10.2.2.2 Schizophrenia

Although schizophrenic patients often suffer from problems of initiating and maintaining sleep in the prodromal phase or during an acute productive phase (in these phases the treatment of schizophrenia is in the prime focus so that sleep-related diagnostic and therapeutic interventions can only be appropriately performed after positive symptoms have subsided), hypersomnia complaints may found in chronic schizophrenic patients with long-term medication with neuroleptics.

Often, those complaints are explained by the sedating effect of the medication and are not properly evaluated. However, experiences from our practice show that sleep-related diagnostic procedures should be initiated in cases of severe daytime sleepiness in patients with schizophrenia.

Case Report

A young schizophrenic patient presented in the sleep clinic because he sometimes fell asleep during occupational therapy sessions.

Because of neuroleptic medication, he has significantly gained weight (which is a frequent side effect), and being asked, he reported increasing daytime sleepiness in the previous weeks. He was not able to provide information about possible snoring at nighttime or the occurrence of nocturnal sleep apnea episodes because he slept alone. Subsequent polygraphy showed a moderate obstructive sleep apnea and daytime sleepiness was significantly improved after starting CPAP therapy.

In addition to developing a sleep-related breathing disorder due to weight gain during treatment with neuroleptics, there is the problem that those substances affect the dopaminergic system. Side effects due to the occurrence of periodic leg movements during sleep causing sleep problems and nonrestorative sleep may result. If possible, reduction of the neuroleptic dose is recommended. As compensation, up to 600 mg valproic acid may be applied at night. Positive effects are reported in the literature about low-dose dopamine antagonists (ropinirole or pramipexole) without re-occurrence of positive symptoms (delusion, hallucinations) in those patients. By increasing the cerebral dopamine concentration, this might be a possible complication in the treatment of schizophrenic patients.

Case Report

A young female patient with borderline personality disorder was presented in the sleep laboratory with disorders of initiating and maintaining sleep. Treatment with a benzodiazepine receptor antagonist (zopiclone) could not improve the complaints, so the patient was treated with a neuroleptic (Pipamperone) at night. Despite subjective improvement of sleep, the patient reports significant hypersomnia complaints.

Polysomnographic measurements indicated a very high index of periodic leg movements during sleep that subsided after discontinuing of the neuroleptic. That is, the hypersomnia complaint has occurred as a side effect of the neuroleptic medication that was originally applied as sleeping aid.

Treatment with trimipramine led to a positive effect on sleep quality and restorative sleep.

Because of possible side effects of many psychopharmaceuticals (gain in weight, periodic leg movements during sleep), it is necessary that patients who receive long-term medication and report hypersomnia complaints undergo sleep diagnostics.

10.3 Questions

? 1. Please indicate the most important organic diseases that must be taken into consideration in the differential diagnosis of sleep disorders.

? 2. What are the most important mental disorders that play a major role in the differential diagnosis of insomnia, hypersomnia, and parasomnias?

Sleep Disorders in Children

A. A. Schlarb and B. A. Stuck

B. A. Stuck et al., *Practice of Sleep Medicine*, https://doi.org/10.1007/978-3-030-17412-5_11

Sleep disorders in childhood occur rather frequently. Many typical sleep disorders of adults are already prevalent in childhood or adolescence; others occur typically or exclusively in childhood. Insomnia disorders with difficulties of initiating and/or maintaining sleep are particularly frequent in preschool and primary school children as well as in adolescents. Parasomnia complaints such as night terror (pavor nocturnus) and nightmares are also frequently observed in children. The treatment of sleep disorders in children and adolescents is different from that of adults and should be adjusted according to age. This chapter also discusses sleep-related breathing disorders in children, with a special emphasis on pediatric obstructive sleep apnea. Even if the clinical presentation and the pathophysiology of obstructive sleep-related breathing disorders in children and adults are very similar, their treatment differs in various aspects.

11.1 Sleep Disorders in Children and Adolescents

For the development of children and adolescents, sufficient duration of sleep is essential. Thus, besides nutrition and physical activity, as well as regeneration, sleep is considered as a pillar of health. Many children and adolescents, however, do not sleep sufficiently. Other activities in the evening, such as watching television, playing computer games, or being active in social media, often deprive them of sleep without intention. However, lack of sleep has significant consequences for the psychological and physical development of children and adolescents as well as for their performance in school.

11.1.1 Sleep and Sleep Development of Childhood and Adolescence

11.1.1.1 Development of Sleep

The sleep of newborns is clearly different from that of an adult. After only about 6 months, however, the infants adapt, and their sleep becomes more and more slowly similar to that of an adult. Thus, in newborns the difference is seen between active sleep (AS), which is interpreted as an immature type of the so-called rapid eye movement (REM) sleep, and the quiet sleep (QS) that corresponds to the later deep sleep. Those phases that cannot be clearly assigned are defined as indeterminate sleep (IS).

In infants a few weeks old, active sleep represents the highest percentage of their overall sleep time, approximately 60%. This percentage is reduced in the course of development; at the age of 6 months, active sleep amounts to about 25% of the overall sleep and further decreases thereafter. ◘ Figure 11.1 graphically displays the changes.

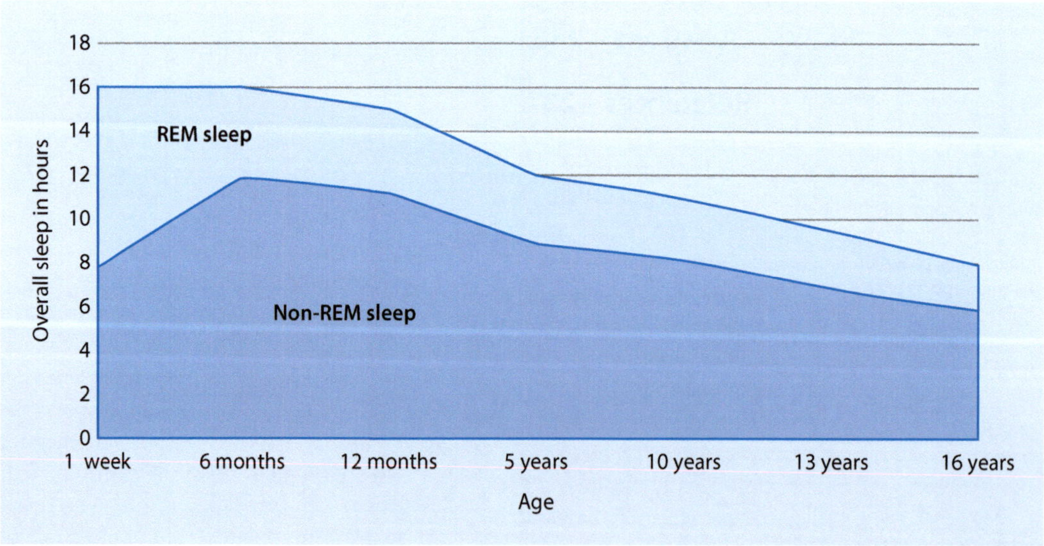

◘ **Fig. 11.1** Development of sleep duration and distribution of rapid eye movement (REM) sleep and non-REM sleep depending on age (adapted from to Roffwarg et al. 1966)

As well as sleep duration and the sleep architecture, the length of a sleep cycle also changes. In infants, it is much shorter, 45 to 60 min, compared to adults whose sleep cycle encompasses 80 to 120 min. Furthermore, the respective sleep time until the next longer wake phase amounts to only 2 to 4 h. The following figure depicts the described changes (◘ Fig. 11.2).

Sleep develops from the polyphasic sleep rhythm to the biphasic rhythm and finally to the monophasic sleep rhythm (◘ Fig. 11.3). With maturation and alteration of the sleep–wake rhythm of the child, erroneous associations of initiating or reinitiating sleep may be learned. Instead of sleep-related self-regulation, the infant learns that sleep is only possible under certain circumstances and strongly requests these for initiating or reinitiating sleep (e.g., in the parent's arms, in the presence of one parent, one parent sitting at the bedside, or falling asleep with a baby bottle).

11.1.1.2 Sleep Duration

The following graph shows approximately how much sleep is needed on average, depending on age (◘ Fig. 11.4). Young children, of the age of 3 to

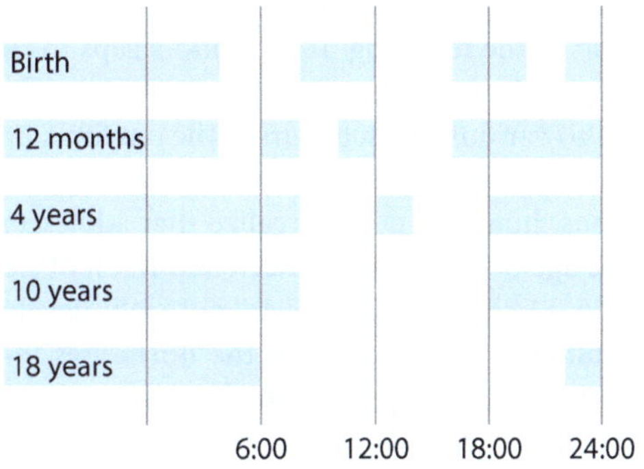

◘ **Fig. 11.2** Age-dependent changes of the distribution of sleep and wake episodes during 24 h (based on Borbély 2004)

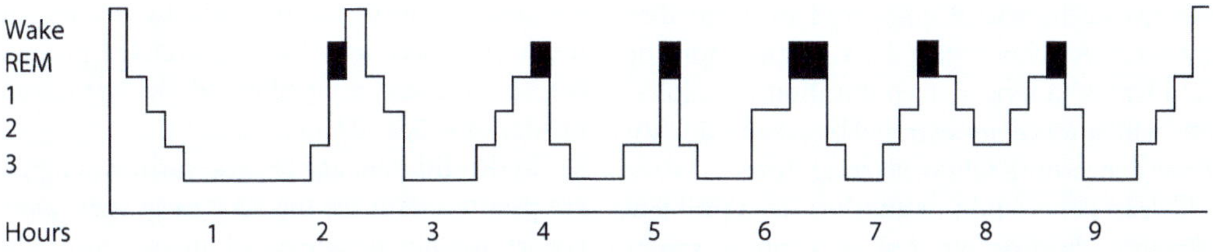

◘ **Fig. 11.3** Exemplary display of the sleep architecture in childhood

◘ **Fig. 11.4** Reported sleep duration according to the study results of an investigation of childhood and adolescent health in Germany, depending on the age of the children and adolescents, based on parents' reports or self-reports, respectively. *Dotted lines* represent standard deviation (SD) (according to Schlarb et al. [22])

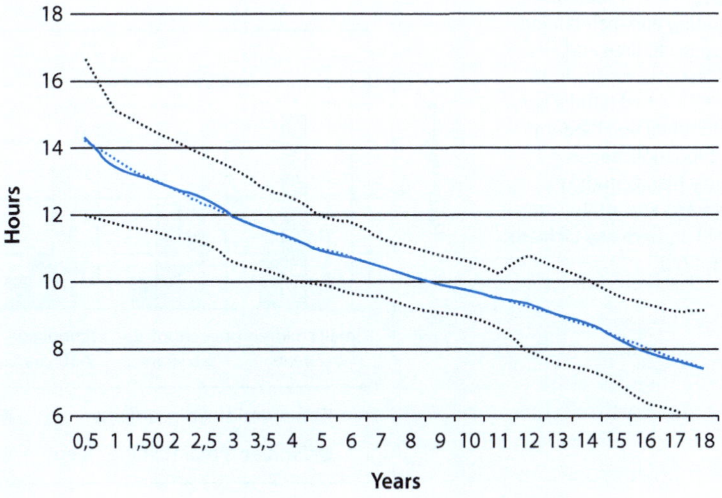

4 years, need about 11.5 h of sleep; the necessary sleep time at night continuously declines to approximately 10.5 h until the age of 7 years. During primary school, the average sleep duration decreases again, to 9.5 h, until the age of 10 years. The sleep profile of children reveals that a deep sleep phase takes place directly before waking up in the morning. If the child sleeps insufficiently, this deep sleep phase is omitted, which leads to various impacts during the daytime.

Many adolescents and adults, as well as pediatricians, however, do not realize that adolescents at the age of 13 years also need about 9 h of sleep (Fig. 11.4). During puberty, not only developmental changes are seen on the hormones level; melatonin as a sleep-inducing hormone is generally released later. Adolescents become tired later in the evening and thus go to bed later. However, school still starts early in the morning, and the consequences of short sleep duration are reported as reduced daytime alertness of adolescents. Thus, because of their delayed sleep onset, many adolescents do not get enough sleep and show poorer performance in school compared to when they are rested. A school start later in the morning would lead to a longer sleep duration for adolescents, which was demonstrated by several investigations concerning school starting times.

If sleep deprivation or another sleep problem is present, children often show daytime symptoms that are similar to attention deficit disorders. In addition, some become aggressive, and others have significantly impaired school performance. As well as neurocognitive limitations, however, a permanent lack of sleep also seems to be associated with the sequelae of a delayed cerebral maturation so that the development of behavioral control and emotion regulation may be impaired or delayed. Other studies reveal that children and adolescents suffering from sleep deprivation or sleep disorders have altered cortisol release and respond to stressing events with an increased or reduced cortisol reactivity compared to healthy individuals. Thus, sleep deprivation and sleep complaints may even change the hormone balance.

Practical Tip

To assess the individually needed sleep duration, a sleep diary should be conducted for about 14 days during the holidays. The child or adolescent should be allowed to sleep as long as desired during this period.

For assessment of the individually needed sleep duration as well as other sleep-related problems, see also the recommendations for further diagnostics in ▶ Sect. 11.1.6.

In the different age phases, various symptoms are predominant. At the very early ages, parents report mainly problems of maintaining sleep, but at the time of entering school problems of initiating sleep more prevalent (Fig. 11.5). Because sleep problems in childhood and ado-

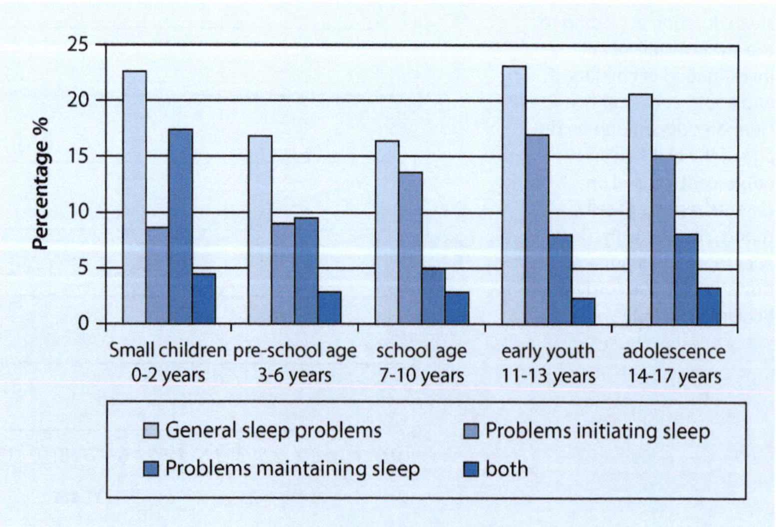

Fig. 11.5 Problems of initiating and maintaining sleep in children and adolescents: results from the KiGGS trial (Studie zur Gesundheit von Kindern und Jugendlichen in Deutschland; Study on children's and adolescents' health in Germany (Schlarb et al. [22])

lescence are more likely to chronify, an early intervention is reasonable and necessary.

11.1.1.3 Parents' Behavior and Impact of Children's Sleep Disorders on Parents

Not only does the child experience the consequences of sleep deprivation or sleep complaints, but the family is also usually involved. After the child's birth, parents generally show changed sleep patterns. Mothers have reduced overall sleep time in comparison to the last third of their pregnancy; for both parents, time awake at night and the incidence of waking up in the nighttime are increased compared to the period of pregnancy. However, this is especially true for the mothers and less so for fathers. Parents frequently suffer greatly because of the infant's sleep problems, which is seen in the increased depressiveness of mothers of young children as well as from their own sleep deprivation. The severity and persistence of infant sleep problems are influenced by the mother's perception to set limits to the child's actions. Other factors are the child's nervous temperament, anxiety of the mother, ambivalent bonding, and intensive active calming such as immediately taking the baby from its bed when awake. Those factors may negatively influence the self-regulation of the sleep–wake rhythm of the child. Thus, during pregnancy, as a prevention not only sleep-related education but also the parents' sleep-related cognitions are discussed to strengthen the parents' ability to handle possible infant sleep problems (see ▶ Sect. 11.1.9).

To what extent parents influence their child's sleep, in particular in early childhood, by their behavior becomes clear by the early application of active calming that may clearly affect the child's sleep. It is thought that too rapid active intervention of the patients in problems of initiating sleep or waking up at nighttime may impede the child's development or consolidation of self-soothing competence. In contrast, autonomy-enhancing educational strategies, emotional availability, and rituals when going to bed have a calming effect and lead to a high quality of sleep for the child. Thus, the availability of sleep-related educational strategies for parents an important aspect of healthy sleep behavior in young children.

If the child suffers from sleep problems or disorders, most often the parents also experience significantly impaired sleep. They wake up more frequently at night and often report insufficient and disturbed sleep. Parental sleep deprivation is then often associated with increased stress experiences, a deteriorated state of physical health, as well as an increased risk to develop anxiety disorder or depression, which applies especially for mothers.

As well as the consequences for physical and psychological health, parental partnership is also often affected by these sleep problems. Satisfaction of the partners' relationship is considered to be less when their child does not sleep well. Often, conceptions of the couple regarding the correct strategy for the child's sleep problems differ, which may lead to nighttime disagreements. Thus, unsatisfactory relationships and problems or conflicts of the couple as well as aggression in the partnership are often associated with infant sleep problems.

It should also be taken into consideration that interaction problems with the child occur because the sleep deprivation of the parents may also impair their educational competence, and as a consequence, anger and feeling upset as well as helplessness may come up. In addition, the impaired educational competence of the parents not only becomes apparent at night but is also obvious during the daytime.

11.1.2 Sleep Disorders of Childhood and Adolescence

The most important sleep disorders in childhood and adolescence include insomnia, parasomnia, sleep-related movement disorders, sleep–wake rhythm disorders, and sleep-related breathing disorders. In this chapter, these diseases are presented with a special focus on insomnia complaints. In this context, it should be noted that earlier chapters are dedicated to parasomnia (see ▶ Chap. 7), movement disorders (see ▶ Chap. 8), and sleep-related breathing disorders in childhood (see ▶ Sect. 11.2).

Frequent Disorders in Childhood and Adolescence

- Insomnia (disorders of initiating and maintaining sleep)
- Nightmares
- Night terror (pavor nocturnus)
- Sleep-related movement disorders
- Sleep-wake rhythm disorders
- Sleep-related breathing disorders

11.1.2.1 Insomnia in Childhood and Adolescence

Acute Insomnia/Short-Term Insomnia

According to ICSD-3, a short-term insomnia with problems of initiating or maintaining sleep in children and adolescents is generally classified as pathological and sleep disturbed when the duration of initiating or reinitiating sleep is extended (orientation value, 20–30 min), when the child resists going to bed at the scheduled time, wakes up early in the morning, or needs the parents' help to go to sleep, and when all these concerns have appeared several times per week (at least three times per week) during the past months. The child or adolescent suffers from impairment during the day such as fatigue, daytime sleepiness, concentration or memory problems, or problems with school performance, and emotional irritability, behavioral problems (e.g., hyperactivity, impulsiveness, aggressiveness), reduced energy or motivation, an increased number of accidents, or dissatisfaction with sleep. The reported sleep problems, however, cannot be explained only by insufficient possibilities (e.g., there is not enough time to sleep) or adverse circumstances (e.g., insecure, bright, loud, or inappropriate environment).

Diagnostic Criteria of Insomnia in Childhood and Adolescence

- At least one of the following symptoms must be present several times per week:
  - Prolonged duration of initiating or reinitiating sleep.
  - Resistance when going to bed.
  - The child needs parental help or support to initiate or reinitiate sleep.
  - Impaired daytime alertness such as sleepiness, hyperactivity, behavioral disorders, or learning difficulties is observed.
- The sleep problems are not caused by insufficient possibilities or adverse circumstances.
- The sleep problems cannot be explained by another sleep disorder, medical, neurological, or psychological disease, drug intake, or substance abuse.

Chronic Insomnia

If these sleep problems and their consequences persist over 3 months, chronic insomnia is diagnosed. The DSM-5 also includes the age-specific problems of children and adolescents and states that the problems have to occur at least three times per week during 3 months (DSM-5, 2013).

11.1.2.2 Sleep-Related Movement Disorders in Childhood

Periodic movement disorders such as stereotypic head banging, head rolling, or body rolling in particular occur in childhood. The movements start shortly before falling asleep or during sleep and are sometimes accompanied by noises. For diagnosis, video clips recorded by the parents, for example, with a smartphone, may be helpful by showing typical movement behavior. If possible, an examination should be performed in the sleep laboratory (see ► Chap. 2). In severe cases, behavioral therapy is indicated.

In the context of restless legs syndrome (also known as Wittmaack-Ekbom syndrome), children or adolescents report uncomfortable movement sensations of the legs (for further description of the symptoms and treatment recommendations, see ► Chap. 8). The resulting sleep deprivation generally leads to daytime sleepiness, symptoms of hyperactivity, and cognitive performance impairment such as difficulties with concentration.

11.1.2.3 Sleep–Wake Rhythm Disorders

The key problem of sleep–wake rhythm disorders is the discrepancy between one's inner clock and environmental time. The child or adolescent is able to sleep, but not at the "normal" times. Children and adolescents then have respective problems with getting up at "normal times" (i.e., at 7 AM). One frequently observed consequence is the absence from school or sleeping at school and a lack of attention. In adolescence, such a shift may be caused mainly by activities in social networks, phone calls, or meeting friends late in the evening. Because of the blue-light portion of computer screens, for example, release of the sleep-inducing hormone melatonin is delayed. Furthermore, often the production of the stress hormone cortisol is changed, which is associated with later sleep onset. Based on this rhythm alteration the symptoms of adolescents are frequently called social jetlag.

Delayed Sleep Phase Syndrome

Affected children or adolescents show relevantly delayed times of going to bed and arising for at least 3 months, accompanied by an inability to fall asleep or to wake up at a desired or requested time. If the child or the adolescent is allowed to follow his/her individual need or rhythm of sleep, sleep quality and age-related sleep duration improve with a continuously delayed 24-h sleep–wake pattern. The sleep-related problems should be documented by means of sleep diaries and, whenever possible, actigraphy, each for at least 7 and more than 15 days, respectively. Delay of the normal sleep phases is then detected. Workdays or schooldays as well as holidays have to be taken into consideration in this diagnostic phase. Effects of such sleep problems are often absence from school or relevantly reduced school achievements.

Advanced Sleep Phase Syndrome

This syndrome is defined by advancing the main sleep phase for at least 3 months relative to the desired or requested sleep and waking time. This diagnosis becomes apparent by chronic or recurrent difficulties to stay awake until the desired or requested time, associated with an inability to sleep until the desired or requested wakeup time. Further criteria and procedures regarding the diagnosis correspond to the delayed sleep phase syndrome.

Irregular Sleep–Wake Rhythm

The patient or contact person reports a pattern of irregular sleep and wake episodes during the 24-h day that persists or recurs for at least 3 months. Insomnia symptoms are observed at the planned time of sleep onset (mostly at night) or excessive sleepiness occurs during the day. Further criteria and procedures in the context of diagnosis correspond to the delayed sleep phase syndrome.

In particular, adolescents and young adults such as university students suffer from these disorders of the sleep phases, especially from the problems of delayed sleep phases. One risk factor in this context is media consumption or the possibility of organizing one's rhythm freely (studies). The structured and stepwise adaptation to the appropriate time of going to bed is the procedure of choice. Such elements are implemented, for example, in the training concept for adolescents.

11.1.2.4 Hypersomnia

Even if night sleep is perceived as restorative by children and adolescents, they fall asleep during the day without wanting to do so or being able to avoid sleep. The symptoms are mostly associated with significant negative effects on school and leisure time. The main characteristic is an excessive daytime sleepiness with sleep attacks. If no physiological origin is found for the sleep problems, the exclusion of psychological disorders also is recommended.

Two subtypes of childhood hypersomnia are differentiated:

- Idiopathic hypersomnia with long sleep durations
- Idiopathic hypersomnia without long sleep durations
  - In general, these disorders occur rarely compared to insomnia or nightmares. ▶ Chapter 5 covers hypersomnia complaints more comprehensively.

11.1.2.5 Sleep Disorders and Psychological Disorders

Sleep problems or disorders also appear in the context of or in comorbidity with psychological disorders. Frequently, sleep problems play a key role in cases of anxiety disorders, depressive disorders, attention deficit disorders, and even in conduct disorders (CD). Up to 52% of the children and adolescents with insomnia also have psychological diseases. Such comorbid symptoms should imperatively be taken into account because they most frequently enhance the symptoms and significantly impair the quality of life of the child or adolescent.

Anxiety Disorders and Sleep Problems

Children suffering from anxiety disorders and children with separation anxieties display sleep problems more frequently. Emotionally unsure children often need their parents to initiate or reinitiate sleep at night. With their distress associated with the separation situation, the children experience a physiological arousal, which then significantly impairs reinitiating sleep. Typically, those sleep problems are observed in the context of anxiety disorders between the ages of 6 and 20 months. The child tries to avoid being alone and thus also sleeping alone. About 90% of the children with separation anxiety display at least one sleep problem.

Depression and Sleep Problems

Another group of internalized disorders that are often associated with sleep complaints in childhood are depressive diseases. Although such disorders only rarely occur in early childhood, many adolescents show severe symptoms of depression. Often the affected children or adolescents report sleep problems. Besides difficulties of initiating and maintaining sleep, often also an increased need for sleep is observed with the simultaneous perception of not feeling rested. Adolescents report typical concerns and negative cognitions frequently. However, those cognitions and feelings are not limited only to sleep but are comprehensive with regard to the future, the world and environment, and one's own self (cognitive triad). Increasingly occurring nightmares are considered as an important factor for the development of suicidal thoughts and suicide attempts of adolescents.

Posttraumatic Stress Disorders and Sleep Problems

Experiencing traumatic events leads to severe symptoms, not only in adults. Younger children of preschool age generally show not only clear avoidance and anxiety behavior but also especially frequent nightmares and sleep disorders, in particular disorders of initiating and maintaining sleep. Approximately 70% of the children and adolescents with PTSD suffer from recurrent nightmares. Both sleep disorders (insomnia and nightmares) are attributed to changed hyperarousal that counteracts relaxing and thus also falling asleep.

Attention-Deficit/Hyperactivity Disorder and Sleep Problems

Parents of children suffering from attention-deficit/hyperactivity disorder (ADHD) often report the high level of activity of their children and respective problems in the context of going to bed. Furthermore, these children frequently suffer from daytime sleepiness and insomnia symptoms. Besides these problems, increased snoring is observed in some of those children (2.2 times more frequently than in healthy individuals). Occasionally a correlation of lack of sleep, daytime sleepiness, hyperactivity, and inattentiveness is discussed because tired children show similar behavior as children with ADHD symptoms. The vicious circle of sleep pressure (◘ Fig. 11.6) tries to describe this dynamism. In comparison to healthy children, children with ADHD often suffer from continuously recurring sleep–wake problems with alternating problems of initiating sleep, sleep duration, and sleep efficiency. Considering the subtypes of ADHD, children with hyperactive-impulsive symptoms show the most severe sleep complaints, whereas children with predominantly inattentive behavior rather suffer from daytime sleepiness, nightmares, and unwillingness to go to bed. Children with mixed symptoms (hyperactivity and inattentiveness), however, more frequently suffer from sleep-related breathing disorders. Both subtypes (hyperactive and mixed symptoms) are often accompanied by waking up early in the morning in contrast to attention-impaired children.

Emotion Regulation and Sleep

Lack of sleep is often attended by a depressed mood and reduced capacity of adaptation in the context of emotional events. A higher level of daytime sleepiness in children is associated with negative emotional reactivity, low frustration level, as well as less positive emotional reactivity. Children who are sleep deprived, or sleep less than they need, are more irritable and more rapidly frustrated. Sleep deprivation not only reduces the positive affections of children and adolescents but also increases anxiety. Good quality of sleep, however, is associated with emotional balance.

Aggression and Sleep

Not only sleep deprivation but also insomnia symptoms and nightmares are closely related to the increased aggressive behavior of children and adolescents. Children sleeping less than needed and suffering therefore from sleep deprivation, cannot control their frustrations very well, and are more likely to show aggressive symptoms in cases of frustration. Although this is expressed in children as crying and tantrum, older children

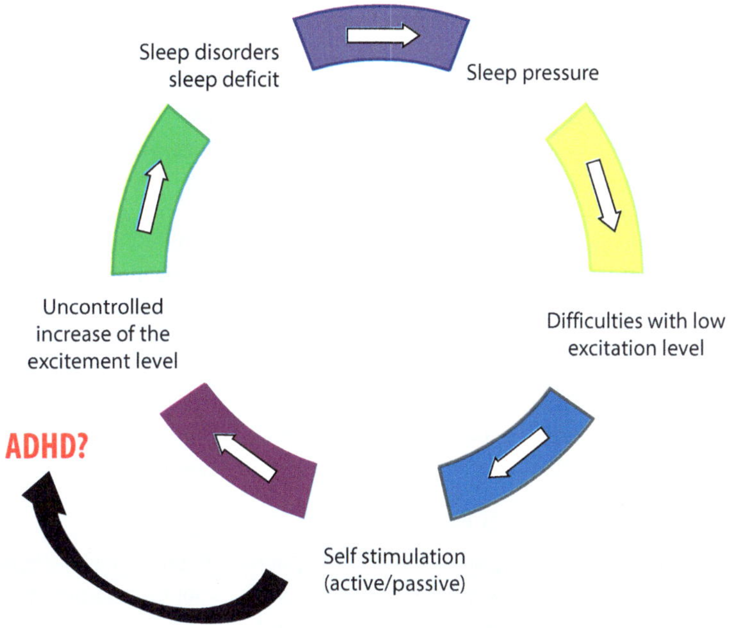

Fig. 11.6 Vicious circle of sleep pressure in children and adolescents suffering from attention-deficit/hyperactivity disorder (ADHD) symptoms (adapted from Rabenschlag 2001)

are often aggressive toward their peers or may damage objects. Auto-aggressive behavior, up to even suicidal developments, may be summarized under this phenomenon. These behaviors predominantly occur in adolescence.

Autism and Sleep

Autism, a severe development disorder displayed by deficits of social interaction and communication as well as limited repetitive behavioral patterns, is a rare disease with relationship to anxiety or depressive disorders. Children with autism spectrum disorders clearly suffer more frequently from sleep problems than healthy individuals, with a prevalence of 80%. The most frequent disorders are insomnias (80%) and parasomnias (53%). A higher portion of sleep problems is generally associated with reduced daytime alertness and functionality, with more externalized problem behavior, and with more, and more severe autism symptoms.

11.1.2.6 Sleep Disorders and Other Comorbid Disorders

Epilepsy and Sleep

Children and adolescents with epilepsy often suffer from sleep problems. Most frequently, these children and adolescents suffer from sleep-related breathing disorders, waking up at night, and excessive daytime sleepiness. A higher rate of parasomnias, shorter sleep duration, reduced efficiency of sleep, and sleep-related anxiety are also found to a larger extent in epileptic children. The consequences of sleep deprivation or daytime sleepiness can be seen in relationship to epileptic seizures. Furthermore, these sleep problems are closely related with the degree of seizure control.

Headaches and Sleep

Children who are affected by headaches also suffer from sleep problems more often than do healthy children. In addition, further psychological complaints and stress contribute to the maintenance of both problems. Some findings seem to confirm that both groups of complaints are based on common metabolic anomalies and neuroendocrine particularities, so that combined treatment of headaches and sleep seems to be reasonable. Although little is known about the effect of headache treatment on sleep problems or of sleep treatment on headaches in children, an implementation of this correlation in the therapy seems to be reasonable.

Atopic Dermatitis and Sleep

Atopic dermatitis (AD) or atopic eczema mostly occurs in early childhood and is associated with reduced quality of life for the affected children.

Children and adolescents with neurodermatitis suffer from sleep disorders more frequently than healthy peers. Several trials could show that children with atopic dermatitis often have a prolonged sleep-onset latency. Furthermore, they frequently reveal a reduced sleep duration and efficiency; that is, they sleep too little and the quality of their sleep is impaired. Also, sleep fragmentation often enhances the present symptoms of AD. In this context, it must be taken into account that the severity of the disease has a direct impact on the child's sleep. This kind of sleep impairment is then closely related to manifold impairments during daytime so that these children frequently report attention problems, problems with school achievements, and further consequences.

Functional Abdominal Pain and Sleep

The correlation of ambiguous abdominal pains and sleep has been investigated less intensively and does not seem to be so important as that of headache diseases and sleep in children and adolescents. Of children and adolescents who suffer from recurrent abdominal pain (RAP), only about 25% perceive their sleep as good, whereas nearly 90% of healthy individuals are satisfied with their sleep. Furthermore, children with RAP often (about 30%) report that abdominal pains occur before falling asleep or that they wake up at night because of these pains. These children suffer more severely from sleep problems, insomnia symptoms, and nightmares as well as increased daytime sleepiness compared to healthy children. It must be taken into consideration that objective data (actigraphy) do not reflect these observations. Overall, children with RAP have a significantly higher risk to develop sleep disorders. The inverse correlation is also true: children who regularly do not sleep well have a 2.8-fold risk to develop regular stomachaches than children with a high quality of sleep.

Chronic Inflammatory Bowel Disease and Sleep

Chronic inflammatory bowel diseases (IBD) are also associated with poorer quality of sleep. So far only a few trials have been published on Crohn's disease or ulcerative colitis and sleep in children and adolescents. These study results, however, indicate that according to the parents' reports, affected children and adolescents suffer significantly more often from sleep problems, nightmares, an increased need for sleep, and more daytime sleepiness compared to healthy peers. About 20% of adolescents with chronic IBD report sleep problems, and approximately 40% of them additionally suffer from anxiety problems and depressive symptoms, whereas only 16% of adolescents with chronic IBD without sleep problems reveal such emotional difficulties.

In summary, it can be stated that sleep disorders and comorbid disorders interact. As shown by the aforementioned comorbidities, these types of sleep disorders in these combinations tend to chronify. Sleep disorders in children and adolescents accompanied by psychological disorders such as depression, anxiety, ADHD, or also headaches, recurrent abdominal pain, irritable bowel syndrome, or chronic inflammatory bowel diseases are frequently observed and seem to reciprocally influence each other. An existing sleep disorder may increase the risk of psychological or somatic complaints by fourfold to even sevenfold.

11.1.3 Etiology and Pathophysiology

Sleep disorders in children and adolescents are influenced by various *multifactorial influencing factors*. Depending on the appearance of the disorder, sleep disorders have rather a physiological origin, or they result from manifold psychological and family-related influences. Children with chronic diseases (e.g., atopic dermatitis, rheumatic diseases, chronic headaches, chronic inflammatory bowel disease) are subject to other influencing factors compared to those with psychological disorders (anxiety disorders, ADHD, CD) or those without additional diseases. This correlation must be considered in the context of diagnosis and treatment. Furthermore, *age* is crucial concerning the influencing factors with regard to the origin and maintenance of sleep disorders. Factors such as the elimination of daytime sleep phases, immaturity of vigilance transitions, or physiological and development-associated changes of the NREM quantity of sleep may lead to increased occurrence of parasomnia in children 3 to 7 years old (see ▶ Chap. 7).

In young children with problems of initiating and maintaining sleep, for example, other factors may be effective compared to adolescents who also suffer from multiple puberty-associated factors. ◘ Figure 11.7 displays a model of influencing factors for children of young ages.

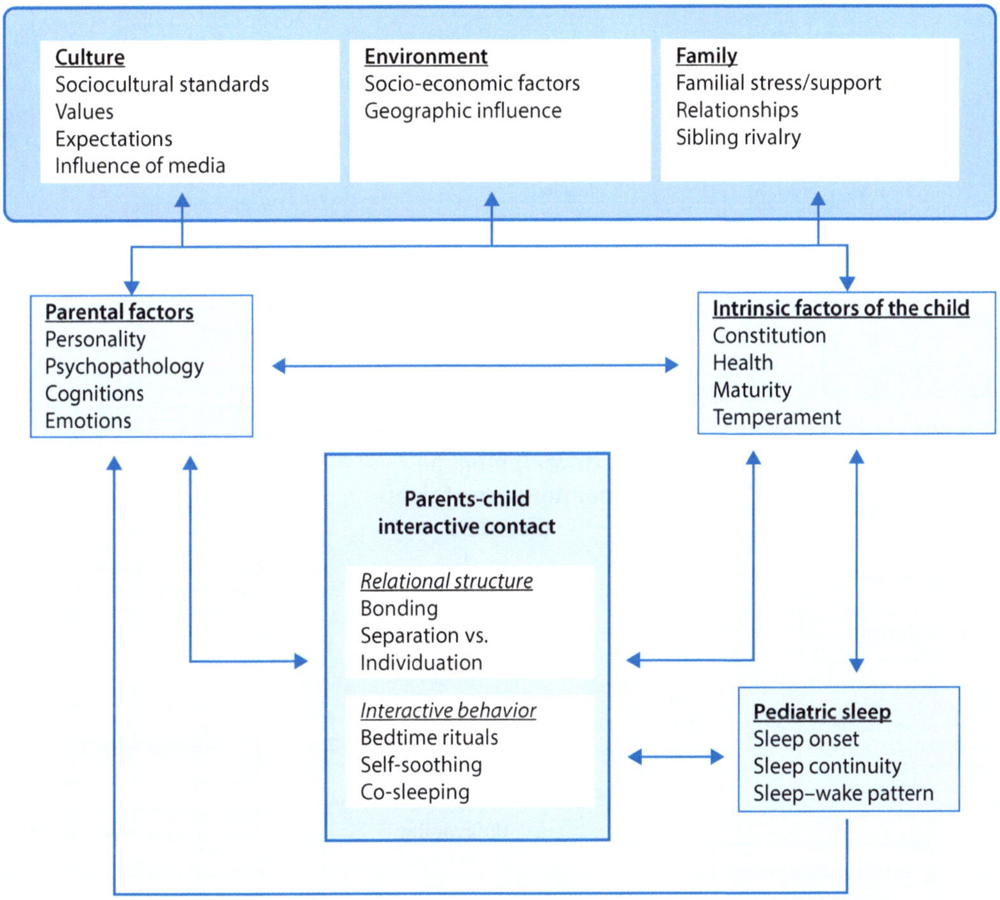

Fig. 11.7 Adapted model of sleep–wake regulation according to Sadeh and Anders [10], as well as Cattarius and Schlarb (2016)

A specific model for adolescents, however, should emphasize other factors. The model displayed in the following figure takes this requirement into account (Fig. 11.8).

11.1.4 Epidemiology

Between 15% and 25% of preschool children and schoolchildren are affected by problems of initiating and maintaining sleep. About 25% of all children suffer from sleep disorders in the course of their childhood or adolescence. Problems of initiating and maintaining sleep (insomnias) are the most frequently observed disorders. Approximately 20% of the children have general sleep complaints, about 17% of young preschool children suffer from complaints of maintaining sleep, and about 14% of the schoolchildren have difficulties with initiating sleep. Often the parents are involved in dynamic of the sleep disorders of younger children, because the children need their parents to reinitiate sleep, whereas adolescents often lie awake in their beds at night or occupy themselves with media such as smartphones. About 10% to 30% of adolescents suffer from acute insomnia; about one third even suffer from several insomnia symptoms. Findings with regard to a gender-specific risk to develop insomnia are often contradictory. Trials oriented at sexual maturity show no differences between boys and girls (before the onset of menarche) regarding insomnia. With the onset of menstruation, the risk for girls increases threefold. With increasing age, adolescents show more preference for late evening hours and going to bed later as a consequence of puberty, but this is often associated with increased daytime impairment.

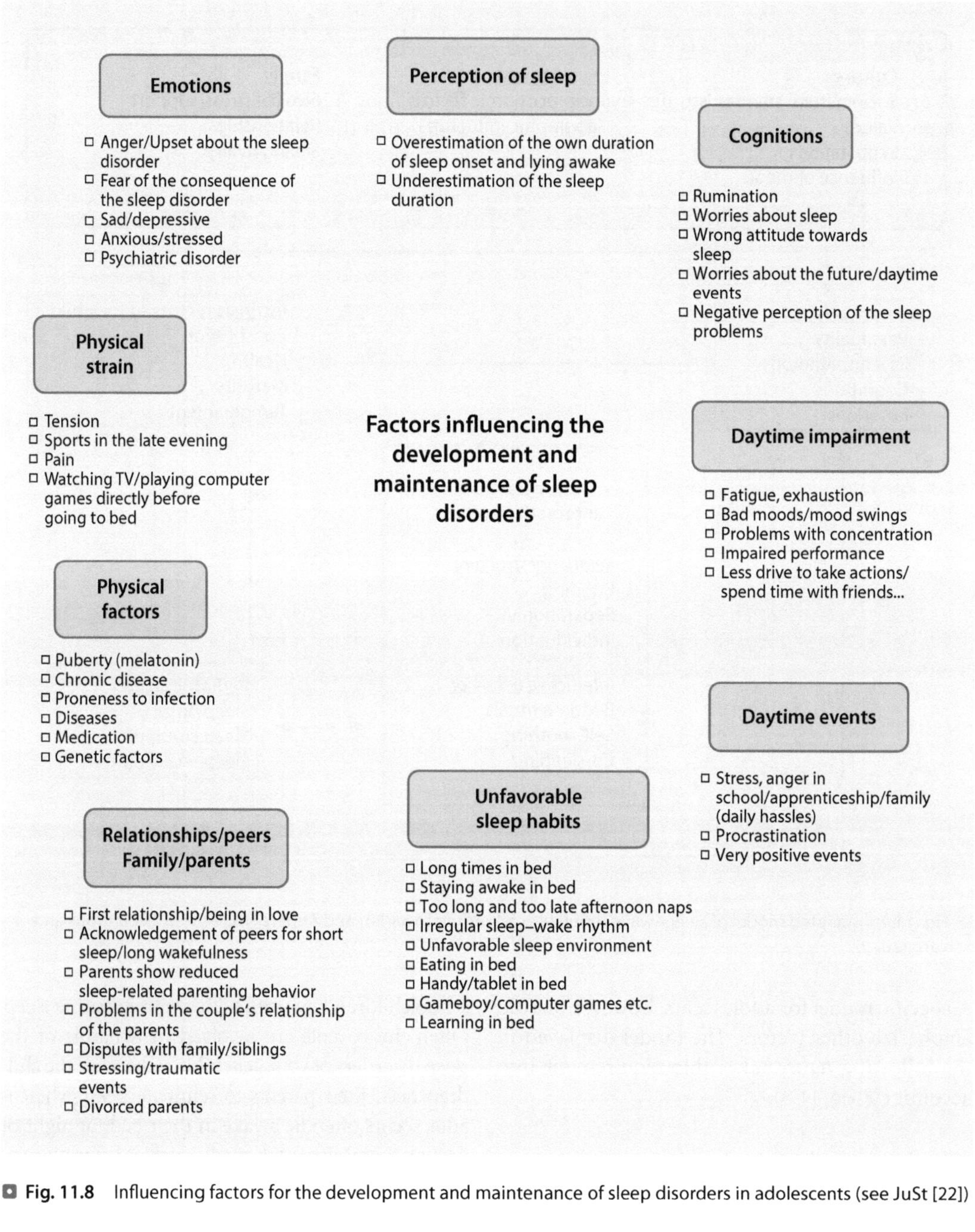

Fig. 11.8 Influencing factors for the development and maintenance of sleep disorders in adolescents (see JuSt [22])

Symptoms such as excessive daytime sleepiness may also indicate other existing sleep problems or insufficient sleep. Between 16% and 40% of adolescents suffer from such daytime sleepiness. About 35% of adolescents have difficulty in waking up in the morning, and up to 67% report sleep deprivation.

In particular, adolescence is closely related to onset of the circadian rhythm disorder of the delayed sleep phase type (delayed sleep phase disorder, DSPD). Between 0.5% and 7% of adolescents suffer from this disorder. In addition, DSPD in adolescence often leads to the development of insomnia problems. On the other hand, about 10% of adolescent insomnia patients meet the diagnostic criteria of DSPD.

11.1.4.1 Chronification

The frequent assumption that children or adolescents would "grow out" of their sleep disorder is only true to a limited extent because more than

80% of children and adolescents report insomnia symptoms in their histories. Sleep disorders also often have an intermittent course in childhood and tend to resist; several studies even report a persistence of nearly 50% up to adult age. Furthermore, long-term trials confirm that early sleep problems are correlated with later emotional and behavioral problems in adolescence.

Thus, age-appropriate tools are important for early diagnosis that allow asking specific questions to patients in early ages. Not only may a lack of sleep or too much sleep have respective consequences, a therapist for children and adolescents also should be aware that a sleep disorder may be apparent. Therefore, the following paragraph focuses on the possibilities of diagnosing sleep disorders in children and adolescents.

In childhood and adolescence, sleep problems are also widely distributed and have a great impact on the development of children and adolescents. These problems:

- Frequently occur very early.
- Tend to chronify.
- Are risk factors for the physical, emotional, cognitive, and social development of children and adolescents.
- At the same time aggravate already existing medical, psychiatric, psychosocial, and developmental problems and disorders.
- Have a significant influence on the whole family, especially when occurring in children.

11.1.5 Clinical Presentation

Sleep deprivation, insomnia symptoms or insomnias, and nightmares are very frequently observed in children and adolescents and are associated with relevant impairments during the daytime. Young children especially only rarely complain about impaired sleep quality or even daytime sleepiness; rather, such impairment during the daytime is perceived by adolescents or adults. So, most often the parents are addressed in the context of diagnosing sleep problems in early ages. As previously described, children who suffer from sleep deprivation or sleep difficulties often display symptoms of ADHD; therefore, a differential diagnostic examination is essential. Also, the long-term sequelae of sleep deprivation and sleep disorders are not actually known to the children or adolescents: they do not reflect or realize that they remain clearly below the performance level they would be normally able to achieve and that they experience more disputes and conflicts with peers or family members. Even adolescents are not conscious of the consequences of persisting sleep deprivation, especially in puberty. They do not classify their mood swings as sequelae of lacking sleep or poor sleep hygiene.

Practical Tip

Sleep deprivation and sleep disorders in children are often expressed by hyperactive and inattentive behavior during the day. In children who present with the suspected diagnosis of ADHD, sleep deprivation, insomnia, or another sleep disorder should always be excluded by differential diagnosis and assessed (e.g., by means of sleep diaries or questionnaires).

11.1.6 Examination Procedures

11.1.6.1 History Taking

At the beginning, comprehensive *sleep history taking* by means of sleep protocols and age-appropriate screening questionnaires for children and parents is important to diagnose sleep disorders. In cases of several sleep-specific differential diagnostic questions, an interview may also be performed (see following). Together with the *clinically physical and psychological examination*, the patient's history helps in discovering comorbidities or underlying disorders. A video clip displaying the child's sleep behavior may also contribute to better findings. With only low light (e.g., a bedside lamp), informative sequences may be recorded that allow differentiating between pavor nocturnus disorder and possible epileptic seizure. In adolescents, questions about stimulant intake, and in children and adolescents also questions about drug intake, must be asked, because various pharmaceuticals may lead to sleep problems such as difficulties in initiating and maintaining sleep.

11.1.6.2 Sleep Protocol

To assess sleep deprivation as well as different events during sleep, taking a sleep protocol may be helpful. A 24-h protocol is suitable for infants and children; a normal protocol is suitable that refers to the problems of initiating and maintaining sleep whereas a detailed assessment of the day is not required. In young children, the parents should additionally record a sleep protocol from their own sleep to assess the consequences for parental sleep. Adolescents, however, are mostly better able to report about their sleep than their parents. Therefore, in these ages the adolescents are mostly a better source of information. However, it must generally be taken into consideration that the assessment by the children in comparison to those of the parents may vary, so an evaluation from both the child's and the parents' perspective seems to be reasonable.

By applying screening questionnaires, sleep-related information can be retrieved rapidly and effectively.

11.1.6.3 Questionnaires on Parents' Information

Children's Sleep Habits Questionnaire (CSHQ)

The CSHQ is a questionnaire for parents of preschool and primary school children (4–10 years) intended to screen typical, clinically relevant sleep problems in this age group: difficulties of going to bed, delayed sleep onset, insufficient sleep duration, sleep-related anxieties, waking up at night, parasomnias, sleep-related breathing disorders, and daytime sleepiness. An overall "sleep disturbance score" is calculated as well as eight subscale scores. The original questionnaire in English was evaluated in a clinical and a nonclinical sample.

Sleep Disturbance Scale for Children (SDSC)

The SDSC is a short screening questionnaire intended to identify sleep disorders in children and adolescents. This questionnaire can be completed by the children or adolescents as well as by the parents. Twenty-six items should be answered on a gradual Likert scale (rarely, once or twice per month; sometimes, once or twice per week; frequently, three to five times per week; always, nearly every day). The subscales of "disorders of initiating and maintaining sleep," "arousal disorders," "disorders of the sleep–wake transition," "sleep-related breathing disorders," "excessive sleepiness," and "excessive sweating" allow a good overview of the most frequent sleep disorders. In healthy samples, the internal consistency is in a good area, whereas clinical samples are found in the satisfactory range. With a T value greater than 70, the score is considered as suspicious. The cutoff for the scales of "disorders of initiating and maintaining sleep" amounts to a raw value of 17, for "arousal disorders" to 7, for "sleep-related breathing disorders" to 14, and for "excessive sleepiness" to 13; a higher score corresponds to greater severity of the disorder.

11.1.6.4 Questionnaires for Self-Reporting

Children's Sleep Comic (CSC)

The children's sleep comic (CSC) is a tool for self-reporting and assesses sleeping habits and age-typical sleep problems in young children. The CSC was conceived for children between the ages of 5 and 10 years and was validated based on other tools such as the Children's Sleep Habits Questionnaire (CSHQ) and the Diagnostic Interview of Pediatric Sleep Disorders (DIKS, Diagnostisches Interview Kindlicher Schlafstörungen). The internal consistency is rather high. The comparison with respective diagnoses according to DIKS showed significant correlations. The children's sleep comic may be applied as a reliable tool for self-assessment as well as maintaining the contact to the child and his/her sleeping habits.

Sleep Self-Report (SSR)

The Sleep Self-Report (SSR) is a validated tool to assess pediatric sleep disorders from the child's perspective between the ages of 7 and 12 years. Because many items correspond to the version of the questionnaire for parents, a comparison between the answers of the parents and the children is possible. The cutoff is reached at 25 (sensitivity, 73%; specificity, 64%); a conspicuous stanine value of 8 is applicable as of a SSR total score of 31. However, to fill in the questionnaire, the child should be able to read and write.

Screening of Pediatric Sleep Disorders (PSS-J)

The screening of pediatric sleep disorders for adolescents (PSS-J) is a short screening tool for diagnosis of possible sleep problems in adolescence. The PSS-J consists of seven screening items with detailed questions for better clarification of the respective problem area. Based on the criteria mentioned in the PSS-J, the diagnosis may very rapidly reveal the symptoms of a sleep disorder.

Epworth Sleepiness Scale for Children (ESS-C)

Originally, the Epworth Sleepiness Scale is a self-reporting scale validated for adults for monitoring daytime sleepiness (see ▶ Chap. 2). The ESS version for children and adolescents (ESS-C) has been adapted for the age group of 6- to 19-year-old individuals. It encompasses seven items. On a four-point scale with the gradation of 0 (I never drop off), 1 (I rarely drop off), 2 (I frequently drop off), and 3 (I nearly always drop off), the children and adolescents estimate their likelihood to fall asleep in the listed situations. A verification of the psychometric properties of the ESS-C is currently not available. The cutoff for adolescents (age group between 13 and 19 years) amounts to a sum score of 13 points. Higher values have to be considered as noteworthy.

Nightmares Effects Questionnaire (NEQ)

Nightmares in adolescence may sometimes have massive impacts on daytime alertness. The Nightmares Effects Questionnaire (NEQ) assesses the effects of nightmares on the daytime alertness of adolescents and adults. The NEQ includes more than 30 items to evaluate the daytime impairment, which is characterized by six factors: (1) emotion regulation, (2) stress and aggressiveness, (3) depression, (4) attentiveness/concentration, (5) anxiety, and (6) hyperactivity. The NEQ has high reliability and may be considered as an excellent tool for assessment of daytime impairments resulting from nightmares in adolescents and adults.

11.1.6.5 Interviews

Furthermore, several standardized interviews are available as comprehensive and very exact procedures:

Diagnostic Interview of Pediatric Sleep Disorders (DIKS)

Based on the criteria of the ICSD-3, the DSM-5, and the ICD-10, an interview was developed for sleep disorders in preschool childen and schoolchildren between the ages of 5 and 10 years that is based on the parents' report. Based on the parents' reports, discrimination is possible among the most frequent sleep disorders.

Sleep Inventory for Children and Adolescents (SI-KJ)

The sleep inventory for children and adolescents (SI-KJ) encompasses the age group of 5 to 10 years. Based on four different tools, detailed diagnostics of sleep problems and sleep disorders in children and adolescents are possible. The sleep inventory takes into account the child's own as well as the parental perspective.

Diagnostic Interview of Adolescent Sleep Disorders (DIAS)

The interview is also based on criteria of the ICSD-3, DSM-5, and ICD-10 and can be applied either from the self-reporting perspective or from the perspective of the parents. Therefore, it consists of two versions. The age relationship refers to adolescents between 11 and 21 years. Frequently observed sleep disorders are assessed and can be examined by differential diagnostics.

In general, the interviews have a high content validity.

For assessment of further effects such as behavioral problems, further instruments such as questionnaires on behavioral disorders in children and adolescents may be reasonable in addition to the application of sleep-specific tools to evaluate the daytime impairment or psychological problems. Besides the Child Behavior Checklist (CBCL) in the version for parents and the derived questionnaires for self-report of children/adolescents (YSR) and for teachers (TRF), also the Strengths and Difficulties Questionnaire (SDQ) as well as other tools may be applied.

11.1.6.6 Test Psychological Examinations

To differentiate a possible psychological or cognitive impairment, a test psychological examination (performed by psychologists, psychotherapists for children and adolescents, or psychiatrists for children and adolescents) may be recommended. Such an examination should be planned if hints are found of a cognitive or psychiatric disorder (e.g., anxiety disorder, ADHD). Comprehensive diagnostics are necessary because psychiatric diseases may be associated in particular with disorders of initiating and maintaining sleep and nightmares, and sometimes also sleep-related breathing disorders. Intelligence tests (Wechsler Intelligence Scale for Children, WISC) as well as attentiveness tests (e.g., pediatric version of the test battery on attention, KiTAP; TAP for adolescents; and the d2 test of attention) may reveal daytime impairments as well as comorbid symptoms/disorders.

11.1.6.7 Physical Examination

To exclude physical origins for sleep problems of children and adolescents, a comprehensive physical examination is essential. In this context, possibly the melatonin level (in case of suspected sleep–wake rhythm disorders) or also the iron level (in case of suspected restless legs syndrome in childhood) should be measured (see also ▶ Chap. 2).

11.1.7 Sleep Medical Diagnostics

11.1.7.1 Actigraphy

An actigraph may be applied to measure physical activity and to identify disorders of the sleep–wake rhythm or movements during sleep (see ▶ Chap. 2). In infants, the actigraph is placed at the lower leg; older children wear the actigraph at the wrist. It may be useful to assess the sleep for several days to identify recurrent patterns. Attention must be paid that the evaluation software is specially developed for children because they move significantly more during sleep and thus produce other patterns. Evaluations performed by software designed for adults would result in erroneous sleep and wake times. However, for extensive sleep medical examination of children, inpatient polysomnography is also required.

11.1.7.2 Polysomnography

If a sleep-related breathing disorder is assumed, or any other rather organic sleep disorder, a pediatrics sleep laboratory should be involved, and polysomnographic examination should be initiated. In particular in cases of suspected periodic leg movements during sleep/restless legs, epileptic seizures at night, narcolepsy, disorders of the sleep–wake rhythm, or chronified insomnia, in general examination in a sleep laboratory is recommended. For diagnosis of nonorganic insomnia as well as nightmare disorder or pavor nocturnus, PSG usually is not necessary.

The basics of performing and evaluating polysomnography are described in ▶ Chap. 2. In the context of childhood and adolescence, however, the following particularities have to be observed with regard to technical performance and the subsequent evaluation because polysomnography examinations of infants, children, and adolescents are clearly more difficult and should meet special requirements. Children are often much more irritated by the unfamiliar environment than adults so placing the necessary measuring instruments may be problematical. Therefore, a comfortable and friendly atmosphere should be created. The applied sensors have to be adapted to the children and their smaller body surface without disturbing them in their sleep behavior. Sometimes the electrodes have to be placed closer to each other (e.g., to assess leg movements). Technically, the application of high-resolution digitization parameters for assessing and displaying the measured signals is important for examinations in children because, in comparison to adults, children have a clearly higher breathing and heartbeat frequency. Furthermore, the EEG amplitudes are more variable in this young age group. The electrodes should be placed according to age. For 2-year-old children, the following structure is recommended because of the asynchronously occurring sleep spindles: F4-M1, C4-M1, O2-M1, F3-M2, C3-M2, O1-M2, C4-Cz, and C3-Cz (see also ▶ Sect. 2.6). However, the feasibility is essential for the measurement so that for routinely performed measurements possibly only C3-M2 and C4-M1 should be measured in children younger than 2 years to minimize the stress for these young patients. In addition, young children react strongly to the sensors for measuring oral and nasal breathing, so it is probably suitable to limit the measurements to the oronasal thermistor or nasal suction pressure. According to the recommendations of the American Academy of Sleep Medicine (AASM), the measurement of suction pressure should be preferred for the identification of hypopnea.

Because children might react strongly to unfamiliar environments, an examination during two nights is recommended. If after the first night clear results have already been obtained, assessment on a second night can be omitted.

Limb movements as well as an overall high movement frequency are typical for children. Phases with such movement artifacts lasting more than 15 s are a frequently observed phenomenon, but they are not regularly associated with a transition to another sleep stage. In children with ADHD or with sleep-related breathing disorders, movements lasting more than 10 s are often observed and are typical for the disorder.

With regard to the evaluation of the breathing pattern, the child's age should be considered because the breathing frequency is modified depending on the development. According to the criteria of the AASM, at least two skipped breaths related to the previous breathing pattern allow the assumption of obstructive apnea if the amplitude of the oronasal airflow is reduced by 90% or more as well as a continuous or even increased effort is measured for breathing. However, only in children up to the age of 8 years is such a pattern observed relatively often in the context of movements. Therefore, the measurement of the leg EMG is essential for classification. If the symptoms occur during movement, they should not be considered.

11.1.8 Differential Diagnostics

As already mentioned, sleep complaints or disorders also frequently occur in other psychological or physical disorders. In those cases, it has to be determined if the sleep problems are the focus and have to be treated first, or if the sleep-related difficulties have to be considered in the context of other disorders. Then, the treatment of the underlying disease is indicated together with a referral to a pediatrician, a pediatric psychiatrist, or a pediatric psychotherapist. Hence, it is important that the sleep disorder is included in the therapy and to treat it appropriately.

The Child or Adolescent Should Be Referred to a Sleep Specialist

- In cases of chronified disorders of initiating and maintaining sleep
- If the child/adolescent is not restored when waking up in the morning over a longer time or if it is difficult to wake him/her up
- In cases of relevant daytime sleepiness (falling asleep at school, during trips in buses/cars/trains of less than half an hour)
- In cases of chronic snoring/breathing noise at night or breathing interruptions
- In cases of behavioral disorders at night that cannot be explained otherwise

11.1.9 Insomnia Therapy in Childhood

11.1.9.1 Sleep Education and Sleep Hygiene

Age-appropriate information and psychoeducation is an important component of sleep medical counseling in childhood and adolescence. Information for parents but also for children regarding healthy sleep as well as the consequences of poor sleep quality are important. In particular, providing information about age-appropriate and age-based sleep duration is essential. Furthermore, information should be given about factors influencing sleep, for example, the parental behavior or media consumption, and the importance of a healthy and age-adequate sleep quality environment should be discussed. Often, this information also contains recommendations for good sleep hygiene to improve sleep quality and to achieve a higher sleep duration and efficiency. In this way, the daytime sleepiness of children and adolescents can also be reduced. It must also be taken into consideration that the recommendations regarding sleep hygiene should be adapted to the developmental stage and the cultural values of the children and adolescents as well as their families. The following examples represent age-oriented recommendations.

Sleep Hygiene Recommendations for Preschool Children

- Parents should take turns bringing their child to bed. In this way it can be avoided that going to sleep is associated to a certain person, which promotes the child's autonomy regarding the behavior of sleep onset.
- Daytime activity and physical activity of the day have an impact on the evening tiredness and sleepiness of the child. An active waking time with sufficient physical activity as well as mentally stimulating and creative playing contribute to restorative sleep. These activities, however, should not take place directly before going to sleep.

- Sleep-related self-soothing strategies of the child should be supported.
- When parents have put their child to bed, they should not hurry back and lift him/her up at the slightest noise. Waiting briefly may help the child to apply self-soothing strategies. Of course, it is important the parents let their children know that they are always there if he/she really needs them.

Sleep hygiene recommendations for schoolchildren:
- The parents' bed should only be available as a refuge in exceptional situations (for example, when the child is ill).
- It should be possible that the child perceives his/her room as shelter. The sleep environment should be designed according to the anxieties and preferences of the child if they have sleep-improving properties (calm, quiet, dark, etc.).
- At least 2 h before going to bed, watching TV and playing computer games should be discontinued. There must be enough time for the child to process the daytime noises and images. In this way, events that have happened during daytime can be discussed and may lose their probably stressing character.

Sleep hygiene recommendations for adolescents:
- Sun or light in the morning: allow the sun in the morning to shine into the room and to expose the room to as much daylight as possible; this helps getting awake and fit. At night, however, the room should be dark so that the body may relax and restorative sleep is possible.
- Avoid a clock at the bedside: removing the clock from the bedside so that the adolescent cannot read the time at night may be helpful in the context of unfavorable sleep-related cognitions.

11.1.9.2 Stimulus Control and Structured Bed Routine

Besides sleep education and sleep hygiene, stimulus control also belongs to the standard elements in the context of treating insomnias in children and adolescents.

The Following Aspects of Stimulus Control and Structured Bed Routine Are Relevant for Children and Adolescents

- Sleeping area: The bed should be used only for sleeping. Activities such as watching movies, listening to music, learning, doing homework, or using other media (e.g., smartphone, tablet) should not be take place in bed and thus not be associated with sleep.
- Time of going to bed: The child or adolescent should go or be taken to bed when he/she is tired.
- Initiating sleep: Depending on the age, it is often recommended that the child or adolescent leave the bed after 15–20 min if not able to fall asleep. Alternatively, the child may apply relaxation techniques or other mental distraction strategies (see below).
- Rhythm: In the morning, the child or adolescent should get up if possible at the same time and in the evening go to bed at approximately the same time.
- Daytime sleep: Daytime sleep should be avoided as of a certain age (about 5 years); this is especially important for adolescents. Sleeping during daytime, too long and too late, may significantly impair night sleep and even support a rhythm shift. If day sleep is necessary, a nap should take place early in the afternoon and not exceed 20–30 min.

These recommendations of stimulus control and bed routine are effective, especially for parents of young children, and may significantly improve the sleep behavior.

11.1.9.3 Extinction

If a child opposes going to bed or wants to come into the parents' bed at night, the procedure of extinction may be suitable and effective. In this context, the parents learn to remain consequent and to effectively ignore the child's disturbing behavior. In case of disturbing behavior of the child (calling for the parents, leaving the bed and asking to be allowed to watch TV or sleep in the parents' bed), the parents do not react with fulfilling the wish. Hereby, it is important that the parents remain consistent until the child's behavior no longer occurs. This result is called extinction when there are no positive consequences concerning problem behavior. Regarding implementation, however, it must be ensured that the parents are confident with this method and that they are certain that their child is not afraid.

11.1.9.4 Positive Reinforcement

A very effective strategy to modify a child's behavior is positive reinforcement. The child is offered an attractive reward for showing a certain desired behavior. For example, the child could receive a small gift in the morning, deposited by the sleep fairy, if he/she has stayed in bed in the evening or has tolerated being brought to bed alternatively by the parents (the mother in one evening, the father in the other evening). The reward, however, can also be immaterial (for example, having special time exclusively with the father). In this context, the difference must be made between short-term reinforcement (direct) or long-term reinforcement (for example, after 1 week or 1 month). In this way, a long-term reward may be agreed on for successfully modified behavior. In particular for young children, however, short-term reinforcement strategies should be applied because their time perception is different from that of older children or adults. Adolescents, however, may well anticipate long-term reinforcement.

11.1.9.5 Relaxation Techniques

In children and adolescents, relaxation techniques may also be applied. It must be noted here that progressive muscle relaxation (PMR) is easy for children and adolescents to learn compared to autogenic training. Techniques that are related to this procedure, such as imaginative techniques or relaxation training are also suitable for children and adolescents as of a certain age. Regarding the implementation, care should be taken for an age-appropriate application. The general rule to be applied is the older the child the more complex techniques can be learned and implemented. Younger children need simpler and easier strategies. In younger children of preschool age, massage techniques and physical relaxation strategies, for example, caressing the back, may contribute to the child's relaxation and encourage sleep. Also, relaxing by singing a song to the child or repeating rhymes as more speech-oriented options may be helpful for some children. Parents should try different strategies to decide which is best suited for their child.

11.1.9.6 Cognitive Restructuring

Concerns, impairing cognitions, and irrational convictions may also develop in children and adolescents with sleep disorders at a certain age (mostly at the beginning of school age). Therefore, the procedure of cognitive restructuring may be applied in an age-appropriate way in cognitive behavioral therapy (CBT). Those unfavorable sleep-related cognitions may increase arousal in children or adolescents and thus contribute to the stability and chronification of sleep problems.

Also in childhood and adolescence, different sleep-related cognitions may be differentiated:

- Unfavorable cognitions about the origins of insomnia: "Mum and Dad have to be by my side otherwise I cannot fall asleep."
- Unfavorable cognitions regarding sleep-encouraging strategies: "I can better fall asleep when I am online in bed and have my smartphone with me."
- Wrong associations regarding the consequences of poor sleep: "If I do not sleep well this night, I will not be able to provide good performances and I will fail in school."
- Unrealistic expectations toward sleep: "I have to sleep well every night, otherwise I will get ill."

11.1.9.7 Imaginative Techniques/ Modern Hypnotherapy

Generally, children and adolescents benefit from pictorial and imaginative techniques. A modification of sleep is possible with such procedures. Hypnotherapeutic treatment of children and adolescents suffering from sleep disorders shows first results based on reports of single cases. Also, imaginary rescripting therapy (IRT) that is applied for treatment of nightmare disorders is included in the group of imaginative therapy approaches (see ▶ Chap. 7). The implementation of this technique in age-appropriate ways shows very good results in the treatment of nightmares. The therapy of PTSD is based on the same procedure.

11.1.9.8 Bedtime Restriction

For children and adolescents who spend too much time in their bed when not using it for sleeping, bedtime restriction may be suitable. First, the time in bed is reduced to real sleep duration the child or adolescent. The aforementioned sleep diary may serve as the basis for the calculation of the actual sleeping time. After 1 week, the sleep efficiency is calculated (see ▶ Chap. 2). Based on the number of hours, the sleep duration is gradually increased if the sleep efficiency amounts to 85% to 90%. Then, the time of going to bed is gradually advanced in the following weeks until the desired sleep duration is reached. The positive outcome of such a procedure is confirmed for cases of insomnia in particular for adults (see ▶ Chap. 3). However, regarding the treatment of children and adolescents, results are still possible.

11.1.9.9 Age-Oriented Interventions

In the following, age-appropriate structured treatment programs are presented, which, according to age, are focused on parents, involve parents and children, or mainly concentrate on adolescents. These three age-oriented treatment programs are predominantly based on cognitive behavioral therapy with insomnia (CBT-I) and imaginative/hypnotherapeutic techniques. The aforementioned techniques (rules of sleep hygiene, relaxation procedures, stimulus control, extinction, or other therapeutic procedures) are generally included.

Not all these procedures are suitable for each age. The younger a child is, the more the parents have to be included and involved in the treatment. Different sleep problems or disorders occurring simultaneously as comorbidities have to be taken into consideration. In this way, a child may suffer from problems of insomnia and at the same time from a sleep-related breathing disorder. Therefore, adequate diagnostics and a structured procedure are essential.

11.1.9.10 Treatment of Infants and Children of Preschool Age

For young children, the aforementioned methods of behavioral modifications such as stimulus control, sleep education, and extinction or restructuring are especially effective approaches. Based on the following case report, symptoms are described that are typical for early childhood. It will become clear that the parents have to be involved in the intervention.

Case Report

A 3-year-old boy called Paul lives together with his younger sister (age 2 years) and both parents in the parental household. Both parents work during the day. They report that Paul has always had rather poor sleep. His birth was highly complicated and they had enormous concern for his health. Several weeks were needed after his birth before they could take him home. They always stayed with him until he had fallen asleep because they were afraid of missing some concern about their child. Thus, he was used to always having his mother or father around him in the evening. By and by, he increasingly required his mother to be present in the evening and meanwhile refuses his father when the father tries to bring him to bed or wants to calm him at night. Each attempt to change the situation is refused by Paul, and he starts screaming and crying until his mother is there.

This case report makes clear that the sleep problems often start with an early disruption or an event. Based on the subsequent educational behavior of the parents regarding sleep, Paul developed a preference, and it is no longer the act of sleeping itself, but he chooses his mother and decides that only she "is allowed" to help him. Hereby the educational problem becomes obvious. If Paul was really afraid, he would also accept his father's presence and would cooperate. The fact that he refuses being consoled by him shows that he wants to influence his parents by applying this behavioral pattern. In the context of such problems, the parents should communicate the altered roles, visualize them, and ignore Paul's moaning and complaining (see further aspects under "Mini-KiSS").

In the context of treating such sleep problems, parents might design a positive *sleep environment* for Paul and modify the evening *bedtime ritual* in a way that it is new for Paul and interesting without stimulating him too much. By means of, for example, photos placed at the door that describe the procedure of going to bed and which the parents have already talked about with Paul during the day, Paul is already prepared for going to bed in another way. Based on the possibility of *extinction*, parents may change their behavior starting at this point. In the photos, the parents have the security of visual support. However, it is important that the parents reflect their previous, unconsciously reinforcing behavior (*cognitive restructuring*). The parents should also apply *positive reinforcement* (sleep fairy in the morning; see mini-KiSS) so that the probability for a change in Paul's behavior increases.

Mini-KiSS Training: Treating Early Childhood Sleep Disorders

Taking into account the aforementioned basics of age-adapted therapy in early childhood, the so-called Mini-KiSS program has been developed and comprehensively evaluated. Based on the structured and manualized procedure, the therapist/physician has good options to treat typical age-oriented problems within six sessions. The age-appropriate treatment program focuses on insomnias, sleep-related anxieties, resistance when going to bed, and nightmares. It is based on training elements such as psycho-education, sleep hygiene, sleep-related educational competences, learning relaxation techniques by parents and child, learning appropriate sleep-related strategies of resolving problems of parents and child, and reduction of dysfunctional, sleep-related as well as general cognition of parents on the basis of CBT-I techniques. To ensure the integration into daily routine, parents receive exercises after each session for training. For physicians/therapists, a comprehensive trainer manual and the respective material for parents are available. ◘ Table 11.1 briefly describes the single sessions and thus allows an overview.

This sleep training includes all relevant topics for treatment of typical and frequently occurring sleep disorders in early childhood, in particular, regarding disorders of initiating and maintaining sleep, nightmares, and sleep-related anxieties.

Such a procedure is well accepted by parents, and according to several studies, it leads to a reduction of sleep problems as well as the improved psychological well-being of the children. Parents also benefit from the training with regard to their own sleep and their psychological situation.

◘ **Table 11.1** Overview about the Mini-KiSS training

Session and purpose		Contents
1	Psycho-education	Introduction, information about sleep: day–night rhythm, function of sleep, sleep disorders, influencing factors regarding sleep, rituals, daily structure, etc., exercises to do at home
2	Thorough checkup of situations and sleep behavior	Correlation of sleep and behavior during the day, vicious cycle of sleep pressure, educational behavior and child's sleep, educational rules for healthy sleep, house of healthy sleep, educational strategies, creative resolution of problems, Kalimba the sleep helper, exercises to do at home
3	Crying, screaming, and stubbornness	Crying and screaming, soothing techniques, stubbornness and childhood aggression, behavioral recommendations, alteration of the sleeping place environment, exercises to do at home
4	Stress and relaxation	Stress and relaxation, escalation trap, stress enhancing factors, mental control techniques, time and attention for the child, time for oneself, imagination exercises, exercises to do at home
5	Anxiety and security	Security and childhood anxieties, help in case of nighttime fears, help for nightmares, stepwise procedure in problem situations, modification of sleep and nutrition, relaxation and massage techniques for the child, imagination exercises, exercises to do at home
6	Concluding session	Temptation to indulge: typical traps regarding sleep behavior, sleep habits, feedback, exercises to do at home

11.1.9.11 Treatment of Schoolchildren

Schoolchildren are cognitively more able to think and worry. Also, anxieties occur frequently at that age. Based on the following case report, typical symptoms are described as well as the procedure in the context of schoolchildren.

Case Report

The 8-year-old Sophie is presented with insomnia symptoms. Her parents report that she frequently needs more than 1 h to fall asleep. Sophie is the oldest of three children; her younger sister Clara shares the bedroom with her, and the youngest sister Marla (4 years) still sleeps in the parents' bedroom. Sophie appears to be thoughtful and very considerate toward her younger sister, who suffers from asthma. She provides toys and entertains her sister during waiting times. In the further course, it becomes obvious that Sophie is highly concerned about her sister's health because Clara has already had to go to hospital several times because of her breathing problems. During KiSS training (see following), it became apparent that Sophie was afraid of falling asleep because her sister presents breathing problems at times. Sophie does not know if she will be woken up at night by her sister's problem, and so she gradually developed the fear of falling asleep. Furthermore, she meanwhile dreams of falling and of monsters, which also cause anxiety.

11

For the treatment of Sophie, different procedures may be suitable. On one hand, Sophie should have a positive *sleep environment* giving her the feeling of safety and courage. The parents may, for example, change her sleep environment with positive elements taken from Sophie's preferred stories or fairy tales. Further, she should learn to *relax* (PMR, magic breath; see KiSS) so that she does not focus on her concerns in the evening but on relaxing her body. A cuddly toy as sleep helper, together with *imagination techniques* and respective bedtime stories, may work as a coping model (see KiSS) as well as being comforting and encouraging for the child. The evenings should be spent in a way that Sophie is able to better cope with the worries and concerns of the day. For this purpose, creative *methods of CBT-I* for children may be helpful (e.g., sorrow box). The evening *bedtime ritual* can be associated with encouraging slogans (CBT-I for children) so that Sophie is in a positive mood and likes going to bed. The parents should further apply positive reinforcements so that Sophie is rewarded when she succeeds in sleeping well and is motivated to implement the strategies she has learned.

For children of Sophie's age – between 5 and 10 years – the sleep training for children was developed as is described in the following. Also here, comprehensive systematic verifications regarding the effectiveness of the therapeutic scheme have been performed so that also KiSS training is displayed as an example for a treatment program for schoolchildren.

KiSS Training: Treating Sleep Disorders in Schoolchildren

KiSS training addresses children between 5 and 10 years of age suffering from insomnia or nightmares. This treatment program also encompasses six sessions for children with sleep difficulties and disorders and is based on the aforementioned techniques (CBT-I and imaginative elements or hypnotherapeutic implications). The treatment program includes three sessions with the children and three sessions with parents: the contents of the sessions are summarized in ◘ Table 11.2. The central element in the children's sessions is the soft toy *Kalimba*, a stuffed leopard, that fulfills several functions: as a model, it is intended to associate properties such as strength, courage, speed, and fearlessness. Furthermore, it is company and an object of protection for the children to feel supported; and finally it serves as a memory keeper for the strategies that have been learned so that the children may easily recall the lessons although they often cannot read or write.

The children's sessions are designed age-appropriately by Kalimba. Folders with drawings of Kalimba support active cooperation during the sessions and serve as memory keepers for exercises to do at home. In this context it must be emphasized that there is no need for children to be able to read or write to memorize strategies and to implement or recall them later. Also, this training includes parents' sessions with psycho-educative elements as well as sleep-related educational situations. In this age group, the focus is placed more on the topic of fears and sorrows because in school age thoughtfulness and concerns may have a sleep-impairing role and thus impede the restorative and sufficient sleep of the child.

Table 11.2 Overview of the KiSS training

Session and purpose		Contents
1	Parents' session 1: psycho-education	Information about the development of sleep disorders (psycho-education); behavioral recommendations, educational strategies for healthy sleep behavior
2	Child's session 1: sleep behavior from the child's perspective	Information about healthy sleep; rules of sleep hygiene; introduction of Kalimba, magic breathing as relaxation technique
3	Parents' session 2: sleep situations	Modifying specific sleep situations, sleep rules, activating resources for resolving problems
4	Child's session 2: modifying sleep behavior	Modifying of sleep-specific behavioral patterns, using Kalimba to cope with fears of sleep
5	Child's session 3: fears and sorrows	Overcoming sleep problems with Kalimba, coping with sorrows and thoughtfulness, learning review
6	Parents' session 3: transfer	Training of the learned strategies, going into detail of specific difficult sleep situations

Also regarding the KiSS-intervention, several studies show a high satisfaction as well as a significant reduction of sleep-related symptoms up to 1 year. Furthermore, the psychological well-being of the children may be improved.

11.1.9.12 Treatment of Adolescents

In adolescence, parents have a relatively less important role regarding sleep than in other age groups, but the changes of puberty, which are also changes sleep and the psychological shifts must be taken into consideration. Furthermore, media have a more and more important role. The following case report tries to demonstrate this phenomenon.

Case Report

The 15-year-old Marius presents to the sleep medical center. He reports that he has often difficulties calming down in the evening and needs quite a long time to fall asleep. He then often switches on the computer to play, increasingly even at night. Then he forgets about the time, but at least it distracts him. Just lying down, he sees his desk and immediately the next exams come to his mind. This stresses him because he could have bad results. Further, he does not get along with his teacher. And altogether, he does not like school at all! In the morning, he has difficulties getting up; he often feels absolutely whacked, and sometimes he is not even able to get up and thus misses school. Of course, the consequences are visible. He has concentration problems and worries that he cannot be promoted because of bad marks. He notices himself that he is mentally distracted and cannot focus. Also, the parents report that he is very tense and aggressive in the afternoon, which has a strong impact on the family life. He sleeps poorly and is afraid of getting addicted to gambling.

This description makes clear that Marius already has many symptoms of insomnia as it is seen in adults (see ► Chap. 2). He often worries in the evening, thinks about the consequences of his sleep problems, and fears sequelae regarding school performance and health. It is obvious that Marius has a typical teen bedroom with his bed, desk, and media, which can sometimes impair good sleep.

In the case of Marius, different aspects have to be taken into consideration. Besides comprehensive and differential diagnostic examination of non-substance-related addiction problems, however, clearly the school-based stress is also the focus. Therefore, the treatment should include an adaptation of the *sleep environment* so that Marius is not confronted with the topic of school in the

Table 11.3 Overview of JuSt training

Session and purpose		Contents
1	Adolescent session 1: psycho-education	Prof. Paul Paulsen as "Sleep Doc," sleep lab, rules and rewarding system, development of sleep disorders (psycho-education), imagination exercises
2	Adolescent session 2: sleep hygiene	Discussion of the exercises, rules of sleep hygiene
3	Parents' session: sleep and parental behavior	Sleep and sleep disorders, consequences of sleep problems, parents' educational behavior and sleep of the adolescent, comfortable sleep environment
4	Adolescent session 3: sleep environment	Stimulus control, sleep rituals, rules of sleep hygiene, imagination exercises
5	Adolescent session 4: fears and sorrows	Dealing with sorrows and thoughtfulness, restructuring of sleep-impairing cognitions, imagination exercises
6	Adolescent session 5: stress	Sleep and stress, techniques for stress reduction, imagination exercises, my private sleep lab, sleep quiz: "Who wants to be a sleeponaire?"

evening. Furthermore, general relaxation techniques should be taught (PMR); it may also be helpful to apply *imaginative procedures* for cognitive relaxation. By means of *cognitive procedures* in the context of insomnia (CBT-I), sleep-impairing thoughts may be identified and modified accordingly. Marius should also imperatively work on *rules of sleep hygiene* with the goal that he no longer plays computer games in the evening or at night. His depressive mood may be treated with the options of *positive psychology*.

JuSt Training: Sleep Training of Adolescents

In analogy to the KiSS training for younger children, the JuSt training here is presented as sleep training for adolescents. Teens already show significantly more sleep-related cognitions so that the treatment of adolescents with insomnia or nightmares is rather similar to that of adults with the respective CBT-I strategies (see ▶ Chap. 2). However, in this training further sleep problems such as sleep–wake rhythm disorders and puberty-related imbalances of the chronotype are focused. It must also be taken into consideration that the strategies elaborated for adults cannot be fully applied in this age group.

Regarding their adolescent children, parents often do not know much about the puberty- and sleep-related changes and the necessary sleep duration (in particular, sleep duration of adolescents amounting to about 9 h; see earlier). In this age group, the parents no longer have a crucial role at bedtime because teenagers mostly go to bed on their own. Also, the treatment program of adolescents encompasses six sessions, but because of the aforementioned aspects, five sessions are conducted for adolescents. During the training, the adolescents meet "Sleep-Doc Prof. Paul Paulsen" in a fictional sleep lab who presents the appropriate strategy for the adolescent (see ◘ Table 11.3).

Also the JuSt is well accepted by adolescents and their parents; after the training significant improvements of the sleep problems are seen. The problems of initiating and maintaining sleep are significantly reduced, and sleep efficiency as well as the overall sleep duration can be increased. In addition, the adolescents report a significantly less important tendency to worrying after the training and are less focused on their sleep problems. Even after 3 months to as long as 1 year, these significant results remain stable, and so a long-term effectiveness may be assumed.

11.1.10 Therapy of Other Pediatric Sleep Disorders

11.1.10.1 Treatment of Delayed Sleep Phase Syndrome

The treatment may be performed by means of so-called chronotherapy. This therapy includes a successive delaying of going to bed by 2 to 3 h per day until an adequate time of sleep onset is reached. This bedtime should be consequently observed. If an adolescent goes to bed at 3 o'clock at night, for example, the timepoint of going to bed should be gradually delayed until the adolescent goes to bed at an adequate time. This procedure takes some days, but the effect is that a certain rhythm is achieved. In this way, a possibly existing absence from school may be eliminated, and a resumption of regular school visits can be started. In the concept of JuSt training, elements to modify the delayed sleep phase syndrome are found (session 3). Regularity of bedtime is an important objective of the treatment and should be emphasized for the adolescents. Hereby, the assessment of the evening activities (e.g., computer games) may be helpful for the identification of possible origins of the delay. Also the application of light therapy with 10,000 lux for 45 min in the morning is recommended by some authors, mostly applied in the inpatient situation. This measure is recommended in particular with the background of comorbid depressive disorders.

11.1.10.2 Treatment of the Advanced Sleep Phase Syndrome

Generally, patients report relevant tiredness in the early evening hours and waking up very early in the morning. This disorder is much rarer in children and adolescents compared to the delayed sleep phase syndrome. The treatment of the advanced sleep phase syndrome should be performed in the opposite direction. Chronotherapy is oriented at the subjective sleep time. Every day, the adolescent should go to bed 2 to 3 h earlier until an adequate timepoint of sleep onset is achieved. Also, this type of therapy has to be planned accurately. It is often performed in a partly or completely inpatient setting because of a frequently existing comorbidity. As already described, several studies show that exposure to light may also be helpful for adolescents with chronotype-oriented symptoms. Application of light in the evening is considered to be effective in cases of advanced sleep phase syndrome. The application of light allows tiredness and sleepiness to start later so that the adolescents go to bed at a later time.

11.1.11 Drug Therapy

The administration of hypnotics leads to short-term improvement of the symptoms, in particular in cases of insomnia disorders; however, in the long term, behavioral therapeutic interventions seem to be superior. Thus, similar strategies apply for children and adolescents as for adults: for insomnia complaints and nightmares, psychotherapeutic procedures, generally based on the aforementioned techniques, are the measure of choice. For adolescents it must be observed that sleep-inducing drugs and hypnotics are applied only with permanent medical supervision.

The administration of melatonin may lead to a significant reduction of the duration of sleep onset, a prolongation of sleep duration, and an improvement of the quality of sleep. In previous trials, melatonin was well tolerated and did not cause severe side effects. Also, in children with ADHD and chronic problems of initiating sleep, different studies showed that the application of melatonin led to a reduction of the latency of initiating sleep and an increased duration of night sleep after an intake during about 4 weeks. Drug therapy with sleep-inducing homeopathic preparations may be started, only after careful decision. This rule is often neglected, and medication is taken because other options are not available. If the therapy with homeopathic drugs is not successful, sleep-triggering non-hypnotics such as low-potent neuroleptics may be prescribed, and only if even this therapy does not have a positive effect, hypnotics may be taken.

11.1.12 Rehabilitation Measures

In cases of high chronification and family impairment or impaired implementation of the sleep medical recommendations by the parents, rehabilitation measures may be suitable.

Practical Tip

Possible indications of sleep medicine regarding pediatric rehabilitation might be, for example:
- Chronic insomnias without CBT-treatment improvements
- Sleep-related breathing disorders
- Sleep-related hypoventilation syndromes
- Sleep disorders caused by other diseases (psychological disorders, chronic organic disorders)
- Hypersomnias, for example, narcolepsy
- Sleep–wake rhythm disorders
- Parasomnias
- Nocturnal movement disorders

Possible objectives of such rehabilitation strategies might be:
- Improvement of sleep hygiene by modifying the context
- Including the family and implementation of sleep-related measures on an inpatient basis
- In cases of sleep–wake rhythm disorders: measures of behavioral therapy for finding a day and night rhythm with specific support
- In cases of sleep-related breathing disorders, possible introduction of weight reduction and nutritional advice
- In cases of comorbid disorders: reduction of comorbidities for improvement of the somatic and psychiatric risk profile
- Improvement or restoration of the limited participation ability and restoration of the psychological balance such as the renewal of the ability to go to school for adolescents

11.2 Sleep-Related Breathing Disorders in Children

In correspondence to sleep-related breathing disorders in adults, sleep-related breathing disorders with and without obstruction of the upper airways are also found in children and they are substantially different with regard to their pathophysiology as well as diagnosis and treatment. The most important sleep-related breathing disorders in children that are discussed here are summarized in Table 11.4.

Table 11.4 Most important sleep-related breathing disorders in children and their incidence (as far as it is known)

Sleep-related breathing disorder	Incidence
Congenital central alveolar hypoventilation syndrome	Very rare[a]
Sleep apnea in infants	
Secondary sleep-related hypoventilation	
Pediatric snoring	4–8 (10–21)%[b]
Pediatric obstructive sleep apnea	1–4%

[a]Approximately 1:200,000 live births
[b]Permanent (occasional) snoring (according to parents' report)

11.2.1 Nonobstructive Sleep-Related Breathing Disorders

11.2.1.1 Congenital Central Alveolar Hypoventilation Syndrome

The congenital central alveolar hypoventilation syndrome or Undine's curse syndrome is a congenital disease that is caused by a disorder of the autonomous central breathing regulation. It is the result of a mutation of the PHOX2B gene, which is also mentioned as an obligatory diagnostic criterion in the ICSD-3. In case of good genotype-phenotype correlation, the number of polyalanine repeat mutations determines the severity of the disease. Because of negligible or completely missing central sensibility toward hypercapnia or hypoxia, severely affected children experience increasing hypoventilation and hypoxia during wakefulness; in even all affected children, it is observed during sleep. Also during wakefulness, these children show no respiratory response to hypercapnia, but in wakefulness they are able to control their breathing consciously. Also, in cases of combined hypercapnia and hypoxia, almost no arousal reactions are observed during sleep.

The congenital central alveolar hypoventilation syndrome occurs very rarely; an incidence of about 1 in 200,000 live births is assumed. The following possible origins of the breathing disorder have to be excluded before the diagnosis can be made:
- Neuromuscular diseases
- Pulmonary diseases

- Cardiac diseases
- Metabolic diseases
- Brainstem lesions

Children with congenital central alveolar hypoventilation syndrome become suspect as newborns with cyanosis and hypoxia and have to undergo postpartum intubation. In rare cases, so-called late-onset congenital central alveolar hypoventilation syndrome, the typical symptoms occur with delay in the course of further childhood development. With attempted weaning from the respirator, extended phases of hypoventilation occur, with hypercapnia and hypoxia.

Nearly all patients need lifelong ventilation therapy. In the course of further development, breathing becomes more stable in some children, at least during wakefulness, so that treatment is only required during sleep. The treatment consists of invasive ventilation via a tracheostoma or noninvasive ventilation therapy. Alternatively, a diaphragmatic pacemaker may be discussed for stimulation of the phrenic nerve at a later time. The children should be diagnosed and treated in a specialized institution. By means of appropriate therapy, these children may reach adult age.

11.2.1.2 Primary Sleep Apnea of Infancy

In early infancy, a series of phenomena are found that are explained by the immature condition of the infantine respiratory center. From the sleep medical point of view, the two most important ones are these:

- Primary sleep apnea of prematurity
- Primary sleep apnea of infancy

Apparent life-threatening events (ALTE) may appear in the context of those breathing disorders; however, their origins may be manifold. Apparent life-threatening events have several aspects in common with sudden infant death syndrome. The risk factors, however, are significantly different, so currently they have to be regarded as two distinct phenomena. The diagnosis and treatment of these phenomena is a primary responsibility of neonatologists and pediatricians.

The respiratory events in the context of the above mentioned sleep-related breathing disorders may be central, mixed, or also obstructive; however, the central genesis is typical. Regarding the definition of respiratory events, certain particularities have to be observed as they are explained more in detail in the section on obstructive sleep apnea in children (see ► Sect. 11.2.2). In this context, in particular the time-related criteria of apnea or hypopnea in children must be mentioned that are seen in relation to two previous breathing cycles of normal respiration.

The incidence of central breathing disorders in premature babies and newborns is directly dependent on the age of gestation. These disorders can mostly (but not only) be registered during sleep. Numerous external influences may trigger the occurrence of apnea. The breathing disorder ceases with maturation of the respiratory center; only in rare cases, for example, an intervention with pharmaceuticals is required.

Infant apnea manifests in the first 2 years of life. Also in this field, a correlation with the incomplete maturation of the central nervous respiratory regulation is assumed. Furthermore, a gastrointestinal reflux is correlated with the occurrence of apnea. Infant apnea often remains asymptomatic, but it may also lead to apparent life-threatening events. In this context, a series of differential diagnoses have to be observed, in particular infections of the airways and congenital syndromes (e.g., Arnold-Chiari malformation, Prader-Willi syndrome), but also syncope, breath-holding spells, convulsions, or diseases of the central nervous system.

11.2.1.3 Sleep-Related Hypoventilation Syndrome

Some types of sleep-related hypoventilation syndromes in adults may manifest in children in a comparable way. In cases of secondary sleep-related hypoventilation syndrome, hypoventilation becomes obvious because of the lower respiratory drive and the decreasing muscle tone during sleep. Underlying diseases include the following:

- Obstructive and nonobstructive pulmonary diseases (e.g., chronic bronchitis, bronchial asthma)
- Neuromuscular and vascular diseases
- Central nervous diseases (e.g., epilepsy)
- Morbid obesity

Diseases that manifest typically in childhood and that in the further course may lead to secondary sleep-related hypoventilation include the following:

- Cystic fibrosis/mucoviscidosis
- Neuromuscular diseases such as Duchenne muscular dystrophy

Obesity hypoventilation syndrome in childhood is rare; however, it is possible in adolescence and early adulthood. Similar to the findings in adults, the pathophysiological mechanism consists of a reduction of the thoracic and abdominal respiratory excursion caused by obesity. Additionally, obstructive sleep-related breathing disorder may be observed that is often caused by an obstructive component from adeno-tonsillar hyperplasia besides the obesity-based obstruction of the upper airways observed in these children.

The diagnostics of sleep-related hypoventilation syndromes in children are comparable to those of adult patients.

Also in children, the treatment should be based on the therapy of the underlying disease. If it is not or only insufficiently possible to treat the underlying disease, ventilation therapy at night may be required, probably also timely limited or intermittent, that might be performed as noninvasive CPAP ventilation or with bilevel devices. In cases of advanced neuromuscular diseases, often tracheostomy may be necessary in the further course for (initially nocturnal) ventilation therapy. Alternatively, also the nighttime application of oxygen may be discussed in the context of nonobstructive pulmonary diseases. The basics of ventilation therapy are comparable to those of adult patients. Particularities with regard to ventilation therapy in children are described in more detail in the following part of this chapter (see ► Sect. 11.2.2). The treatment of pediatric sleep-related breathing disorders should be imperatively performed in close cooperation with the institutions that are treating the underlying disease.

11

11.2.2 Obstructive Sleep-Related Breathing Disorders

In this context, the ICSD-3 mentions only *pediatric obstructive sleep apnea*. Snoring in children is not explicitly listed, but it is found, as is also snoring of adults, in its own paragraph on isolated symptoms and normal variants in the chapter of sleep-related breathing disorders.

The transition between these two phenomena, however, is fluid, and the determination is not always reliable in clinical routine; but there is often no imperative necessity for clear definition. Furthermore, relevant overlapping is seen especially in the context of (surgical) therapy. Thus, both phenomena are described together in this chapter.

11.2.2.1 Definitions

A clear definition of pediatric snoring does not exist. From a practical point of view, pediatric snoring is diagnosed in general when relevant respiratory noise is reported by parents or guardians, and further examination (history and polysomnography) does not reveal any hint for pediatric obstructive sleep apnea. The definition of pediatric obstructive sleep apnea is based on the patient's history and polysomnographic criteria.

Diagnostic Criteria of Pediatric Obstructive Sleep Apnea According to the AASM

- Presence of at least one of the following symptoms:
  - Snoring
  - Strained, paradox, or obstructive breathing during sleep
  - Sleepiness, hyperactivity, behavioral problems, or learning difficulties
- The polysomnographic monitoring reveals one or both of the following particularities:
  - One or more obstructive apnea phases, mixed apnea, or hypopnea per hour of sleep
  - Signs of obstructive hypoventilation, defined as hypercapnia ($PaCO2 > 50$ mmHg) during at least 25% of the total sleep duration in combination with at least one of the following phenomena:
    - Snoring
    - Flattening of the inspiratory nasal pressure graph
    - Paradoxical thoracoabdominal movements

As already mentioned, pediatric snoring may occur episodically and first manifest or increase/aggravate in particular in the context of an acute infection. In clinical routine, the persistence of the complaints over a certain period of time, for example, during 4 weeks, has to be confirmed. In its international classification of sleep disorders, however, the AASM does not include such a time criterion.

It can be easily seen that the definition is highly complex, and the diagnosis of pediatric obstructive sleep apnea according to the criteria presupposes a polysomnographic examination. However, in most healthcare systems, comprehensive polysomnographic examination of all children suffering from snoring or all children with suspected pediatric obstructive sleep apnea is not possible. With this background, it was implemented, for example, in German-speaking countries to confirm the indication of therapeutic measures in snoring children primarily based on medical history, clinical examination and questionnaires and to request previous polysomnographic diagnostics only when the children belong to defined risk groups.

11.2.2.2 Etiology and Pathophysiology

Corresponding to the obstructive sleep-related breathing disorders in adults, in pediatric patients suffering from obstructive sleep-related breathing disorders an increased resistance of the upper airway is also observed, with consecutive respiratory strain and sometimes reduction of airflow. The pathophysiological explanation models in this context mostly correspond to those of adults (see ▶ Chap. 4). Also, in this way, hypotonia of the upper airway dilating muscles during sleep finally induces the nocturnal breathing disorder.

Although in adults functional aspects have a major role, the anatomical factors leading to mechanical obstruction of the airway, such as *congenital malformations* or *syndromic diseases*, are predominant in children.

Malformations such as micrognathia, retrognathia, or midface hypoplasia are often associated with obstructive sleep apnea in children.

Furthermore, obstructive breathing disorders at nighttime are often observed in children with trisomy 21, which can be explained by the macroglossia and the frequently accompanying obesity. More rare syndromes are, for example, Pierre Robin sequence, Crouzon syndrome and Apert syndrome, Goldenhar syndrome, or achondroplasia, which are associated among others with malformations of the mandible and often with severe obstructions of the upper airway. Of course, hyperplasia of the lymphatic tissue in all these children, as is physiologically observed in this age group, may contribute to deterioration or manifestation of the nighttime breathing disorder.

The predominant significance of *adeno-tonsillar hyperplasia* in the pathophysiology of pediatric obstructive sleep apnea becomes evident with the incidental association between adeno-tonsillar hyperplasia and sleep-related breathing disorder in children and the high effectiveness of surgical removal or reduction of the mentioned structures. Furthermore, numerous studies with imaging procedures revealed that the primary location of obstruction in children is generally found in the area of the pharyngeal or palatine tonsils, mainly where these structures overlap. In many studies, an increase of the mentioned lymphatic structures correlated not only with the occurrence but also with the severity of the sleep-related breathing disorder.

First of all, adeno-tonsillar hyperplasia in children is a physiological reaction and not pathological per se. Depending on the severity of the hyperplasia of the pharyngeal and palatine tonsils, symptoms may be completely missing or manifest only in the context of aggravating factors such as infection of the upper airway. On the other hand, such hyperplasia of the mentioned lymphatic organs may lead to massive obstructive sleep apnea. Also in this case, anatomical variants or comorbid disorders such as concomitant obesity may deteriorate the disease or favor its manifestation.

Unfortunately, obesity is increasing, even in children. Similar to observations in adults, obesity leads to fat deposits in the parapharyngeal soft tissue and thus to stenosis of the upper airway. In the future, an increasing number of sleep-related breathing disorders in children may be expected.

Practical Tip

Enlarged palatine and pharyngeal tonsils are the most important origin of pediatric obstructive sleep apnea. Often pediatric obesity is an aggravating factor, with increasing incidence.

Based on the described pathophysiological aspects, some authors request a classification of pediatric obstructive sleep apnea into three types:

- In *type I*, the adeno-tonsillar hyperplasia is in the focus.
- Pediatric obesity is predominant in *type II*, with less severe hyperplasia of the lymphatic system.
- Children with complex craniofacial or neuromuscular malformations are classified as *type III*.

From a didactical point of view, this classification seems to be reasonable; however, in practice it could not prevail.

Further factors contributing to sleep-related breathing disorder in children are *neuromuscular diseases* that may aggravate the hypotension of the pharyngeal dilators observed during sleep and *laryngopharyngeal reflux* that may enhance the airway obstruction via reflux-induced swelling of the mucosa.

In rare cases, surgical corrections of the palate as necessary for the treatment of cleft palates may contribute to postoperative occurrence or aggravation of nocturnal airway obstruction. Also, children suffering from laryngomalacia may present with primary or accompanying sleep-related breathing disorders.

11.2.2.3 Epidemiology

Snoring at night is widely observed in children. A recent epidemiological survey revealed that the incidence of permanent snoring in children reported by their parents amounts to 4% to 8% depending on the age, whereas the prevalence for occasional snoring is given as 10% to 21%. Because no standardized definition exists for snoring, these data, however, are not reliable.

The transition to obstructive sleep apnea is fluent, and the available literature regarding the distribution of obstructive sleep apnea in children can only be compared to a limited extent because different criteria for performing and evaluating the basic assessment procedures were applied.

However, it seems to be confirmed that obstructive sleep apnea has the highest prevalence in the age group of children between 2 and 8 years corresponding to the phase of lymphatic hyperplasia. Data in the literature regarding the incidence in otherwise healthy children amount to 1% to 4%, whereby boys seem to be affected more frequently than girls. The incidences in younger children or adolescents are unknown. The relationship between children with habitual snoring and children with obstructive sleep apnea amounts to 3:1 and 5:1, respectively. In correspondence to adult patients, the prevalence of obstructive sleep apnea in children is higher in the Afro-American population compared to Caucasian people.

However, with regard to the incidence of pediatric obstructive sleep apnea, it must be considered that the prevalence of the disease is significantly higher in high-risk cohorts. Based on polygraphic and polysomnographic trials, it can be expected that up to two thirds of the children with trisomy 21 are affected by obstructive sleep apnea.

In past decades, a change in the population of children suffering from obstructive sleep apnea could be observed. The incidence of children with concomitant obesity has significantly increased. Because of this development, an increasing number of cases of pediatric sleep apnea and an increasing number of complex cases that are difficult to treat must be expected.

11.2.2.4 Clinical Presentation

In both manifestations, that is, pediatric snoring and pediatric obstructive sleep apnea, *snoring* as defined by breathing noise during sleep noticed by an observer, is the leading symptom.

The fact that snoring might not be observed, however, does not exclude obstructive sleep apnea. Frequently, parents describe strained breathing, wheezing, or simply an intensive breathing noise. The assessment of what a normal breathing noise in children is and what acoustically indicates an increased breathing strain, however, is certainly subject to the individual estimation of the observer, and some parents are more attentive or even more anxious than others.

With increased airway obstruction, generally also the snoring noise increases, or irregularities of breathing are observed as well as hints of hypopnea or apnea. However, it must be mentioned that children much more rarely show the pattern of obstructive apnea that is typical for obstructive sleep apnea in adults. If parents report classic apnea at night, often a severe pediatric sleep apnea is already present.

As indications of airway obstruction or increased breathing efforts, indrawing of the intercostal space or paradoxical breathing during sleep may become apparent. In cases of longer-lasting pediatric obstructive sleep apnea, the presentation of funnel chest may result. To reduce the airway resistance, children often adopt unfamiliar body positions during sleep; for example, they stretch their arms over their heads or prefer sleeping in an upright position. These children frequently sleep restlessly and often change body position. Further symptoms in this context are sweating at night, headaches in the morning, and prolonged or recurrent enuresis during sleep.

Practical Tip

Frequently, particularities of sleep behavior besides the respiratory disorder are found in children with obstructive sleep apnea: these include restlessness, sweating, or unusual sleeping positions that frequently change. The parents should be actively interviewed regarding those factors.

Comparable to adult age, in children respiratory obstruction during sleep also leads to the observation that sleep is not restorative even if the corresponding arousal reactions and fragmentations of the sleep profile are less significant than in adults. The consequences may be *impaired well-being* or *limited performance* during the day. Sometimes excessive daytime sleepiness can be observed, although this phenomenon is usually not reported spontaneously by children. If respective questionnaires or objectifying examinations such as a multiple sleep latency test (MSLT; see ► Chap. 2) are considered, signs of hypersomnia are frequently found, even if they are not as severe as it is typical for obstructive sleep apnea in adults.

Often children try to compensate their tiredness or sleepiness by *increased activity*, so hyperactivity or aggressive behavior may also indicate nocturnal breathing disorders. For this reason, the workup of pediatric hyperactivity and accompanying behavioral difficulties should include the differential diagnosis of sleep-related breathing disorder and also sleep disorders (see ► Sect. 11.2). Finally, more and more data are available confirming that obstructive sleep apnea also impairs the quality of life in children.

Practical Tip

Obstructive sleep apnea in children often manifests clinically by behavioral difficulties and hyperactivity, whereas daytime sleepiness relatively rarely is the complaint. So, in children with relevant behavioral difficulties sleep-related breathing disorder should be considered as a differential diagnosis.

Furthermore, pediatric obstructive sleep apnea may also lead to *cognitive deficits* and *deterioration of the school performance*. Particularly critical in this context is the fact that recent trials could also document behavioral difficulties and poorer school performance in children when these children only snore, that is, even when no other hints of obstructive sleep apnea were present. Thus, it can also be expected that isolated nocturnal snoring in children may already indicate a pathologically increased airway obstruction. This symptom may further lead to relevant impairment of the daytime vigilance and cognitive performance of the children, even if no other changes of nighttime breathing can be identified with the currently available methods. Those correlations especially make clear why strict differentiation between pediatric snoring and pediatric obstructive sleep apnea is not possible from a clinical point of view.

Finally, relevant *cardiovascular sequelae* and *metabolic changes* may also result in children:
- Sinus arrhythmia
- Pulmonary hypertension
- Pulmonary heart disease
- Systemic arterial hypertension
- Increased insulin resistance

Metabolic changes most often occur when additional obesity is present.

Relevant growth and development disorders may also be a sequela of an existing sleep-related breathing disorder. Even if the corresponding values are still in the normal range, nearly all children experience a development boost after successful therapy.

11.2.2.5 Examination Procedures

The basics of every diagnostic procedure consist of comprehensive *history taking* in which the aforementioned symptoms and hints have to be directly addressed, and the *clinical examination* that includes the assessment of size and weight as well as the general development status of the child.

In the clinical examination, the described anatomical predictors of pediatric sleep apnea have to be addressed. In the first place, these include possible obesity of the children as well as externally visible hints and malformations such as are typical for the mentioned syndromes and that are often associated with obstructive sleep apnea. However, adeno-tonsillar hyperplasia is certainly most significant, so that an intensive inspection of the oropharyngeal space is the standard examination for all children with suspected nocturnal breathing disorder. In this context, the size of the tonsils has to be examined, which might have impressive extensions up to so-called kissing tonsils, especially in pediatric patients (see ◘ Fig. 11.9). Further, enlarged adenoids have to be identified. Typical signs of pharyngeal obstruction in childhood in this context include:

11

- Increased or exclusive oral respiration
- Adenoid facies
- Closed nasality
- Frequent infection of the upper airways
- Persisting nasal secretion
- Eustachian tube dysfunction
- Otitis media with effusion (OME) with associated hearing loss

In addition, parents should be asked about hearing loss and probable existing delay of language development, and if necessary, middle-ear ventilation should be examined by means of otoscopy or ear microscopy as well as tympanometry.

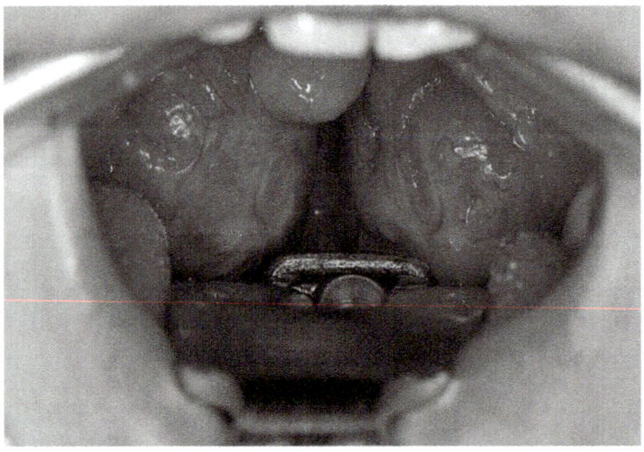

◘ **Fig. 11.9** Tonsillar hyperplasia in children

Furthermore, a series of questionnaires exist to assess typical symptoms of pediatric sleep apnea. From the authors' point of view, the subscale for sleep-related breathing disorders of the Pediatric Sleep Questionnaire (PSQ-SRBD subscale) seems to be the most suitable. By means of this questionnaire, patients with pediatric sleep apnea can be identified with high reliability.

Further technical examination procedures for assessing the upper airway of pediatric patients with obstructive sleep apnea include endoscopic or radiological examinations as well as the assessment of the collapsibility of the airway. These techniques, however, have a key role in the scientific evaluation of the disease or in the context of specific questions and are currently not part of routine diagnostics.

11.2.2.6 Sleep-Related Medical Diagnostics

Objectifying sleep medical examination in the sense of *polysomnography (PSG)* is still the gold standard in the diagnostics of pediatric sleep apnea. Polysomnographic examinations in children are associated with higher staff-related and organizational efforts; they require the relevant technical equipment and specific experience.

Because of the described particularities, out of center sleep testing generally does not seem to be sufficient in children because of the low sensitivity to exclude a relevant sleep-related breathing disorder. Although a recent comparative study showed that pediatric obstructive sleep apnea in older children (in this context, >10 years) can generally be diagnosed by means of outpatient recording polygraphic examinations in infants and preschool children are almost nonsignificant or can only be used in cases of clearly pathological findings. In a recently published position paper, the American Academy of Sleep Medicine draws the conclusion that a home sleep apnea test for diagnosing pediatric sleep apnea cannot be recommended. Alternative examination procedures such as home *audio or video recordings* or an isolated nocturnal *pulse oximetry* are not sufficiently sensitive, and at best they can only provide diagnostic hints.

Regarding polysomnographic examinations in children with suspected obstructive sleep-related breathing disorder, a series of particularities should be observed. In the context of evaluating respiratory events it must be considered that for the definition of obstructive apnea no comparable rigid time limits (e.g., 10 s) exist, but the duration of the respiratory event relative to the duration of two previous cycles of regular respiratory activity is considered as a measure. If two cycles of unimpaired inspiration and expiration are measured in the PSG, for example, with 6 s, a subsequently occurring respiratory event (e.g., apnea) is registered when it lasts longer than 6 s.

In analogy to the adult age, the breathing disorder may manifest as a typical cyclic sequence of apneas or also be associated with longer episodes of partial airway obstruction in the sense of obstructive hypoventilation with hypercapnia and desaturation. Furthermore, respiratory-related arousals are found more rarely in children because of their higher arousal levels. The hypnogram is generally less remarkable than in adults. If airflow limitations, apneas or hypopneas occur in children, they are frequently associated with significant desaturations because of the high breathing rate and low functional reserve.

CO_2 measurement at nighttime is generally not required if it is the case of routine diagnostics of obstructive sleep-related breathing disorders, even if the ICSD-3 defines obstructive hypoventilation as an alternative diagnostic criterion regarding the presence of hypercapnia. For differentiation against a respective nonobstructive breathing disorder, it may be very useful.

In addition to diagnostics of obstructive sleep-related breathing disorder, a *video documentation* at nighttime may be suitable to identify the described secondary signs of airway obstruction such as oral respiration, jugular or thoracic indrawings, or exceptional sleeping positions. During the night of documentation, it may also be helpful to observe the child in his/her sleep at the bedside to identify the presentation of the breathing disorder. In particular, the acoustic aspects of breathing disorders can be better assessed in this way compared to merely technical monitoring.

Practical Tip

The criteria for definition of respiratory events in children are significantly different in some aspects from those for adults. Under no circumstances can the evaluation and assessment criteria of polysomnography in adults be transferred to children.

According to the criteria of the AASM, polysomnography is required for diagnosis of pediatric sleep apnea. If in otherwise healthy children with clear history, typical symptoms, and apparent adeno-tonsillar hyperplasia are presented, objectifying sleep medical examinations before introduction of antiinflammatory or surgical therapy are not routinely required and from a practical point of view are not always possible. In these cases, the symptomatic adeno-tonsillar hyperplasia is the leading diagnosis and thus indication for therapy.

An indication for polysomnography, however, is obvious in the following constellations:

- Children with more complex craniofacial malformations or syndromic diseases
- Children with neuromuscular diseases
- Children with severe obesity
- Before introduction of ventilation therapy
- In cases of nondirective clinical findings (missing adeno-tonsillar hyperplasia)
- In cases of persisting complaints after surgical therapy

Case Report

A young mother presents her 4.5-year-old son Ian who, according to the parents, has been snoring increasingly in the course of the previous 6 months. Being asked, the parents report that they have observed breathing interruptions in the past weeks. In the morning, the bed is rumpled, and the boy wakes up at night again and again. During the day, according to the mother, Ian can barely be kept under control, and in kindergarten which he previously has attended without any problems, more and more conflicts with other children must be managed. Furthermore, he often suffers from a common cold and would then breathe only through the mouth and even hear poorly. Previous medical checkups were all unremarkable; the boy has a good health status.

The clinical examination reveals a slender boy who is otherwise regularly developed. The most prominent findings are massively enlarged palatal tonsils and relevantly enlarged adenoids appearing in the examination of the nasopharynx. Ear microscopy shows a retracted eardrum with middle-ear effusion; the tympanogram appears flat on both sides.

The diagnosis of bilateral adeno-tonsillar hyperplasia with middle-ear effusion is made as well as the suspicion of pediatric obstructive sleep apnea, which is confirmed by a conspicuous score in the respective questionnaire (PSQ-SRBD). Based on the clear symptoms, polysomnography is not performed, and adenotomy and tonsillotomy with insertion of tympanostomy tubes are indicated. Surgery and postoperative healing take place without complications.

In a follow-up examination, the mother reports the nighttime breathing disorder has ceased, with a relevant improvement of his well-being during daytime. In the months after the intervention, her son has experienced a physical development boost, and the problems in his social environment have significantly improved. Under these circumstances, postoperative control-PSG is not performed.

11.2.2.7 Differential Diagnoses

In the clinical routine, a differentiation of *nonobstructive sleep-related breathing disorders* may be difficult, especially when in the individual case such a breathing disorder is associated with an obstructive component or overlapping is observed.

11

In the context of central sleep apnea, classically thoracic and abdominal breathing excursions are missing; in cases of hypoventilation syndromes, however, typically snoring or hints of paradox breathing are not found. In particular, in severely obese children signs of airway obstruction as well as hypoventilation are observed.

If nocturnal snoring is observed in children, it nearly always indicates airway obstruction or increased airway resistance. It is then important to identify the severity and the clinical relevance of the airway obstruction. The clear differentiation of obstructive sleep apnea from *snoring* may be difficult even with PSG because the transitions are fluent.

Peculiar nocturnal movements or positions must sometimes be differentiated from pediatric *parasomnias* (see ▶ Chap. 7). In the context of hypersomnia without any hint of obstructive sleep-related breathing disorder, other origins of hypersomnia have to be excluded, as, for example, *restless legs syndrome*, *periodic limb movements* (see ▶ Chap. 8), or *narcolepsy* (see ▶ Chap. 5). A differentiation of nocturnal *epilepsy* may further require the performance of a complete sleep EEG.

If behavioral difficulties are the leading symptom, differential diagnostics of neurological and psychiatric diseases may be indicated.

11.2.2.8 Treatment

In analogy to the treatment of obstructive sleep-related breathing disorders in adults, the treatment of children may also be classified into conservative, device-related, and surgical concepts.

Conservative Treatment

Regarding all overweight or obese children suffering from snoring or obstructive sleep apnea, a reduction of body weight should be achieved, and the parents should be informed about the significance of obesity for the development of pediatric breathing disorders (as well as other problems and diseases, of course). It seems to be necessary not only to state an appeal but also to give specific recommendations. Because the therapy of pediatric obesity, in particular, severe obesity, is highly complex and not every sleep professional acquires the relevant experience, it is recommended to obtain an overview of the locally available sites and institutions that might offer or provide the required therapeutic concepts. Those sources may include specially trained and experienced pediatricians but also training programs of the health insurance.

In the past years, the data regarding topical nasal steroids significantly improved so that their effectiveness in the context of pediatric snoring as well as pediatric obstructive sleep apnea is meanwhile confirmed. Because of the high tolerance, a conservative treatment attempt is generally justified and often achieves a successful outcome. In cases of severe symptoms, severe tonsillar hyperplasia, or hearing loss existing for a longer time because of an impaired Eustachian tube ventilation, however, surgical therapy should not be delayed.

If the respiratory situation is aggravated by infections, the timely restricted application of decongesting nose drops or spray, adapted to the child's age, may also be indicated. In particular for persisting problems, it must be discussed if *adenotomy* performed on an outpatient basis cannot be preferred.

Device-Related Therapy

For treatment of obstructive sleep apnea in children, different orthodontic treatments are available; however, they have not all been scientifically verified to date. Hereby, the (forced) *rapid palatal expansion* is of particular interest, which consists of the expansion of the still open midpalatal suture by means of an intraoral distractor that may be applied in children. The phase of active expansion generally takes only a few weeks ("rapid" palatal expansion). Afterward, the phase of consolidation follows. By means of this technique, the maxilla and thus the midfacial structures may be expanded relevantly in the transversal axis. The children's airways may be significantly enlarged in this way, and the existing sleep-related breathing disorder is improved.

In cases of respective conspicuities such as retrognathia, dental malposition, maxillary constriction (narrow, high palate), or midfacial hypoplasia, a specific *orthodontic consultation* and *examination* should be performed. This examination is particularly important when no adeno-tonsillar hyperplasia is found or the breathing disorder persists after surgical therapy.

Nocturnal positive airway pressure therapy for obstructive sleep-related breathing disorder alone is only rarely required in children because in this age group the alternative (especially surgical) therapies are very effective. Frequently, ventilation therapy is necessary when the children suffer from severe malformations that cannot be corrected currently or in the long term. Further, severe obesity with respective hypoventilation and airway obstruction may require ventilation therapy in individual cases.

The implementation of ventilation therapy is performed in analogy to the adult treatment in form of a nocturnal continuous positive airway pressure (CPAP) therapy that is generally applied nasally also in children. Even if the introduction of ventilation therapy in children requires particular experience and intensive counseling, generally the compliance is not poorer than in adults. It is certainly most decisive that parents or reference persons of the child can be convinced of the necessity of the treatment and commit themselves accordingly.

Regarding the application of CPAP therapy in children, however, one must bear in mind that this therapy may lead to midfacial growth retardation or impairment of the child's cranium, which may further aggravate the underlying sleep apnea. The necessity of CPAP therapy in children should be regularly checked, and the fitting of the mask should be adjusted at regular intervals.

Practical Tip

Because of the problems of long-term ventilation therapy in children (e.g., with regard to the development of midfacial hypoplasia), the necessity of ventilation therapy or the possibility of applying alternative measures in children should be regularly verified.

Surgical Therapy

In contrast to the adult age group, the surgical therapy of obstructive sleep-related breathing disorders of infancy is not controversially discussed, and because of its high effectiveness, it is meanwhile widely distributed. The most important surgical intervention is at the same time one of the most frequently performed operations in children: the (partial) *resection of the pharyngeal and palatal tonsils*.

The success rates regarding polysomnographically confirmed elimination of respiratory events amount to 75 to 100%, according to the scientific literature, and also the respective improvement of the already described clinical symptoms seems to be evident even if the perceived clinical improvement does not always correlate with the polysomnographic outcome. Because of the effectiveness of the intervention, (adeno-)tonsillectomy is internationally considered as the standard procedure for therapy of pediatric obstructive sleep apnea in cases in which hyperplasia of the pharyngeal and palatal tonsils is found in the clinical examination and no contraindications exist. In a large patient population of more than 450 children suffering from obstructive sleep apnea, a recent randomized trial performed in the US compared the outcome after tonsillectomy with a wait-and-see strategy. This elaborate project allowed important insights in the surgical therapy of pediatric obstructive sleep apnea and could confirm that surgical therapy is highly superior to wait and see with regard to the normalization of polysomnographic parameters. However, it became also clear that in the control group that did not undergo therapy, an important percentage of the children experienced a normalization of the sleep laboratory findings during the evaluation period of 7 months, which confirms the frequently self-limiting character of the disease in the context of physiological hyperplasia of the palatal tonsils in this age group. Furthermore, it became evident that even tonsillectomy does not always lead to healing of the breathing disorder. In particular, children with severe sleep apnea, obesity, or craniofacial malformations may expect postoperative persistence of the disease, which confirms the necessity of clinical and in cases of doubt also objectifying control, in particular in this last-mentioned cohort. The indication to perform tonsillectomy has to be made in a highly differentiated way and further has to take into account the severity of the disease, expected course of the disease, clinical complaints, risks that are associated with the intervention, and the parents' hopes and expectations.

> **Practical Tip**
>
> Surgery of the tonsils, if needed also in combination with adenotomy, is the most important therapeutic measure in the context of pediatric obstructive sleep apnea, in particular with existing hyperplasia of pharyngeal and palatal tonsils. Because of the high effectiveness, it is the treatment of first choice even when aggravating factors such as obesity or craniofacial malformations are also found.

In some European countries, partial resection of tonsils (tonsillotomy) is recommended or even exclusively performed as an alternative to tonsillectomy, mentioning the reduced postoperative risks and the lower postoperative morbidity. If tonsillotomy is really comparable to tonsillectomy regarding its therapeutic effect in the context of pediatric sleep apnea, cannot be estimated based on the reduced data available and generally depends on the surgical technique used. Besides adeno-tonsillectomy, a series of other surgical procedures must be mentioned even if they are not frequently used. For children with severe retrognathia, as is typical for certain malformation syndromes, distraction osteoneogenesis may be helpful and avoid ventilation therapy or tracheostomy of these children. Tracheostomy is necessary only in exceptional cases or for bridging airway obstructions that otherwise cannot be directly eliminated. With this indication, it is highly effective. Also, children with a breathing disorder resulting from laryngomalacia may benefit from relevant surgical interventions (e.g., supraglottoplasty).

11.3 Questions

1. Please describe the similarities and differences of the clinical symptoms of sleep disorders in children and ADHD disease.
2. Please list questionnaires that assess sleep disorders in children from the parents' and the children's perspective.
3. Which interventions should be applied for treatment of insomnia in children and adolescents?
4. Which interventions should be applied for treatment of nightmares in children and adolescents?
5. Please describe the similarities and differences of the clinical symptoms of obstructive sleep apnea in adults and children.
6. Please explain the polysomnographic criteria of obstructive sleep apnea in children.
7. Please list the most important origins of obstructive sleep apnea in children.
8. Please characterize the most important therapeutic options in the context of pediatric obstructive sleep apnea and list the indications for these procedures.
9. Please explain practical problems that occur in the differentiation of pediatric snoring and obstructive sleep apnea.

References

1. American Academy of Pediatrics, Section on Pediatric Pulmonology, Subcommittee on Obstructive Sleep Apnea Syndrome. Clinical practice guidelines: diagnosis and management of childhood obstructive sleep apnea syndrome. Pediatrics. 2002;109:704–12.
2. American Academy of Sleep Medicine. International classification of sleep disorders, 2. Aufl. Diagnostic and coding manual. Westchester: American Academy of Sleep Medicine; 2005.
3. BORBÉLY AA. Sleep mechanisms. Sleep and Biological Rhythms. 2004;2:67–68.
4. Cattarius B, Schlarb AA. Gegenseitige Beeinflussung von Eltern und Babys in ihrem Schlafverhalten. Somnology. 2016;20(3):189–198.
5. Capdevila OS, Kheirandish-Gozal L, Dayyat E, Gozal D. Pediatric obstructive sleep apnea. Complications, management, and long-term outcome. Proc Am Thorac Soc. 2008;5:274–82.
6. Fricke L, Lehmkuhl G. Schlafstörungen im Kindes- und Jugendalter. Ein Therapiemanual für die Praxis. Göttingen: Hogrefe; 2006.
7. Fricke-Oerkermann L, Plück J, Schredl M, et al. Prevalence and course of sleep problems in childhood. Sleep. 2007;30:1371–7.
8. Fricke-Oerkermann L, Frölich J, Lehmkuhl G, Wiater A. Schlafstörungen – Leitfaden Kinder- und Jugendpsychotherapie. Göttingen: Hogrefe; 2007.
9. Handwerker G. Epworth-Sleepiness-Scale für Kinder (ESS-K). In: Schulz H, editor. Kompendium Schlafmedizin, III-2.3.7.1. Landsberg/Lech: Ecomed; 2002.
10. Kirk V, Baughn J, D'Andrea L, Friedman N, Galion A, Garetz S, Hassan F, Wrede J, Harrod CG, Malhotra RK. American Academy of Sleep Medicine position paper for the use of a home sleep apnea test for the diagnosis of OSA in children. J Clin Sleep Med. 2017;13:1199–203.
11. Roeser K, Schwerdtle B, Kübler A, Schlarb AA. Further evidence for the JuSt program as treatment for insomnia in adolescents: results from a 1-year follow-up study. J Clin Sleep Med. 2016;12:257–62. https://doi.org/10.5664/jcsm.5496.
12. Roffwarg, H. P., Muzio, J. N., & Dement, W. C. (1966). Ontogenetic development of the human sleep-dream cycle. Science, 152(3722), 604–19.
13. Sadeh A, Anders TF. Infant sleep problems: origins, assessment, interventions. Infant Ment Health J. 1993;14:17–34.
14. Schlarb AA. JuSt-Therapeutenmanual: Das Training für Jugendliche ab 11 Jahren mit Schlafstörungen. Stuttgart: Kohlhammer; 2012.
15. Schlarb AA. Just – Begleit- und Arbeitsbuch für Jugendliche, Das Training für Jugendliche ab 11 Jahren mit Schlafstörungen. Stuttgart: Kohlhammer; 2012.
16. Schlarb AA. Mini-KiSS – Begleit und Arbeitsbuch für Eltern, Das Elterntraining für Kinder bis 4 Jahre mit Schlafstörungen. Stuttgart: Kohlhammer; 2013.
17. Schlarb AA. Mini-KiSS, Therapeutenmanual. Das Elterntraining für Kinder bis 4 Jahre mit Schlafstörungen, 1. Aufl. Stuttgart: Kohlhammer; 2013.
18. Schlarb AA. KiSS – Begleit- und Arbeitsbuch für Eltern und Kinder, Das Training für Kinder von 5 bis 10 Jahren mit Schlafstörungen. Stuttgart: Kohlhammer; 2014.
19. Schlarb AA. KiSS-Therapeutenmanual. Das Training für Kinder von 5–10 Jahren mit Schlafstörungen. Stuttgart: Kohlhammer; 2014.
20. Schlarb A, Brandhorst. Mini-KiSS online: an internet-based intervention program for parents of young children with sleep problems; influence on parental behavior and children's sleep. Nat Sci Sleep. 2012;4:41–52. https://doi.org/10.2147/NSS.S28337.
21. Schlarb A, Gulewitsch MD. Wenn der Sandmann kommt. Wirkt Hypnotherapie bei Kindern mit Schlafstörungen? Hypnose-ZHH. 2010;5(1+2):189–98.
22. Schlarb A, Hust C, Hautzinger M. Insomnie bei Jugendlichen. Psychologische Einflussfaktoren und Empfehlungen zur Diagnostik im pädiatrischen Alltag. Pädiatrische Praxis. 2009;74:419–30.
23. Schlarb AA, Schwerdle B, Hautzinger M. Validation and psychometric properties of the German version of the children's sleep habits questionnaire (CSHQ-DE). Somnologie. 2010;4:260–6.
24. Schlarb AA, Liddle CC, Hautzinger M. JuSt: a multimodal program for treatment of insomnia in adolescents: a pilot study. Nat Sci Sleep. 2011;3:13–20.
25. Schlarb AA, Gulewitsch MD, Weltzer V, Ellert U, Enck P. Sleep duration and sleep problems in a representative sample of German children and adolescents. Health. 2015;7:1397–408.
26. Schlarb AA, Zschoche M, Schredl M. Der Nightmare effects questionnaire (NEQ). Somnologie. 2016;20:251–7.
27. Schwerdtle B, Kanis J, Kahl L, Kubler A, Schlarb AA. Children's sleep comic: development of a new diagnostic tool for children with sleep disorders. Nat Sci Sleep. 2012;4:97–102. https://doi.org/10.2147/NSS.S33127.
28. Schwerdtle B, Kanis JA, Kübler A, Schlarb AA (2014) The children sleep comic – a new self-rating tool for childhood insomnia. J Sleep Res:315.
29. Schwerdtle B, Kanis JA, Kubler A, Schlarb AA. The children's sleep comic: psychometrics of a self-rating instrument for childhood insomnia. Child Psychiatr Hum Dev. 2016;47:53–63. https://doi.org/10.1007/s10578-015-0542-2.
30. Stehling F, Keull J, Olivier M, Große-Onnebrink J, Mellies U, Stuck BA. Validation of the screening tool ApneaLink® in comparison to polysomnography for the diagnosis of sleep-disordered breathing in children and adolescents. Sleep Med. 2017;37:13–8.
31. Stores G, Wiggs L. Sleep disturbances in children and adolescents with disorders of development: its significance and management. London: Mac Keith Press; 2001.
32. Stuck BA, Götte K, Windfuhr JP, Genzwürker H, Schroten H, Tenenbaum T. Tonsillectomy in children. Dtsch Arztebl Int. 2008;105:852–60.

33. Wise MS, Nichols CD, Grigg-Damberger MM, Marcus CL, Witmans MB, Kirk VG, D'Andrea LA, Hoban TF. Executive summary of respiratory indications for polysomnography in children: an evidence-based review. Sleep. 2011;34:389–98.

34. Zschoche M, Schlarb AA. Is there an association between insomnia symptoms, aggressive behavior, and suicidality in adolescents? Adolesc Health Med Ther. 2015;6:29–36. https://doi.org/10.2147/AHMT.S76511.

GPSR Compliance

The European Union's (EU) General Product Safety Regulation (GPSR) is a set of rules that requires consumer products to be safe and our obligations to ensure this.

If you have any concerns about our products, you can contact us on ProductSafety@springernature.com

In case Publisher is established outside the EU, the EU authorized representative is:

Springer Nature Customer Service Center GmbH
Europaplatz 3
69115 Heidelberg, Germany

Batch number: 10732801

Printed by Printforce, the Netherlands

S

T

U

V

W

O

P

Q

R

Index

Supplementary Information

B. A. Stuck et al., *Practice of Sleep Medicine*, https://doi.org/10.1007/978-3-030-17412-5